Overcoming Attention Deficit Disorders in Children, Adolescents, and Adults

Overcoming Attention Deficit Disorders in Children, Adolescents, and Adults

FOURTH EDITION

Dale R. Jordan

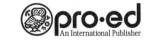
pro·ed
An International Publisher

8700 Shoal Creek Boulevard
Austin, Texas 78757-6897
800/897-3202   Fax 800/397-7633
www.proedinc.com

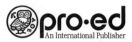

© 2006, 1998, 1992, 1988 by PRO-ED, Inc.
8700 Shoal Creek Boulevard
Austin, Texas 78757-6897
800/897-3202   Fax 800/397-7633
www.proedinc.com

The following figures are from or adapted from *Overcoming
Dyslexia in Children, Adolescents, and Adults,* by D. R. Jordan,
2002, Austin, TX: PRO-ED, Inc. Copyright © 2002 by PRO-ED, Inc.
Reprinted or adapted with permission.
1.1, 1.2, 1.3, 1.4, 1.5, 1.6, 1.7, 1.8, 1.9, 1.11, 1.12, 1.13, 1.14, 1.15, 1.16,
2.1, 2.2, 2.3, 2.4, 2.5, 3.5, 5.1, 6.2, 6.6, 6.13, 6.14, 6.15, 6.20, 6.22, 6.26,
6.27, 6.28, 6.29, 6.30, 6.33, 8.1, 8.2, 8.3

Library of Congress Cataloging-in-Publication Data

Jordan, Dale R.
　　Overcoming attention deficit disorders in children, adolescents, and adults /
　　Dale R. Jordan.—4th ed.
　　　　p.　cm.
　　Rev. ed. of: Attention deficit disorder. 3rd. c1998.
　　Includes bibliographical references and index.
　　ISBN 1-4164-0056-7 (pbk. : alk. paper)
　　1. Attention-deficit hyperactivity disorder.　2. Attention-deficit disorder in
adolescence.　3. Attention-deficit disorder in adults.　I. Jordan, Dale R. Attention
deficit disorder.　II. Title.
RJ506.H9J67 2005
618.92'8589—dc22

　　　　　　　　　　　　　　　　　　　　　　　　　　　　　　　　2004027738

Art Director: Jason Crosier
Designer: Nancy McKinney-Point
This book is designed in Minion, Nexus Serif, and Gill Sans.

Printed in the United States of America

1　2　3　4　5　6　7　8　9　10　　09　08　07　06　05

Dedication

*To Dr. Sam Oliphant, whose wisdom
and compassion have brought
new vision and hope to many
who could not see the way.*

Contents

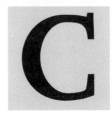

Contents

Is Attention Deficit a Personality Difference or a Mental Health Disorder?

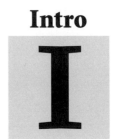

The children and adults who carry [the ADHD Edison gene] have and offer multiple gifts, both individually and as members of our society. Sometimes these gifts are unrecognized, misinterpreted or even punished, and as a result, these exceptional children end up vilified, drugged, or shunted into Special Education. The result is that they often become reactive: sullen, angry, defiant, oppositional, and, in extreme cases, suicidal. Some [ADHD] Edison-gene adults face the same issues, carrying the wounds of school with them into adulthood, often finding themselves in jobs better adapted to stability than to creativity.... [ADHD] Edison-gene children and adults are by nature: enthusiastic, creative, disorganized, non-linear in their thinking, innovative, easily distracted ... capable of extraordinary hyperfocus, understanding of what it means to be an 'outsider,' determined, eccentric, easily bored, impulsive, entrepreneurial, energetic.... All of these qualities lead them to be natural explorers, inventors, discoverers, leaders....

—Thom Hartmann in *The Edison Gene: ADHD and the Gift of the Hunter Child,* 2003

There [is] storytelling about ADHD ... [that] ADHD children are just leftover hunters from the Pleistocene era of human evolution and there's really nothing wrong with them. They're just the good old hunters from our caveman days being forced to live in a world of farmers and education.... That is a silly little idea for building self-esteem in ADHD children, and I don't happen to believe that you should be building self-esteem by lying to people, by practicing small deceits, by creating little stories about the origin of a disorder so that you can craft it as if it wasn't a disorder.

—Russell Barkley at the Schwab Foundation for Learning Conference on ADHD, 2000

ix

We are, without question, engaged in a debate over how to look at people, the world, and life. It's a very old debate with occasional new twists. The battle lines are roughly drawn between the empirical, hard-facts scientific approach on one hand, and a more humanistic, intuitive, even spiritual approach on the other hand. This debate strikes home for people with attention deficit disorders because it is shaping the prevailing view and attitudes about the nature of ADD. Not so coincidentally, it is also shaping our views about the nature of people who happen to have ADD.

—Peter Jaska, president, National Attention
Deficit Disorder Association, May 1, 2000

These sharp differences in point of view about why some individuals do not or cannot pay attention mark the ongoing debate about the nature of attention deficits in the classroom and on the job. When I entered this arena as an elementary classroom teacher in 1957, we had no information about what came to be called LD (learning disabilities or learning differences). No one had a clue about why most individuals paid good attention, while other equally intelligent persons did not. For 47 years I have been part of the effort to understand learning differences and how they impact personal lives, relationships, and achievement. With dismay I have witnessed intelligent professionals within many disciplines almost come to blows in the strength of their disagreement over what causes learning difficulties, what to call various types of learning struggle, and what should be done about them at home, at school, and at work.

The fervent differences between the views of Thom Hartmann and Russell Barkley represent opposite ends of the spectrum of professional thought about attention deficit syndromes, now called ADHD (Attention-Deficit/Hyperactivity Disorder) and ADD (Attention-Deficit Disorder without hyperactivity). Hartmann is a self-identified "Edison-gene hunter" whose lifestyle is marked by intense intelligence, hyperfocus on everything that occurs around him, incredibly productive creativity, very high energy level, and little requirement for sleep. In the classroom, he is restless, quickly bored, aggressively aware of everything around him, and impatient with slower-paced group processes. Barkley has equally intense intelligence and nonstop creativity. Yet in the classroom, he is fully focused for long periods of time, rarely bored with the learning process, and often unaware of what happens nearby. His impatience flares when others disrupt his thoughts and distract his attention. Through their excellent writing skills and gifts for research, Hartmann and Barkley have shaped the debate over the nature of paying attention to learn, to work, and to be. Hartmann defines his kind of restless, quickly bored, easily distracted attention patterns as a unique gift that requires a different curriculum and workplace environment for fulfill-

Introduction

ment. Barkley defines ADHD/ADD as a mental health disorder that requires medical intervention to fix this psychiatric/neurological dysfunction.

Which position is correct? Or is there a middle ground that can guide us in helping poor-attention individuals overcome their disruptive patterns well enough to fit into today's academic and workplace environments?

> In my work I've met hundreds of Edison-trait children and adults who also have ADHD. Because their problems with inattention, impulsivity, or hyperactivity are extreme and interfere with their daily lives, they qualify for the technical diagnosis of ADHD … I've also met hundreds of Edison-trait children and adults who don't have ADHD; because their problems with inattention, impulsivity, or hyperactivity do not interfere with their daily lives, they do not qualify for an ADHD diagnosis. In diagnostic terms, *interference with daily living* is the critical line that separates personality and pathology.
> —Lucy Jo Palladino, in Hartmann, 2003, p. xiv

Mrs. Jolly's Classroom

The scope of today's concern over paying attention can be illustrated by visiting Mrs. Jolly's third-grade classroom. This year she has 22 pupils whose ages range from almost 8 years old to just past 9. Her room is large enough to let her cluster students in different-sized work groups, depending on the kinds of projects she is supervising. Mrs. Jolly's desk is centered at the front of the classroom so that she can see each child at all times. Behind her desk is a brand-new electronic White Board, a gift from a grateful father whose child Mrs. Jolly guided through a difficult academic year. This White Board is a "digital chalkboard" that actually is a large display screen connected to Mrs. Jolly's laptop computer. Anything she types can be displayed on the White Board. Every morning the White Board displays the day's assignments and special language activities for her students to copy. The other walls are covered with colorful posters and student art. The classroom is carpeted, and each bank of overhead fluorescent lights is controlled by a rheostat that lets Mrs. Jolly decrease or increase level of light in different parts of the room. Students sit at flat-topped tables that nest together to create workplaces for group activities. Mrs. Jolly is proud to have a large aquarium with many kinds of water creatures. In a corner at the back is a comfortable cage where Zeke, a huge gray rabbit, resides. Between the aquarium and Zeke's cage is an indoor garden where seedlings sprout into plants as part of the third-grade science curriculum.

Visitors peeking into Mrs. Jolly's classroom are delighted by this friendly, comfortable, inviting learning environment. They seldom notice Mrs. Jolly's frustration, which is triggered by three pupils whose behavior disrupts the class throughout the day. Without their teacher's constant supervision, Luis, Anna, and Jacob rarely pay attention or stay on schedule with assignments and learning new skills.

Luis is a happy, outgoing youngster just past his eighth birthday. He is slender with an athletic quickness that takes him all around the room in the blink of an eye. He seldom stays in the same place very long. Mrs. Jolly never knows where to look for Luis. Within moments after she leaves his group, he is out of his chair to sharpen his pencil. On the way, he stops to check on Zeke and inspect the seedlings just starting to sprout in the garden center. All at once his attention leaps to the aquarium, where he must investigate the new guppies. Out of the corner of his eye, Luis notices Robert's new sneakers and goes to have a look. Suddenly an outside noise catches his attention, and he is at the window peering out. "It's the garbage truck," he tells the class. "There's a new man driving the truck today." By then Mrs. Jolly has left her instruction group to lead Luis back to his table and start him again on today's math lesson, which he begins to do rapidly with no mistakes. Figure I.1 shows his typical "grasshopper" performance on worksheets. When he reaches the fifth line, Luis hears a nearby sound that he turns to investigate. As he turns, he sees something new on the White Board. Out of his seat again, he glides toward the front of the room to investigate. On the way, he hears Mrs. Jolly ask a question to the reading group she is directing. Luis blurts out the answer, then adds additional information he learned last night watching the History Channel. He does

9 + 1	2 + 2	6 + 4	5 + 1	0 + 7	9 + 9	7 + 3	1 + 6	2 + 5	5 + 4
10	4			7					
9 + 4	2 + 0	8 + 7	4 + 1	6 + 6	7 + 8	3 + 2	9 + 8	0 + 8	4 + 6
	2			12					
5 + 2	3 + 9	0 + 6	8 + 1	3 + 3	7 + 4	7 + 0	1 + 5	6 + 7	2 + 3
		6	9	6		7			
1 + 0	5 + 5	7 + 6	3 + 4	2 + 6	9 + 5	7 + 2	4 + 9	0 + 3	6 + 8
1	10							3	
8 + 2	3 + 5	1 + 7	0 + 0	6 + 2	5 + 7	1 + 4	8 + 6	2 + 9	5 + 0
	8	8	0						5

FIGURE I.1. This worksheet is typical of the "grasshopper" work style of individuals with hyperfocused ADHD. They cannot stay focused on the central task without their attention jumping to something seen in the periphery of their visual field. Their visual focus jumps rapidly from place to place without following the linear structure of the worksheet.

Introduction

not see his teacher's frown at this interruption or notice the reading group's negative reaction to his unwelcome contribution. Before Mrs. Jolly has time to call his name and ask him to return to his seat, Luis notices some loose papers on her desk and begins to arrange them properly. By now Mrs. Jolly has him by the arm, firmly moving him back to his workplace while lecturing him about minding his own business.

As she turns back to the reading group, Mrs. Jolly notices that Anna is off in a daydream, her eyes gazing into the distance. She has not realized that she has dropped her pencil on the floor. With a sigh, Mrs. Jolly moves over to touch Anna's shoulder as she quietly calls her name. With a start, Anna "wakes up" and is momentarily puzzled about where she is. It takes several seconds for her to become fully aware that she is in the classroom. For a moment, she gazes at the doodles she had done a few moments ago (see Figure I.2). As she turns back to her language worksheet, Anna cannot

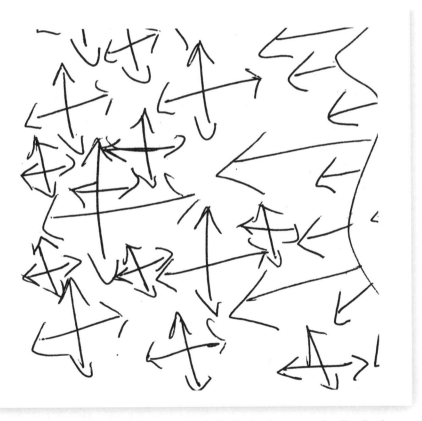

FIGURE I.2. As daydreaming begins, ADD individuals often create doodles that later they do not remember doing. Random doodles like this appear on their workpages whenever boredom triggers make-believe daydreaming or magical thinking.

find her pencil. Suddenly Luis is by her side, handing her the pencil he had found on the floor. It takes more than three minutes for Mrs. Jolly to return Luis to his seat and get Anna going again with her assignment. Meanwhile, the reading group has become restless and has begun talking loudly enough to disrupt the whole class. With all the patience she can muster, Mrs. Jolly must get everyone's attention, repeat instructions to get the groups back to work, and tour the room to make sure everyone is on the right track. By the time the teacher has restored order, Anna is "stargazing" again, off in her silent, private world of make-believe.

Now Mrs. Jolly's attention turns to Jacob, who has begun chewing his pencil and tearing his spelling worksheet into pieces. He is humming his favorite song while rhythmically kicking the legs of his table. His three table-mates have their hands in the air. "Mrs. Jolly," Jo calls out. "Make him stop kicking the table." "Mrs. Jolly," Jim chimes in. "Make him stop sing-ing that song!" As the teacher crosses the room toward Jacob, Luis is up again peering out the door to see what is happening in the hallway. "It's Mr. Bobbit changing a fluorescent light tube," he tells the class. At Jacob's table, the criticisms from his workmates trigger a moderate tantrum as he defends himself: "I'm not doing anything!" he declares. "Make them stop picking on me!" Then he slams his math book to the floor with a thud. As his tantrum increases, Jacob bursts into tears and wads up the rest of his worksheet, which he tosses across the room. Then he leaps from his seat, knocking his chair backwards, and stomps across the room to the library center, where he turns his back on the class. Figures I.3, I.4, and I.5 show Jacob's dyslexic and dysgraphic struggle with encoding any type of writ-

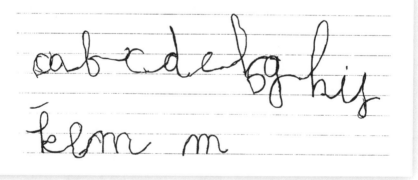

FIGURE I.3. Chapter 6 describes the tag-along layers of dyslexia and dysgraphia that often hide below the surface of ADHD or ADD. Dysgraphic struggle to write is a major source of frustration for this 8-year-old boy in third grade. He also is moderately ADHD.

Introduction

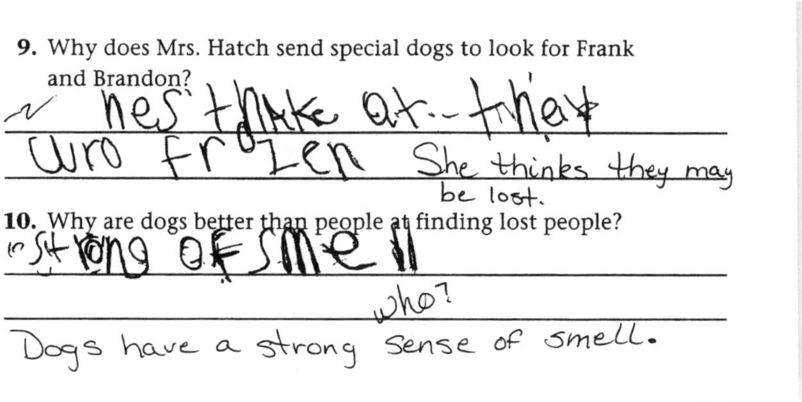

9. Why does Mrs. Hatch send special dogs to look for Frank and Brandon?

[handwritten student response] nes thnke at...they wro frozen *[teacher's note]* She thinks they may be lost.

10. Why are dogs better than people at finding lost people?

[handwritten student response] st ong of smell *[teacher's note]* who? Dogs have a strong sense of smell.

FIGURE I.4. On a better day when ADHD was not a major issue for Jacob, he did his best to do this writing task. Dysgraphia and dyslexia make it impossible for him to write legibly or neatly in confined spaces on worksheets. As he finished Item 10, he burst into a frustrated tantrum and threw his paper to the floor.

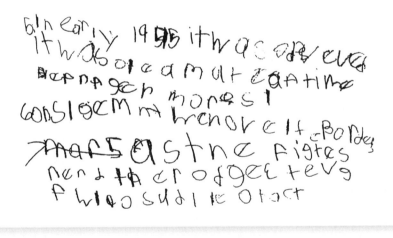

FIGURE I.5. If Jacob tries to write without lines to guide his penmanship, he loses control of spacing between words and lines. This dictated spelling test was unreadable, even though he had done his very best.

ten work. Figure I.6 shows his dyslexic decoding patterns as he works with printed words. Mrs. Jolly intercepts Luis, who is on his way to find out what is wrong with Jacob. As she passes Anna's workplace, Mrs. Jolly notices that the daydreaming girl is creating an elaborate doodle that reveals where she has gone in her magical thinking (see Figure I.7).

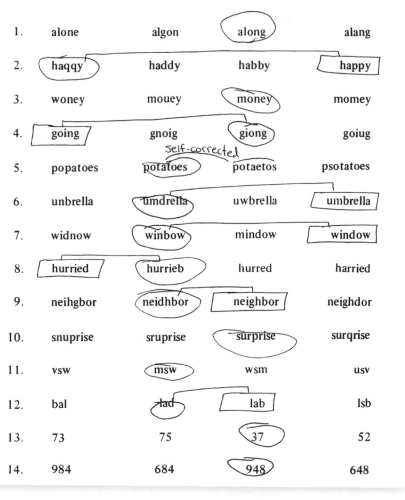

1.	alone	algon	(along)	alang
2.	(haqqy)	haddy	habby	[happy]
3.	woney	mouey	(money)	momey
4.	[going]	gnoig	(giong)	goiug
5.	popatoes	(potatoes) *self-corrected*	potaetos	psotatoes
6.	unbrella	(umdrella)	uwbrella	[umbrella]
7.	widnow	(winbow)	mindow	[window]
8.	[hurried]	(hurrieb)	hurred	harried
9.	neihgbor	(neidhbor)	[neighbor]	neighdor
10.	snuprise	sruprise	(surprise)	surqrise
11.	vsw	(msw)	wsm	usv
12.	bal	(lad)	[lab]	lsb
13.	73	75	(37)	52
14.	984	684	(948)	648

FIGURE I.6. *Identifying Children with Specific Language Disability,* Form C, by B. H. Slingerland, 1984, Cambridge, MA: Educators Publishing Service. Copyright 1984 by Educators Publishing Service. Reprinted with permission.

Are These Children ADHD?

As Mrs. Jolly and the parents of Luis, Anna, and Jacob seek answers for these puzzling behaviors, they face the dilemma of whom to believe. As they read Thom Hartmann's many publications, they recognize Luis as an "Edison-gene hunter" whose natural talents cause him to be a misfit in a mainstream classroom. Does he need medication, or will accommodations that fit his differences level the playing field enough to let him succeed in

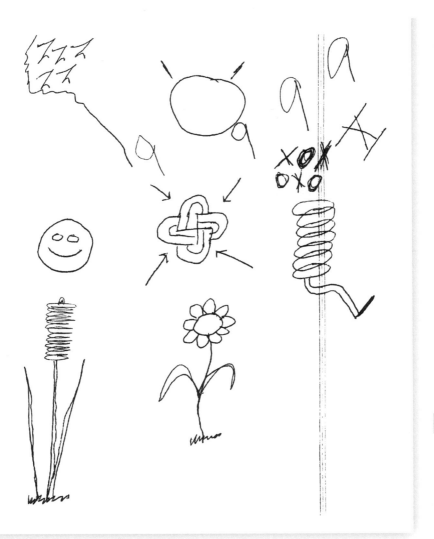

FIGURE I.7. During a prolonged daydream cycle one day at school, Anna doodled this elaborate imaginative scene. Much of her classroom time is spent doing this kind of ADD magical thinking. From *Jordan Dyslexia Assessment/Reading Program* (2nd ed., p. 71), by D. R. Jordan, 2000, Austin, TX: PRO-ED, Inc. Copyright 2000 by PRO-ED, Inc. Reprinted with permission.

the left-brain linear curriculum of our public school systems? As they read the splendid research of Russell Barkley and other scientists, Mrs. Jolly and Jacob's parents recognize the boy's overlapping symptoms of ADHD, dyslexia, and emotional instability. Does Jacob require medication, diet control, and special accommodations to treat his mental health challenge? In seeking answers for Anna's chronic, deep-seated, daydreaming inattention, are Mrs. Jolly and the parents dealing with severe ADD? If so, is medication required to treat this form of attentional disorder?

All of these questions and issues are explored in the following chapters. In Chapter 1 readers will review neurological development from conception into adulthood to see where attention deficits originate throughout the human brain. Chapter 2 explores the critical issue of executive function, along with its counterpart executive dysfunction. Chapters 3 and 4 investigate the challenges of ADHD and ADD in the classroom and the workplace. Chapter 5 describes the many faces of ADHD and ADD that bring conflict and disruption into the classroom, family life, and the workplace. Chapter 6 presents the profiles of other kinds of learning differences that often imitate ADHD and ADD. Chapter 7 explains why diet is critical for many individuals with attention deficits, along with the role that medication often plays in overcoming ADHD and ADD. Chapter 8 presents accommodation and compensation strategies that help persons overcome ADHD and ADD. Finally, Appendixes A and B present the helpful *Jordan Executive Function Index* for children and adults, while Appendix C presents the *Jordan Attention Deficit Scale*. Appendix D points readers to sources of help and information about attention deficit issues.

Introduction

How Differences in Brain Structure Foster ADHD and ADD

❤ ❤

Genetic Blueprints Determine Brain Structure

The human brain may be the most complex living thing on earth. Genetic codes carried by each parent's DNA determine how a child's brain will be structured. Brain imaging research conducted in the 1990s, during what is known as the "Decade of the Brain," determined that 97 percent of the brain's structure is preprogrammed before conception occurs (Damasio 1994, 1999; Eliot, 1999; O'Rahilly & Muller, 1996). Each brain's genetic blueprint is something like a prefabricated building kit that arrives with all the parts ready to assemble in precise order. The owner of this new building has only limited ability to modify the design of the prefabricated package. In a smiliar way, inherited genetic codes determine such physical traits as left or right handedness, color of eyes, shape of ears, tallness, balding hair patterns, and family-related talents. Genetic codes predispose offspring to have certain kinds of allergies and tendencies for specific health problems. Some family blueprints also predict certain types of learning differences, such as dyslexia, ADHD, or ADD.

The Gene for ADHD

During the 1990s, several human genome research teams identified a specific gene, called DRD4, that is most closely associated with the hyperactivity, high-risk/sensation-seeking behavior, and hyperfocused curiosity that signify ADHD. First, scientists found the D4 gene that influences the activity of dopamine. Along with the neurotransmitter norepinephrine, dopamine helps to govern how the thalamus and sensory cortex respond to stimulation. Further research revealed a variation of this gene called DRD4. DR refers to "dopamine receptor," while D4 names the gene that is in charge of how dopamine crosses synapse junctions between neurons. In continued research, scientists discovered a family of DRD4 gene variations called *alleles* that are linked to various subtypes of attention deficit differences (LaHoste et al., 1996; Rowe et al., 1998; Smalley et al., 1998; Swanson et al., 1998). This genetic evidence verifies an older notion that attention deficit runs in families.

How Neurogenesis Builds New Brains

At the moment of conception, an astonishing creative explosion occurs as sperm unites with the ovum. For the next nine months, new cells burst into being at the rate of 250,000 per minute in a genetically determined process called *neurogenesis*. From the moment of conception, many specialized chemical compounds explode into being. Each of these chemical formats is designed to attract specific types of new cells, the way magnets attract iron filings. With incredible speed, cascades of new cells follow their calling to become specialized parts of the new fetus. This swift migration of new cells brings together the ones that are genetically programmed to build all of the different organs that make up the human body. Figure 1.1 shows that by day 25 of gestation, this lightning-swift cell generation process has produced a recognizable embryo that soon will be transformed into a human fetus. By day 28 we can recognize the beginning of the spinal cord, limb buds soon to become arms and legs, cell clusters that will develop into eyes, and folds of cells that will become the higher brain hemispheres.

Neurons and Dendrites

Some of the earliest new cells are destined to become neurons that will be bundled together to build the living brain. Figure 1.2 shows how each new neuron pops into existence equipped with an already-active *growth cone* that puts out thread-like *dendrites,* much like roots sprouting from new seedlings. Instantly each dendrite seeks out other dendrites that are destined to create regions of the new brain. The role of dendrites is to bring new information into cell bodies. Figure 1.2 also shows how neurons mature as they bond with other neurons. Soon complex connecting links called *axons*

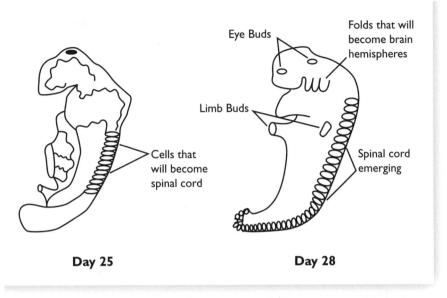

FIGURE 1.1. During the 4th week after conception, the first structures of the brain stem emerge. At the same time, the first formations of the arms, eyes, and higher brain appear.

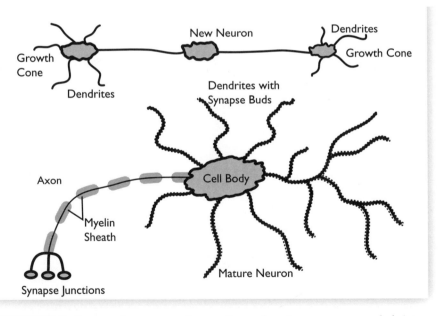

3

FIGURE 1.2. Between the moment of conception and age 2, new neurons explode into existence at the rate of 250,000 per second. Many neurons do not become fully mature until adolescence.

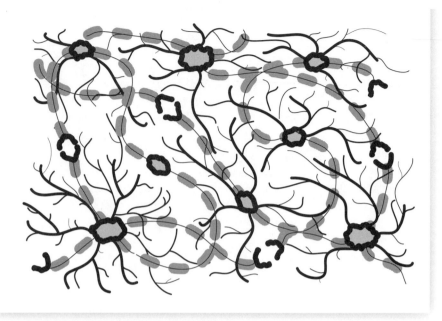

FIGURE 1.3. In the early stages of fetal development, an enormous surplus of neurons and dendrites emerges. This produces an entangled mass of neurons and dendrites as each neuron unit has the potential to connect with all others. This illustration is derived from the research of J. Leroy Conel in *The Postnatal Development of the Human Cerebral Cortex,* Volumes 1 and VIII (1930), Harvard University Press.

emerge. Axons carry information from one cell body to the next. This process of neurogenesis creates billions of neuron clusters called *dendrite trees,* as shown in Figure 1.3. By the time an infant is born, the new brain will contain 100 billion neurons with more than 3 trillion possible connecting points called *synapse buds.*

How the Brain Is Formed and Shaped After Birth

Of course, genes are important, but anyone who has ever studied nerve cells can tell you how remarkably plastic they are. The brain itself is literally molded by experience: every sight, sound, and thought leaves an imprint on specific neural circuits, modifying the way future sights, sounds, and thoughts will be registered. Brain hardware is not fixed, but living, dynamic tissue that is constantly updating itself to meet the sensory, motor, emotional and intellectual demands at hand.

—Lise Eliot, 1999, p. 4

Dendrite Pruning and Stimulus

This chapter began with the statement that before conception occurs, 97 percent of brain structure is predetermined by the genes a person inherits. This scientific fact is called *nature*. Yet, as Lise Eliot, author of *What's Going On in There,* explains, how the human brain finally is formed and shaped is largely influenced by what happens to the brain after the genetic factors are in place. This 3 percent influence on brain structure is called *nurture*. Thus, the quality of a child's environment has the potential ability to modify nature in influencing who each person is and what each individual becomes.

As the explosive creation of new brain cells continues following conception, far too many dendrites emerge. The developing brain becomes filled with overlapping clusters of neurons and dendrites, as Figure 1.3 illustrates. Midway through the first trimester of fetal development, a remarkable process called pruning begins to thin out these thickets of excess neurons and dendrites. Before the end of the first trimester, the first molding and shaping of the emerging brain begins. For the rest of this individual's life, the structure of the brain will change in response to the kinds of stimulus the person encounters. This continual reshaping of the brain is called *plasticity*. The chemical process of pruning melts away neurons and dendrites that do not respond to the stimulus of new experiences. Figure 1.4 shows how

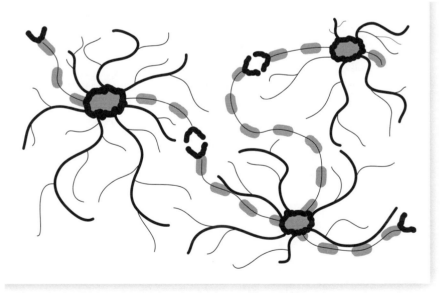

FIGURE 1.4. The neuron and dendrite connections that remain after pruning become the brain centers where specific skills are learned and new memories are formed. Throughout each person's life, these neural units continue to change as new knowledge modifies earlier neuron/dendrite formations.

Differences in Brain Structure

the remaining neurons that do respond become strong and dominant. As the brain continues to be stimulated by repeated experiences, dominant neuron trees take charge of whatever activity each region of the brain is destined to control. Until the moment of death, this is how the plasticity of the brain permits every person to learn new things and make adjustments in memory.

Incomplete Pruning and ADHD

At this very early stage of brain development, the roots of ADHD, ADD, and dyslexia are taking shape. A major factor in learning differences is incomplete pruning throughout the left brain. Children, adolescents, and adults who are dyslexic, ADHD, or ADD have inherited the tendency for pruning to lag behind schedule. When too many excess dendrites and neurons survive, it is difficult for the maturing brain to maintain full attention or to process language symbols fluently (Eliot, 1999; Jordan, 2002).

The Three-Part Brain

Between the moment of conception and birth, the three-part brain comes into being. Just as a three-story house is constructed according to a plan, the fully formed human brain is formed in a genetically determined sequence. The first part of the brain to emerge, called the brain stem, governs automatic body functions such as digestion, heartbeat, blood pressure, and breathing. Next appears the midbrain, which governs all body functions related to emotions and feelings. Finally emerges the higher brain, which is the home of conscious thought, long-term memory, and all other functions of intelligence.

The Brain Stem
Figure 1.5 shows the very early appearance of the "basement level" of the brain, which is called the *reptilian brain,* the *ancient brain,* or the *brain stem.* Figure 1.1 shows that the first recognizable structure in the fetus is the string of cells that soon become the spinal cord. By day 25 of fetal development, the process called *synaptogenesis* is creating new synapse junctions that allow the spinal cord to emerge. Between the 4th week of pregnancy and age 2, synaptogenesis produces new synapse junctions at the incredible rate of 1.8 million per second (Carlson, 1994; Eliot, 1999; Huttenlocher, 1990; Jacobson, 1991; Jordan, 2002). By day 28, this explosion of neuron connections prepares the spinal cord to begin filtering the sensations that reach

the new embryo through the mother's placenta and the amniotic fluid. For the rest of this person's life, all new data will pass through the brain stem on the way to the midbrain and higher brain. From this very early stage of development, the brain stem stands guard over the individual's emotional and physical safety.

Fight-or-Flight Reflex

By the 5th week after conception, the spinal cord and other members of the brain stem shown in Figure 1.5 have formed a safeguard team designed to test each new event or experience for safety. By the 6th week of gestation, new sensations that touch the embryo trigger nervous-like reactions that later will become *startle reflexes* when the person is surprised. Currents within the amniotic fluid cause emerging eyelids to flutter. Loud noises or events that startle the mother cause the tiny limb buds to twitch and rotate. Emerging taste buds where the tongue will be react to strong flavors in the mother's diet that enter the amniotic fluid from the mother's bloodstream. These extremely early reactions to new events are the beginning of the lifelong *fight-or-flight reflex*, which plays a major role in how people

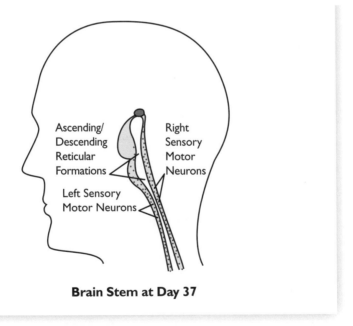

Brain Stem at Day 37

FIGURE 1.5. By the 5th week of fetal development, these regions of the basal brain already are filtering new sensations that reach the tiny fetus through the placenta and amniotic fluid.

Differences in Brain Structure

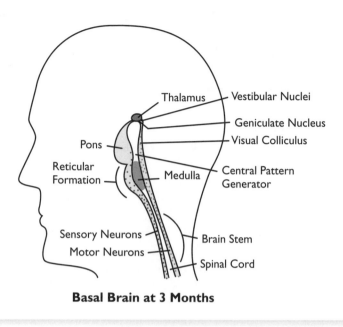

Basal Brain at 3 Months

FIGURE 1.6. By the end of the first trimester of fetal development, these basal brain formations are actively filtering all new sensory information that reaches the fetus through the amniotic fluid and the mother's placenta. For the rest of the individual's life, this fight-or-flight reflex system will safeguard the person's emotional and physical well-being.

with ADHD or ADD cope with surprise and stress. By the 7th week of fetal development, the brain stem structures shown in Figure 1.6 are busy filtering each new event by asking: "Is this safe?" Before the embryo has been transformed into a human fetus, the fight-or-flight reflex is actively testing all new experiences for safety.

The ADHD Brain Is Hypersensitive to Stimulus

At this very early stage of brain development, a fetus that will become a child with ADHD overresponds to stimuli. Inherited DRD4 characteristics are observable in the womb. Later, this individual will have difficulty ignoring what goes on at the edges of his or her environment and will continue to overreact to stimuli. This child will tend to be restless or disruptive in situations that require full attention and an ability to tune out distractions. This individual will be too easily startled, overly sensitive to stressful moments, and overly emotional in handling everyday issues and challenges.

The Basal Brain

By the 6th month of gestation, the basal brain has emerged atop the brain stem, as shown in Figure 1.7. Similar to assembling pieces of a prefabricated building, these genetically programmed regions of the basal brain take shape step by step.

Motor Neurons

By the 7th week of gestation, the *motor neurons* along the left side of the spinal cord take charge of movements of the emerging head and four limb buds. During the second trimester, these motor neurons become linked with the right-brain *motor cortex*, then later with the motor cortex of the left brain. When a fetus has inherited dyslexic traits, these motor neurons develop differently. These genetic characteristics often cause delays in fine

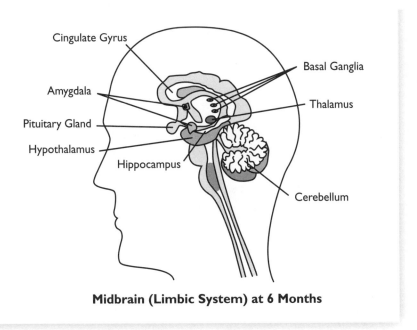

Midbrain (Limbic System) at 6 Months

FIGURE 1.7. By the end of the second trimester of fetal development, these midbrain (limbic system) formations are taking charge of automatic body behaviors, such as heartbeat, blood flow, reaction to skin sensations, sucking reflex, yawning, eyelid flutter, and arm and leg activity. During the first days of infancy, these midbrain regions will work together to govern feelings and emotions, as well as to supervise the first short-term and long-term memories.

Differences in Brain Structure

motor and gross motor development in childhood. Finger movements for handwriting do not become fluent. This person will have poor penmanship, or *dysgraphia* (described in Chapter 6) that never becomes fully neat or legible.

Sensory Neurons

By the 9th week of fetal development, the *sensory neurons* in the brain stem have formed axon links to the cell clusters that are becoming the chin, eyelids, and arms. By the 10th week, sensory and motor neurons are connected to the emerging legs. By the 12th week, these sensory pathways are connected to the entire body surface of the growing fetus. By the 13th week, these sensory neurons are linked to the emerging thalamus (see Figure 1.7), which is one of the lifelong regulators of how the individual responds to feelings, emotions, and stress. As this sensory network takes shape, the fetus begins to respond more actively to stimulus. Eyelids flutter open, then close. Arms and legs stretch and change position. Emerging lips practice opening, closing, and smiling. These repeated motor and sensory actions speed up the pruning process shown in Figures 1.3 and 1.4. When the DRD4 gene and variant alleles exist, the soon-to-be ADHD child often becomes so active in the womb that the mother wonders, "What's going on in there?"

Central Pattern Generator

One of the first motor control regions of the basal brain is the *central pattern generator* (CPG), which becomes active by the 10th week of gestation. The CPG governs rhythmical muscle movements everywhere in the body. Later the CPG links with the cerebellum to provide automatic movement orientation for the whole brain. By the 11th week, the CPG regulates sweeping, rotating movements of the developing arms and legs. Soon the CPG is in charge of back-and-forth and up-and-down eye movements called *nystagmus*. During the last three months of gestation, the fetus begins to have sleep/wake cycles similar to those we see in infants and toddlers. The CPG regulates rapid eye movement (REM) as early as the third trimester of pregnancy. For the rest of the individual's life, the CPG will help to regulate all rhythmical activity, such as breathing, chewing, walking, running, hopping, skipping, and other sports activities. A fetus that has inherited the DRD4 gene tends to develop lifelong overactivity called *hyperactivity*. Children who inherit dyslexic traits often never become well coordinated or graceful in body movements.

Medulla

Figure 1.6 shows the region of the basal brain called the *medulla*. By the 10th week of gestation, the medulla has taken charge of testing each new experience: "Is this safe?" For the rest of the person's life, the medulla will stand guard over emotional and physical safety, ready to trigger the fight-or-flight reflex. When ADHD exists, the individual is always on edge, reacting with overly sensitive emotions before all of the facts are considered. Inheriting the DRD4 gene predisposes ADHD individuals to be impulsive and to have overly emotional reactions. They do not wait to use logic or commonsense reasoning to analyze new situations.

Reticular Formation

During the 16th week of pregnancy, a specialized cluster of neurons emerges just above the medulla. The *reticular formation* plays a lifelong role in how the person interprets and responds to what occurs in the external environment. During the second trimester of fetal development, the reticular formation starts to filter the first sensations of pleasure and pain. Sonograms begin to show the fetus smiling or frowning as the reticular formation becomes more mature. As internal organs take shape within the body of the fetus, the reticular formation participates in regulating rhythms of the heart, digestive tract, and lung activity. During the third trimester, the reticular formation will help to establish sleep/wake cycles and to govern how the taste buds respond to various sensations. In the final weeks of pregnancy, the reticular formation is a major participant in establishing good balance among body functions, called *homeostasis*. For the rest of the person's life, the reticular formation plays a key role in the individual's sense of well-being.

A critical factor for most persons with ADHD is unbalanced emotions and feelings. As Chapter 3 describes, lack of homeostasis creates major lifestyle challenges for individuals who have inherited the DRD4 gene. In these continually frustrated, overly reactive persons, the reticular formation cannot take charge because of differences in neuron development, especially incomplete pruning.

Pons

During week 13 of fetal development, an amazing specialized region called the *pons* emerges at the top of the brain stem. Very quickly, the pons forms

11

axon links with the spinal cord, central pattern generator, reticular formation, and basal ganglia in the midbrain. The pons becomes a major participant in regulating the body's physical activity, including sleep. As newborn infants learn to sleep outside the womb, the pons is the key to deep sleep. As the brain goes through the slowing-down process of falling to sleep, the pons fires a command that paralyzes all of the larger muscles. This process, called *sleep paralysis*, allows the brain to have active, aggressive dreams while the body remains still. A common challenge of ADHD individuals is restless, overly active body actions during deep sleep. Incomplete development of neurons in the pons permits dream content to "leak" into large muscles, causing the sleeping person to thrash about, cry out, or even sleep-walk. This troubled, interrupted deep sleep is disruptive for families and partners. A lifelong issue for sleep-disturbed individuals is chronic fatigue, which becomes a trigger for irritability, quick anger, and aggressive impatience as part of the ADHD profile.

Thalamus

During the 15th week of gestation, twin regions of the basal brain emerge, called the *thalamus*. For the rest of the person's life, the thalamus is a critical relay station between the basal brain, the midbrain, and regions of the higher brain. As the fetus develops during the third trimester, all incoming sensory data is filtered by the thalamus. If the brain stem triggers the fight-or-flight reflex in response to unsafe events, the thalamus "shuts down" higher brain functions until the threat has been resolved. The thalamus is much like the breaker switch panel that safeguards one's home against electrical circuit overloads. When a possibly unsafe event occurs, the thalamus shuts down access to the higher brain. When safety is restored, the thalamus opens access channels to the higher brain. In addition to monitoring personal safety, the twin regions of the thalamus monitor the kinds of information sent on to the higher brain. The left region of the thalamus filters and preorganizes verbal data that is fired up to the parietal and temporal lobes for processing. The right region of the thalamus filters and preorganizes visual and spatial data that is sent on to the somatosensory cortex, the parietal lobe, the temporal lobe, or the occipital lobe. When the thalamus develops normally, children and adolescents arrive at executive function (described in Chapter 2), which overcomes impulsivity with logical thinking and commonsense reasoning.

When ADHD exists, the thalamus cannot maintain complete control over these critical functions. Individuals who inherit the DRD4 gene do not enjoy smoothly functioning thalamus filtering and preorganizing. ADHD allows too much unfiltered, poorly organized data to reach the higher brain, causing the person to live with disorganized mental images, incomplete thought patterns, and inability to wait before acting. Chapter 2 describes the challenge of *executive dysfunction,* which occurs when the thalamus cannot stay in control of new data processing.

The final development of the basal brain occurs during the 5th month of gestation. Three critical regions of the basal brain emerge at the top of the brain stem. Soon these regions will be linked to the developing "second story" of the three-part brain, the midbrain (limbic system), which already surrounds the upper level of the basal brain.

Vestibular Nuclei

At the same time the ear buds are emerging, specialized neurons called the *vestibular nuclei* are forming at the top of the brain stem. These neurons are the first step in developing hearing. During the 7th month of gestation, the vestibular nuclei begin to hear sound patterns, such as the mother's voice, certain ranges of music she listens to, and repeated sounds that trigger sonic vibrations in the amniotic fluid. As they emerge, the vestibular nuclei build axon links to the reticular formation and thalamus to become part of the lifelong fight-or-flight safety system. ADHD often includes hypersensitivity to loud sounds and noise. Individuals who inherit the DRD4 gene tend to overreact to sudden noise. Ironically, these persons often play their music very loudly, creating disruptions and conflict. They also tend to speak too loudly in group situations. Incomplete dendrite pruning in the vestibular nuclei often causes lifelong challenges in how ADHD individuals cope with the noise of their environment and the sounds of language.

Visual Colliculus
During the 7th month of development, the eyes become sensitive to light. Parents viewing ultrasound images of their unborn child often see the eyes squinting as if the baby were staring at bright light. These visual reflexes are governed by the *visual colliculus* at the top of the brain stem. If dyslexia exists along with ADHD, this person will struggle to "see" printed details clearly, especially black print on white background under bright light. This *scotopic sensitivity* is described in Chapter 6 as a tag-along syndrome that often complicates ADHD.

Geniculate Nucleus
The final part of the basal brain to emerge is the *geniculate nucleus.* This highly specialized region of the basal brain plays a critical role in how the person sees and hears. Chapter 6 describes neuron differences that interfere with the work of the geniculate nucleus in seeing classroom details

clearly and in hearing oral language correctly. The lower portion (lateral region) of the geniculate nucleus is designed to process vision details sent to the brain by the retina of each eye. The middle portion (medial region) of the geniculate nucleus is designed to separate human speech from all other sounds, organize speech sounds into correct vowel/consonant sequences, then send that language data to the left temporal lobe, where the higher brain processes language. As I explain in Chapter 6, incomplete neuron development in the geniculate nucleus causes dyslexic struggle with oral language, as well as a visual dilemma called *word blindness*, or *scotopic sensitivity*, which blocks development of reading skills.

Midbrain Limbic System

During the second trimester of gestation, the "second story" of the three-part brain emerges to surround the upper part of the brain stem, as shown in Figure 1.7. This region of the new brain is called by two names, *midbrain* or *limbic system*. By week 15 of fetal development, the midbrain becomes a critical master control center for strong emotions and feelings. At the same time, the limbic system filters and preorganizes incoming verbal and nonverbal information, then decides which new data is sent on to the higher brain. This limbic system clearinghouse is designed to eliminate unnecessary data that would only clutter the higher brain without helping the individual. Several midbrain regions are involved in creating the many enzymes, hormones, and neurotransmitters that make up body chemistry. Chapter 7 describes inherited dietary problems in individuals with ADHD and dyslexia.

Learning Begins in the Midbrain

During the "Decade of the Brain" (the 1990s), brain imaging research revealed that, since the 1600s, Western cultures have been wrong about how educational programs should be designed (Barnard & Brazelton, 1990; Block et al., 1997; Chugani, 1999; Damasio, 1994, 1999; Denckla, 1991; Eliot, 1999; Gilligan, 1996; Huttenlocher, 1990; Jordan, 1998, 2000b, 2002; Killackey, 1995; Lyon, 2000; Penrose, 1994; Ratey & Johnson, 1997; Schacter, 1996; Searle, 1997; Sutherland, 1992; Ungerleider & Haxby, 1994). For centuries, educators have assumed that teaching students involves stuffing their higher brains with facts and new data. This model of education assumes that silent, passive learning that keeps emotions and feelings outside the classroom is the best way to teach and learn. New understanding of how the midbrain starts the learning process shows us that the higher brain is the last part of the central nervous system to deal with new data. Before the higher brain is aware of new information, all incoming data is first processed by the limbic system, which filters the emotions and feelings as the first step in learning. Figure 1.7 shows the family of specialized midbrain regions that are in place by the 5th month of fetal development.

Cerebellum

One of the first regions of the midbrain to emerge is the *cerebellum*. This large member of the limbic system holds half of all the neurons in the entire brain. The cerebellum is the "control tower" that directs all mental traffic coming and going within the brain. The main job of the cerebellum is to interpret for the higher brain every type of muscle movement over the whole body. In partnership with the reticular formation, the cerebellum determines the best possible integration of vision, hearing, body movement, and body motion. No one could walk, lean, run, stand, or turn corners without this constant monitoring by the cerebellum and reticular formation.

Proprioception

Part of this muscle control monitoring is a process called *proprioception*. Inside the cerebellum are specialized neurons called proprioceptors, which link the spinal cord with the higher brain. This proprioceptor network is similar to an antilock braking system that keeps vehicles from skidding on slick pavement. Many times per second, the vehicle's minicomputer adjusts how much pressure the braking system applies to each wheel. In milliseconds each wheel receives slightly more or less pressure to stop. This constantly changing braking pressure keeps wheels from locking so that the vehicle does not skid out of control. In a similar way, proprioceptor neurons in the cerebellum adjust the retraction and extension of muscle fibers in the body. In this way, the cerebellum is the body's command center that "fine tunes" all muscle action to keep body activity well balanced and under control.

In 1985, Martha Denckla began to explain the role the cerebellum plays in paying full attention by preventing random muscle activity that distracts or interrupts higher brain activity. Individuals who inherit the DRD4 gene for ADHD have lifelong difficulty sitting still without jiggling arms and legs, tapping toes and fingers, fiddling with things that make noise, and continually squirming to shift body position. Within their midbrains, incomplete neuron development prevents the cerebellum from staying in charge of muscle activity.

Basal Ganglia

During the 14th week of gestation, triple neuron clusters emerge just above the thalamus. These are the *basal ganglia*, the first brain regions to distinguish between voluntary and involuntary muscle action. Soon the basal ganglia form axon links with the brain stem motor neurons, central pattern generator, cerebellum, and emerging higher brain motor cortex. These team members form a feedback circuit that instantly tells the whole brain what muscle systems are doing. As this feedback circuit matures, the brain develops fluency in voluntary muscle movement. As an infant begins to use large muscles for movement and small muscles for grasping, the child gains fluency in coordinating muscle systems to walk, crawl, run, lift, turn, and lean over without falling. Later this brain feedback circuit enables the child to become fluent at handwriting, keyboard writing, playing musical instruments, and participating in sports activities.

Individuals who inherit the DRD4 gene for ADHD often have trouble with these kinds of coordination activities. Surges of excess energy create spills, accidents, and mistakes in what the person does. Incomplete neuron formations throughout the basal ganglia feedback system causes impulsive, awkward, or disruptive body behavior in many ADHD individuals.

Cingulate Gyrus

Midway through the second trimester of gestation, a long, circular structure emerges above the brain stem. This is the *cingulate gyrus*, which encircles the midbrain as a walking path might encircle a park, following curves and hills and valleys. The cingulate gyrus plays a key role in organizing many factors that will determine the child's future self-image, also called the *self-map*. The cingulate gyrus forms axon links with the hypothalamus, thalamus, and right-brain parietal lobe that shape distinctive traits of the person's body motion, posture, body image (paralanguage habits), speech patterns, and emotional expression that one day will form the person's unique personality. This process of developing the self-map is called the *proto-self*. Like a self-portrait or autobiography, the proto-self allows us to know ourselves for who we really are. The cingulate gyrus also helps the midbrain to filter sensory data and emotions that are linked to pain and pleasure.

Individuals who inherit the DRD4 gene for ADHD often do not develop the ability to see themselves realistically or accurately. As later chapters explain, a major characteristic of ADHD and ADD is make-believe thinking, also called *magical thinking*. Many persons with ADHD or ADD never learn how to separate reality from make-believe. When this strong tendency exists, they grow up with a distorted proto-self that keeps them from seeing themselves accurately. Underdeveloped neurons within the cingulate gyrus foster warped proto-self. In some ADHD individuals, this kind of unreal self-image includes delusional thinking or even paranoia, which prevents these persons from perceiving reality about themselves.

Amygdala

During the 20th week of fetal development, twin clusters of specialized neurons emerge inside the forward curve of the cingulate gyrus. This is the *amygdala,* which quickly becomes the main crossroads of the axon pathways that link the brain stem with the higher brain. Most of the linking pathways in the brain pass through the twin amygdala terminals. The amygdala system regulates automatic decision making and reflexes that do not require conscious thought, such as jerking back from a hot surface, jumping out of the path of a vehicle, or ducking out of the path of an object someone has thrown. Toward the end of the third trimester of pregnancy, the amygdala lobes connect with the emerging *prefrontal cortex* to participate in the left brain's logical thinking and commonsense reasoning.

A major function of the amygdala is to control fear. As dendrite pruning streamlines the amygdala's neuron trees on schedule, young children learn to read danger signals in the environment. The amygdala enables the higher brain to develop a stable balance of emotions called homeostasis, which keeps fear, dread, and anxiety under control. The amygdala becomes the midbrain center of social order by enabling individuals to suppress strong, disruptive, or destructive impulses that trigger inappropriate behavior. The amygdala controls strong emotions such as fear, dread, terror, rage, urge to kill, lust, greed, desire for revenge, and jealousy. As the amygdala becomes more mature, it modifies impulsive urges so that individuals can learn to wait. When neuron development is incomplete, the amygdala cannot fully control a sense of fear, a panic attack, or a fight-or-flight reflex.

Incomplete development of the amygdala presents serious lifelong challenges for many people with ADHD. A major characteristic of ADHD above a moderate level is the person's inability to say no to impulses that release torrents of disruptive emotions and feelings. The ADHD earmarks of impulsivity, lack of logical reasoning before acting, and too-quick emotional reaction to stress arise largely from incomplete neuron formations within the amygdala system.

Hippocampus

Toward the end of the second trimester of pregnancy, just below the lateral loop of the cingulate gyrus, a highly specialized neuron cluster emerges. This cluster, called the *hippocampus,* soon becomes linked with the amygdala, thalamus, and parietal lobes in the emerging higher brain. The midbrain has two major functions: maintaining a healthy emotional balance to enrich a person's life and enabling the higher brain to build a rich "file" of permanent memories. The lifelong role of the hippocampus is to be the starting point for memory. All data that becomes part of permanent (long-term) memory is first filtered and preorganized by the hippocampus. All types of learning differences that create difficulties in building permanent memory stem from incomplete neuron formation within the hippocampus. Chapter 8 describes several promising "brain training" strategies that seem to improve functions of the hippocampus to enhance a person's ability to develop long-term memory. Of all the many faces of learning difference (LD), trouble building permanent memory is one of the most frustrating challenges in the classroom and the workplace.

Hypothalamus and Pituitary

During the 14th week of fetal development, two regions of the limbic system develop side by side. Their lifelong role will be to regulate how the body responds to stress. These are the *hypothalamus* and *pituitary*. Chapter 3 discusses the critical impact that too much stress has on a person's emotional and mental health. The hypothalamus and pituitary govern the production of the stress hormones that spurt into the bloodstream at the first moment of stress. A major hormone in regulating stress is *cortisol,* which is designed to soothe inflamed emotions during fight-or-flight reflex episodes. The hypothalamus and pituitary have the job of keeping stress at lowest possible levels so that the rest of the limbic system and higher brain can function at their best. As Chapter 3 explains, too much stress interferes with paying attention, building permanent memory, and thriving in social development.

The Two-Part Higher Brain

Midway through the first trimester of gestation, the higher brain hemispheres begin to take shape. Genetic programming causes the right brain hemisphere to develop more rapidly than the left brain hemisphere. Partway through its development, the right brain sprouts a thick bundle of neurons called the *corpus collosum,* which becomes a communication bridge between the brain hemispheres. The outer surface of each brain hemisphere is a paper-thin layer of neurons called the *cerebral cortex,* where most of the brain's thinking, learning, and remembering occur. The cerebral cortex is made of three layers of neurons only 3 millimeters thick, less than the distance between two typewritten symbols. By 9 months, each brain hemisphere is complete, with the right hemisphere somewhat larger than the left.

Right-Brain Hemisphere

Figure 1.8 shows the major regions of the right-brain hemisphere at 9 months. If the young child receives safe, culturally rich stimulus during the first 2 years of life, the right brain becomes the control center for positive

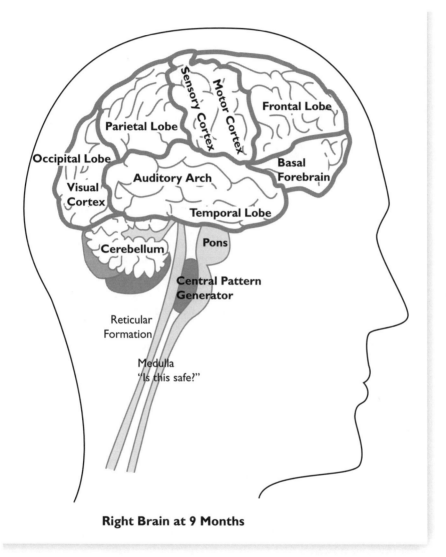

Right Brain at 9 Months

FIGURE 1.8. By the end of the third trimester of fetal development, these right brain regions are in place, ready to enable the newborn infant to interact with the new world of sights, sounds, odors, and skin sensations. During infancy, the right brain matures more rapidly than the left brain as the child responds to all the nonverbal stimulus in his or her environment.

emotion-based thinking, intuition, creativity, and nonverbal problem solving. The right brain is illiterate. It does not learn to read, write, or spell. However, a specialized region within the right parietal lobe learns how to monitor the left brain's language processing. In 1979, Erin Zaidel at the University of California in Los Angeles named this the "Oops Center." As this monitoring center spots left-brain language mistakes (misspellings, errors in using phonics, handwriting glitches, mistakes in math computation), the person often whispers "Oops!" as he or she backs up to correct the error. The major business of the right brain is to imagine, think, plan, create, and make decisions based on feelings, emotions, and intuitive hunches. The right brain is the home of nonverbal talents, such as higher mathematics reasoning, artistic creation, engineering, athletics, musical skills, and expert use of tools.

Motor/Sensory Cortex

The first regions of the right brain to become active are the *motor cortex* and *sensory cortex*. These twin regions of the *somatosensory cortex* work together to control muscle behavior and to interpret sensations that are reported from the brain stem and midbrain. Figure 1.9 shows the sequence of motor development that begins during the third trimester of fetal development. Right-brain motor skills develop in bottom-to-top order, starting with tongue movements and ending with leg movement coordination. As each of these developmental stages occurs, the growing child attains new fine motor skills in the sequence shown in Figure 1.9.

Children with ADHD and dyslexia often do not follow this developmental sequence of motor skills. More than half of all ADHD youngsters also have dyslexic struggle with handwriting, called *dysgraphia,* which is described in Chapter 6 (Barkley, 1990; Jordan, 1996a, 1996b, 1998, 2000b, 2002). Dysgraphia is caused by incomplete neuron formations in the motor cortex region that controls hand motions.

Right Parietal Lobe

As it emerges toward the back of the right-brain hemisphere, the *parietal lobe* becomes a dominant region of the right brain. A major lifelong function of the right parietal lobe is to regulate how individuals perceive their own bodies. This physical self-perception is linked to the midbrain cingulate gyrus, which generates the proto-self (self-image) that each person achieves through repeated emotions and feelings. By the time an infant is born, the right parietal lobe has become the major center for organizing all

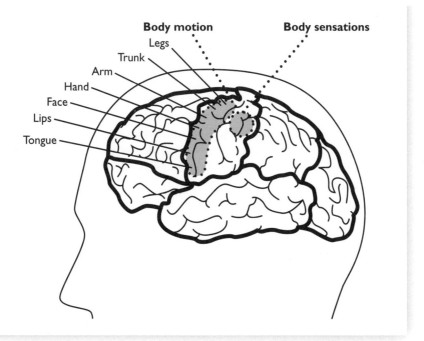

Body motion　　**Body sensations**

Legs

Trunk

Arm

Hand

Face

Lips

Tongue

FIGURE 1.9. Early in the second trimester of fetal development, the emerging fetus begins to make sucking motions with the mouth. As this pre-sucking behavior grows, so do kicking motions of the legs and pushing motions of the arms. Fingers begin to curl into fists, then relax. Toward the end of the second trimester, the fetus makes swimming motions that involve the trunk, arms, and legs. Following birth, the infant's gross motor and fine motor skills emerge in the bottom-to-top sequence shown above.

of the new data the higher brain receives. All new information from the basal brain and limbic system comes first to the right parietal lobe, where it is sorted and evaluated, then is fired on to other higher brain regions for final processing. By age 15, the right parietal lobe becomes a participant in higher nonverbal math concepts. The right parietal lobe plays a major role in vivid imagination and artistic creativity that are expressed in such forms as music, drama, art, fashion design, and architecture. The right parietal lobe regulates body-in-space activity such as moving safely around in one's home, driving through city traffic, or playing sports. Such practical tasks as putting on one's clothes are coordinated by the parietal lobe. This region of the right brain enables the whole brain to assemble visual images, such as seeing a complete clock face, the shape of a tree, or the details of an outdoor landscape. The parietal lobe governs talents for assembling whole structures, such as rebuilding a vehicle engine, tailoring a new garment, or constructing a new building.

Right Occipital Lobe

At the back of the right brain is the *occipital lobe,* where vision for objects occurs. The central region of the occipital lobe is the *visual cortex,* where the brain turns vision energy into mental images. The right occipital lobe translates the outside world into countless mental images. This region of the brain is something like a huge wall covered by thousands of television screens, each showing a small bit of what the person sees. From a distance, this wall of visual images appears to be a whole scene as all of the parts blend into complete images. At lightning speed, the occipital lobe regulates the process called *brain mapping,* which instantly creates new mental images as visual data shifts and changes. This never-ending flow of occipital lobe images keeps track of constantly changing contrasts between light and dark, fluctuations in movement, differences in form and shape, distances between objects, and the figure/ground perception of where objects are. The right occipital lobe specializes in interpreting all of the nonverbal data in our lives, such as recognizing human faces, pictures, designs, and graphic information. However, the right occipital lobe does not interpret the written language symbols we call an alphabet. That visual task, called reading, is done by the left-brain occipital lobe.

Right Temporal Lobe

Just above the right ear is the *right temporal lobe,* which plays a major role in intepreting and governing how we fit into the world around us. The right temporal lobe is the center of time awareness. This region of the brain learns time sequence, such as seconds, minutes, hours, days, months, years, and changing seasons. The right temporal lobe distinguishes between music and environmental noise. This region of the brain processes musical tone, how loudly we speak, and the volume of noise we generate in our lifestyles. When neuron development is incomplete in the right temporal lobe, the person is "tone deaf" to music and cannot hear tonal variations and changes in musical pitch. This neuronal deficit causes monotone singing and flat, monotonous speech that lacks normal inflection and language rhythms, often called *prosidy.* The right temporal lobe governs complex physical activities such as keyboard typing, using tools and machinery, working at a computer, and playing musical instruments.

Right Frontal Lobe

The last regions to develop in the human brain are the large right and left *frontal lobes,* which fill the curved front region of the head. These brain regions become the center for intellectual activity, along with storing important knowledge and information in long-term memory. The right frontal lobe becomes a major control center for positive emotion-based thinking and intuition for solving nonverbal problems.

Right Basal Forebrain

Toward the end of the third trimester of pregnancy, the lower portion of the right frontal lobe becomes the *basal forebrain*. This region of the frontal brain teams with the parietal lobe and cingulate gyrus to govern how a person's proto-self (self-image) is expressed and presented to others. The basal forebrain determines how flexible, spontaneous, and adaptive one's personality becomes. How the basal forebrain develops determines personality styles, such as shyness, boldness, thoughtfulness, or self-focused insensitivity. In Mrs. Jolly's classroom, we met the three different personality styles of Luis, Anna, and Jacob—differences that developed because of how their basal forebrains became "wired."

Right-Brain Style of Learning

Children in all cultures spend the first years of their lives enjoying and expanding their natural right-brain talents and nonverbal abilities. Before children enter the restrictions of formal education, their lives are richly involved in the style of learning called *right-brain circular style*, shown in Figure 1.10. Figure 1.11 summarizes the lifelong roles that the right-brain regions play in the quality and richness of one's life. Youngsters like Luis carry this strong right-brain lifestyle into the classroom. Luis is one of Thom Hartmann's "Edison-gene hunters"—people who flourish with the extraordinary right-brain talents shown in Figure 1.10. These circular-style right-brain attributes often come into conflict with traditional classroom curriculum restrictions.

Left-Brain Hemisphere

The last regions of the brain to mature and become functional are within the left-brain hemisphere, as shown in Figure 1.12. The left brain is the center for language, speech, verbal talent, and logical reasoning. Most individuals have the left-brain neurological potential to master literacy skills (reading, spelling, and writing) if they receive enough neuron stimulus

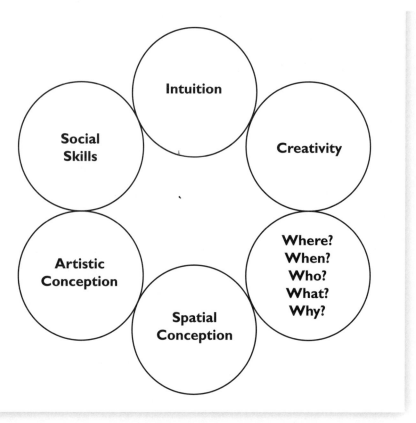

FIGURE 1.10. The right brain is designed to do multitask thinking in which several kinds of thoughts occur simultaneously. This is called right-brain circular style of learning and thinking. The right brain wonders, Where? When? Why? Who? What? at the same time that creative, imaginative ideas occur. The right brain learns to make "educated guesses" that involve intuition at the same time the person reads body language for good social skills.

through several years of literacy skill training. Individuals who are born dyslexic often do not. The left brain specializes in logical thinking, commonsense reasoning, and factual thinking. Chapter 2 describes executive function, which is the final "hardwiring" milestone of the adolescent brain. Through executive function, the left brain maintains whole-brain organization, develops lifelong habits of being methodical, and enables individuals to wait instead of yielding to impulses. If the young child's developing brain is stimulated (nurtured) within a safe lifestyle where the youngster is loved, encouraged, and forgiven, the left brain develops fluent socialization skills along with positive feelings and emotions, such as patience, kindness, generosity, and self-control.

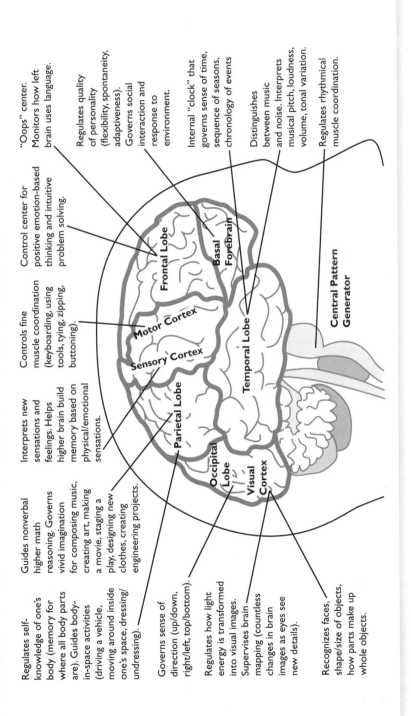

FIGURE 1.11. The business of the right brain is to imagine, think, plan, create, and make decisions based upon feelings, emotions, and intuitive hunches. The right brain is designed to look cautiously for possible dangers or problems. While the left brain urges the person to move ahead into action, the right brain cautions, "Not quite yet. Let's make sure this is safe before we do it."

25

Differences in Brain Structure

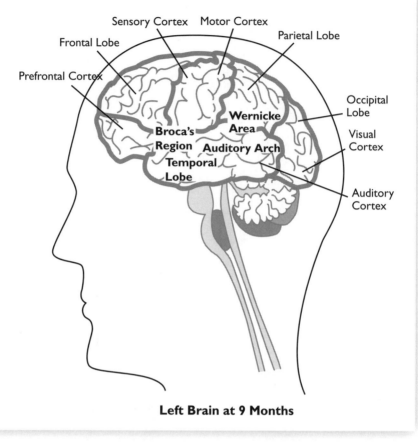

Sensory Cortex   Motor Cortex

Frontal Lobe   Parietal Lobe

Prefrontal Cortex

Occipital
Lobe

Wernicke
Broca's   **Area**
Region   **Auditory Arch**   Visual
                                          Cortex
Temporal
Lobe

Auditory
Cortex

Left Brain at 9 Months

FIGURE 1.12. The business of the left brain is to wait, think things through logically, look at the consequences that likely will occur, and make decisions based upon common-sense reasoning. Over time, the left brain in most individuals gains mastery over literacy skills (reading, spelling, writing). The left brain does not become fully mature until early adulthood.

Left Parietal Lobe

The left parietal lobe guides the visual perceptual process of learning to read math numerals and symbols, along with the verbal process of naming math symbols and labeling objects. This region of the left brain also governs sense of direction (left or right). Figure 1.13 shows where the first steps in reading occur. In individuals who are not dyslexic, specialized neuron clusters within the left parietal lobe learn to decode (interpret) printed or written language symbols. Other neuron formations learn to encode (write) the person's language. At the same time, still other specialized neurons learn how to connect sounds to letters for spelling. The left parietal lobe plays a critical role in learning to read. This region of the brain is where dyslexia first appears as the youngster struggles to "see" printed letters and words in correct sequence. When dyslexia exists, this part of the left brain struggles to remember which way letters face and which direction the eyes should track in reading.

Left Occipital Lobe

At the back of the left brain is the *left occipital lobe,* where the *visual cortex* develops. The right visual cortex specializes in interpreting likenesses and differences of objects. In four out of five individuals, the left visual cortex specializes in decoding written language symbols called the alphabet, as well as math symbols. In four out of five individuals, the left visual cortex

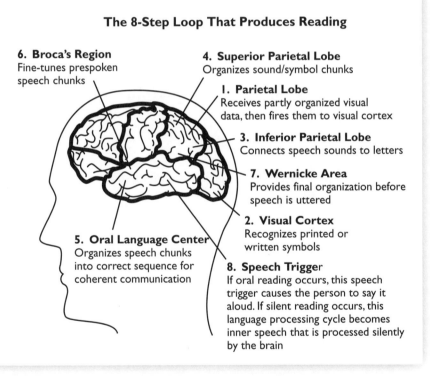

The 8-Step Loop That Produces Reading

6. Broca's Region
Fine-tunes prespoken speech chunks

4. Superior Parietal Lobe
Organizes sound/symbol chunks

1. Parietal Lobe
Receives partly organized visual data, then fires them to visual cortex

3. Inferior Parietal Lobe
Connects speech sounds to letters

7. Wernicke Area
Provides final organization before speech is uttered

2. Visual Cortex
Recognizes printed or written symbols

5. Oral Language Center
Organizes speech chunks into correct sequence for coherent communication

8. Speech Trigger
If oral reading occurs, this speech trigger causes the person to say it aloud. If silent reading occurs, this language processing cycle becomes inner speech that is processed silently by the brain

27

FIGURE 1.13. Brain imaging research by Sally and Bernard Shaywitz at Yale University School of Medicine has described how the left brain reads. This eight-step reading loop emerges gradually as children respond to the stimulus of reading training over time. Those who are dyslexic do not become fluent automatically in this eight-step reading process. This illustration is derived from research reported by Sally Shaywitz in "Dyslexia: A New Model," pp. 2–8, *Scientific American* (November 1996).

has the neurological potential to learn how to decode printed language symbols called the alphabet. As Figure 1.13 shows, the left-brain visual cortex is critical in learning to read. When dyslexia exists, this region of the brain does not develop automatic memory for which direction letters should face. Individuals who are dyslexic face lifelong challenge in interpreting the direction and correct sequence of language symbols in reading, spelling, and writing.

Left Temporal Lobe

During the first years of early childhood, most children follow a predictable developmental sequence that brings them to language-related left-brain milestones at specific ages. Youngsters with ADHD, ADD, or dyslexia do not. Students with these types of LD usually lag behind typical development in the *left temporal lobe,* which plays several critical roles in how language skills become mature and fluent. Figure 1.12 shows the *auditory arch* that links Broca's region with the Wernicke area at opposite areas of the auditory cortex. The Broca region, named after the French neurologist Paul Broca, controls use of words and phrases. The Wernicke area, named for the German neurologist Karl Wernicke, controls fluency in talking, use of grammar, and creativity in word usage. These language team members within the left temporal lobe enable most individuals to learn how to spell, apply rules of phonics, read orally, talk fluently, and use correct syntax and grammar. The left temporal lobe also plays a role in how a person thinks about morality, religious or spiritual issues, and serious reflection. The left temporal lobe teams with the cingulate gyrus and parietal lobes in building one's proto-self (self-image). Finally, the left temporal lobe is the center for musical harmony, tonal variations, and melody.

Prefrontal Cortex

The last region of the higher brain to develop is the *prefrontal cortex,* located just above the left eye. Chapter 2 explains the complex role that the prefrontal cortex plays in the quality of one's life. The prefrontal cortex begins its gradual development during early childhood—a process that continues until the late teens or early 20s. The prefrontal cortex is designed to become the executive in charge of all other brain functions, the way a talented executive takes charge of an organization. Figure 1.14 shows how the mature prefrontal cortex maintains executive function over the whole brain. If a child grows up in an organized, peaceful, emotionally safe environment that is governed by logic and common sense, the prefrontal cortex becomes

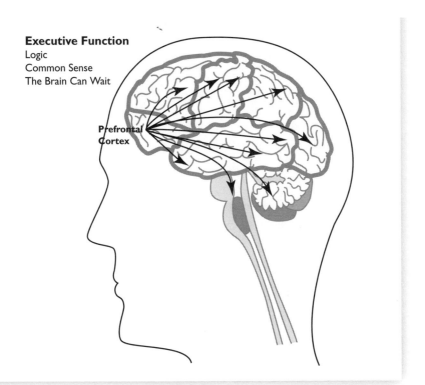

Executive Function
Logic
Common Sense
The Brain Can Wait

Prefrontal Cortex

FIGURE 1.14. At about age 6 the left-brain prefrontal cortex begins to take control of the strong, disruptive emotions that originate in the midbrain. This is called executive function. As the prefrontal cortex continues to mature during adolescence, the child develops greater self-control over impulses. The work of executive function is to enable the brain to wait, to think things through, and to consider the consequences before acting. Executive function applies logic and commonsense reasoning to problem solving instead of allowing midbrain emotions and feelings to govern decisions and actions.

the center of socially constructive emotions and feelings that bring harmony into one's life. A major function of the prefrontal cortex is to enable the limbic system impulses to wait in order to consider consequences before acting. As Chapter 2 describes, one of the major challenges of ADHD is that the person cannot wait but dashes ahead on impulse, then regrets the consequences later.

Left-Brain Style of Learning

In direct contrast to the right-brain circular style of learning (Figure 1.10) is the left-brain linear style of processing shown in Figure 1.15. Inside this left-brain linear box, all details must follow strict left-to-right sequence,

FIGURE 1.15. Virtually all academic curricula and tests are designed to fit inside this left-brain linear box. Details must flow left to right, or the student is wrong. Thoughts must flow left to right, top to bottom, or the student is wrong. Individuals who are ADHD, ADD, or dyslexic do not fit inside this linear box because their natural bent is for circular, not linear, thinking and learning.

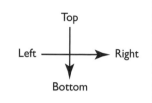

and thinking must flow in a top-to-bottom format. Any deviation from this linear standard is considered "wrong." Since the 17th century, this rigid, inflexible linear box has been the predominant model for classroom learning in most Western cultures. During the 1600s, the French mathematician/ philosopher René Descartes taught the concept that *the brain is a thinking machine that has feelings.* However, Descartes insisted that formal learning must be kept free from emotions and feelings. He taught that the best learners are those who leave emotions and feelings outside the classroom. Descartes believed that the brain is a living machine that processes information the way a mathematician solves algebraic equations, through unemotional logic (Damasio, 1994, 1999).

In 1760, two European leaders, King Frederick II of Prussia and Empress Maria Theresa of Austria, followed the concepts of the German philosopher Ernst Wilhelm von Schlabrendorff in establishing a system of compulsory education that firmly embedded Descartes's left-brain linear philosophy of education. This highly structured linear format for classroom instruction was built upon six principles for formal education: 1) it was compulsory; 2) it was linear; 3) it was timed; 4) it was graded; 5) it was inflexible, with no give-and-take; and 6) its content was controlled (Hartmann, 2003). In many ways, this linear concept of classroom learning continues to dominate American education through such legislative mandates as No Child Left Behind, which requires that all students, regardless of limitations or challenges, take the same standard, timed achievement tests. This left-brain linear mandate is designed to penalize schools that strive to honor different styles through which many students learn and function best.

Descartes's Error

My childhood began during the Great Depression, which devastated American society during the 1930s. My family lived in poverty during most of my formative years. More than 30 percent of adults were unemployed, and there was no social support system to help hungry families get through those hard times. When my parents could not afford food for their three children, my grandmother took me to live in her rural home. That arrangement made it possible for my parents to support themselves and my two sisters. Those years with my grandmother proved critical in my development. My grandmother had little formal education, yet she had learned to read quite well, and the depth of her common sense always amazed me. How did she know all that she helped me to understand? Part of my grandmother's life-shaping influence was to teach me the value of feelings. To this day, I can hear her comments that taught me the importance of feelings: "That feels about empty," she would say as she lifted a jug or box or sack. "That feels about full," she said as she lifted a milk pail. "That feels about right," she commented as she measured cooking ingredients in the palm of her hand. "I feel like a good night's sleep," she yawned at bedtime. "I feel like it's about to storm," she predicted as the western sky darkened in the afternoon. "I feel sorry for them," she said about destitute neighbors whose families were hungry. "I feel happy about that," she smiled over good news from my parents. "I feel like it's time for dinner," she announced at noon after we had worked in the garden all morning. In those days, we ate dinner at noon with supper at sundown.

I grew up with an active understanding that feelings are central to one's life. In 1994, I was intrigued by Antonio Damasio's book *Descartes' Error*, in which he demonstrated that the French mathematician/philosopher had it backwards when he taught that the brain is a thinking machine that feels, but feelings must be left outside of learning. "No," Damasio argued, and I agreed. The brain is a feeling machine that thinks, and feelings must be given first consideration as the brain thinks. In her simple, homespun way, my grandmother had demonstrated for me that, indeed, feelings are at the center of our lives. Formal learning comes later. As Chapter 2 explains, the feelings and emotions of being ADHD or ADD must be acknowledged and dealt with first. Only after those feelings and emotions become safe and comfortable can we begin to educate the higher brain that struggles with ADHD, ADD, or dyslexia.

The Left Brain's Challenge in Becoming Literate

Reading Is Unnatural

> The human brain is not naturally "wired" for reading, spelling, or handwriting. The brain does not come prepared to deal with the inventions of alphabet letters, math numerals, or penmanship symbols.

Differences in Brain Structure

However, in four out of five individuals, the brain is remarkably plastic with the capacity to grow specialized neuron pathways in reponse to the stimulus of learning to read ... one out of five persons never develops the required neuron connections to become competent at reading no matter how much tutoring they receive. Most of these nonreading individuals are dyslexic.

—Dale Jordan, 2002, pp. 81–82

Programmatic research over the past 35 years has *not* supported the view that reading development reflects a *natural* process that children learn to read as they learn to speak, through natural exposure to a literate environment.... If learning to read were natural, there would not exist the substantial number of cultures that have yet to develop a written language, despite having a rich oral language. If learning to read unfolds naturally, why does our literate society have so many youngsters and adults who are illiterate?

—G. R. Lyon, January/February 2000

We have just reviewed 5,500 years of evidence to show that writing systems are inventions, and that humans do not spontaneously and effortlessly develop writing systems or find it easy to learn them. We have seen that the alphabet is a particularly "nonnatural" writing system. Reading is definitely not a biological property of the human brain.

—Diane McGuinness, 1997, p. 117

For the four out of five individuals born with neurological potential to become literate, the stimulus of formal classroom instruction "hardwires" several regions of the left brain for reading, writing, spelling, and language-dependent education. For these neurologically talented persons, the left-brain structures shown in Figure 1.12 become shaped and interconnected to create a complex system that learns and remembers huge amounts of language-related information. For many years, Sally Shaywitz, pediatric neuroscientist at the Yale University Center for the Study of Learning and Attention, has used brain imaging (fMRI) to study how the brain reads. In her book *Overcoming Dyslexia* (2003), she describes the intricate "reading loop" that enables the left brain of 80 percent of the human population to become fluent with literacy skills. Figure 1.16 traces this left-brain process for decoding printed symbols (reading) and encoding language symbols (writing and spelling). This left-brain literacy skill comes only through years of repeated stimulus that, for four out of five individuals, shapes the plastic brain into a "reading and writing" brain.

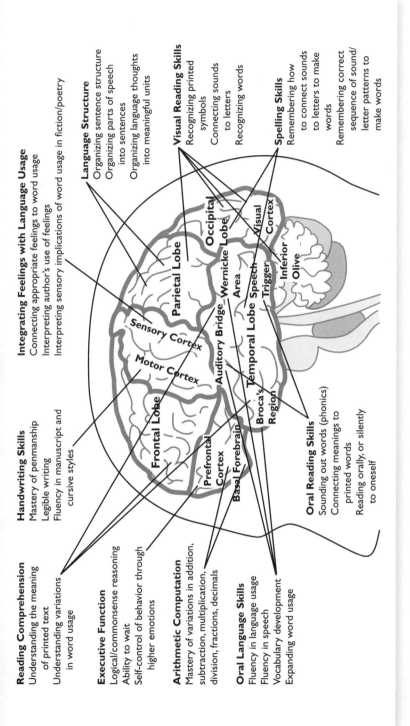

Reading Comprehension
Understanding the meaning of printed text
Understanding variations in word usage

Executive Function
Logical/commonsense reasoning
Ability to wait
Self-control of behavior through higher emotions

Arithmetic Computation
Mastery of variations in addition, subtraction, multiplication, division, fractions, decimals

Oral Language Skills
Fluency in language usage
Fluency in speech
Vocabulary development
Expanding word usage

Handwriting Skills
Mastery of penmanship
Legible writing
Fluency in manuscript and cursive styles

Integrating Feelings with Language Usage
Connecting appropriate feelings to word usage
Interpreting author's use of feelings
Interpreting sensory implications of word usage in fiction/poetry

Language Structure
Organizing sentence structure
Organizing parts of speech into sentences
Organizing language thoughts into meaningful units

Visual Reading Skills
Recognizing printed symbols
Connecting sounds to letters
Recognizing words

Spelling Skills
Remembering how to connect sounds to letters to make words
Remembering correct sequence of sound/letter patterns to make words

Oral Reading Skills
Sounding out words (phonics)
Connecting meanings to printed words
Reading orally, or silently to oneself

Parietal Lobe
Occipital
Visual Cortex
Wernicke Area
Sensory Cortex
Auditory Bridge
Inferior Olive
Motor Cortex
Temporal Lobe Speech Trigger
Frontal Lobe
Broca's Region
Prefrontal Cortex
Basal Forebrain

FIGURE 1.16. In most individuals, these left brain regions do not become fully mature until the early 20s. All of the language-based skills shown above require many years of stimulus through continual practice to become fully fluent and articulate. Chapter 6 describes the many types of learning differences that stand in the way of attaining full left-brain language potential.

Differences in Brain Structure

The Left Brain's Strengths

When all of the left-brain regions mature on schedule, the left brain is capable of extraordinary intellectual work. Figure 1.16 shows the range of skills and talents that the left brain of most individuals potentially is capable of achieving. This chapter began by reviewing genetic research conclusions that 97 percent of what the brain becomes is predetermined before conception. This is called *nature*. What the brain actually becomes is determined by the powerful effect of the kinds of experiences (stimuli) that mold neuronal structures throughout the brain. This is called *nurture*. The following chapters explore the challenges of ADHD and ADD as individuals who are "wired differently" do their best to fit inside the left-brain linear box shown in Figure 1.15.

Executive Function and Executive Dysfunction in ADHD and ADD

~ ~

ADHD probably is not primarily a disorder of paying attention but one of *self-regulation:* how the self comes to manage itself within the larger realm of social behavior. ADHD is … a disturbance in the [person's] ability to use self-control with regard to the future … an inability to use a sense of time and of the past and future to guide … behavior. What is not developing properly … is the capacity to shift from focusing on the here and now to focusing on the future.

—Russell Barkley, 1995, pp. viii–ix

Most ADD [individuals] have the social and emotional maturity of [persons] two-thirds their age. Lack of commonsense is a frequent complaint.

—Christopher Green and Kit Chee, 1994, p. 9

Executive function helps switch a person from the need for immediate action and reward to thought-out responses based on a sense of the past and what the future might hold. Executive function allows an individual to weigh long-term results over short-term consequences.

—Julian Haber, 2003, pp. 200–201

The Concept of Executive Function

One of the most uplifting moments in my professional career occurred in March 1991 at the national conference of the Learning Disabilities

Association in Chicago. On the last day of that inspirational meeting, Martha Denckla, a pediatric neuroscientist at Johns Hopkins University School of Medicine, addressed the crowd of counselors, teachers, parents, and mental health providers. Her presentation was titled "The Neurology of Social Competence." Denckla held the audience spellbound as she reviewed her brain imaging research related to ADHD. In her speech, she challenged the growing movement to use standard test scores with score-discrepancy criteria to identify LD (learning disability) in struggling learners. She drew a standing ovation with her statement: "It is ridiculous to require an arbitrary IQ score for those who struggle to take IQ tests. If the proponents of score-discrepancy need an IQ, then let's give them a universal IQ 90. Now, let's get on with the business of finding out why otherwise bright kids have trouble with learning."

Denckla concluded her presentation with an innovative idea that reverberates today. She proposed the concept of *executive function.* "As I work toward finding out why certain learners struggle," she explained, "I want to know how the prefrontal cortex and the limbic system get along together, or fail to get along. The prefrontal cortex is our executive. It gives logical orders that the rest of the brain is supposed to follow. I contend that a breakdown occurs in executive function when we find attention deficits and learning disabilities" (Denckla, 1991).

That seminal conference presentation started a movement among those of us involved with issues related to ADHD and ADD. I was motivated to develop the *Jordan Executive Function Index for Children* and the *Jordan Executive Function Index for Adults,* which are presented in Appendix A and Appendix B. The term "executive function" has become a universal point of reference as we continue to explore how the brain functions in learning and in social behavior.

The Brain Has Two Centers
for Emotions and Feelings

The Early Childhood Limbic Center

One of the most important publications that resulted from brain research during the 1990s was a book called *Brave New Brain* by psychiatric neuroscientist Nancy Andreasen (2001). Her brain imaging studies have explored the limbic system's role in generating disruptive emotions and feelings linked to various types of mental illness. Her pioneering research demonstrated that the human brain is programmed by genetics to develop two centers of emotions and feelings that are intricate parts of personality, lifestyle, learning style, and balanced mental health called *homeostasis.* For many years, early childhood specialists wondered how the young child's brain generates the strong, basal emotions seen in open display during the stage called "the terrible twos," when self-focused, angry tantrums dominate the lives of many toddlers (Brazelton, 1992; Brody, 1987; Denckla, 1972, 1978, 1985; Eliot, 1999; Hampton-Turner, 1981; Inhelder & Piaget, 1974; Joseph, 1988; Osman & Blinder, 1982; Wacker, 1975). Andreasen's research demonstrated that during a child's early developmental years, as well as in adult mental health challenges, the midbrain (limbic system) controls the person's life through cycles and waves of strong, potentially disruptive emotions and feelings. Figure 2.1 illustrates the wide range of

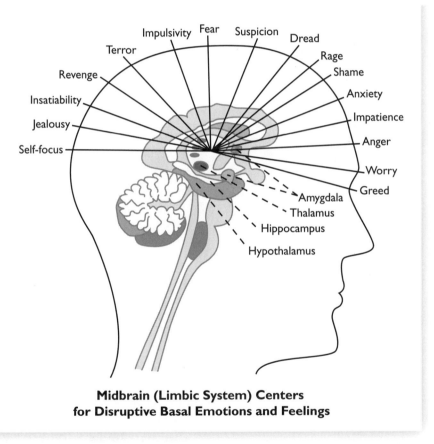

**Midbrain (Limbic System) Centers
for Disruptive Basal Emotions and Feelings**

FIGURE 2.1. From birth to about age 5, most children are driven by strong, often disruptive emotions and feelings that originate in the midbrain. Many parents struggle through the behavior phase called the "terrible twos," when strong emotions control a child's life. When executive function is late emerging, or when it does not emerge at all, some adolescents and young adults are out of control as these basal emotions govern their lifestyle.

Executive Function and Executive Dysfunction

disruptive emotions and feelings that youngsters tend to experience during early childhood, and that adults encounter when emotional homeostasis is lost.

The Higher Brain Takes Charge As the Child Grows Up

Beginning at age 3, most youngsters take their first steps in the developmental process called *socialization*, which gradually replaces disruptive basal emotions with socially constructive emotions and feelings. As the "terrible two's" recede, the lifestyle of most children comes under the control of constructive higher emotions that enable the youngster to become a friendly, thoughtful, self-controlled, and increasingly generous social member. Figure 2.2 shows how this change occurs as executive function emerges during the development of the prefrontal cortex.

> The functioning human brain is like a large orchestra continuously playing a great symphony. We cannot point to any single part, or even combination of parts, and say that it constitutes either the orchestra or the symphony. Violins, violas, cellos, oboes, clarinets, horns, and other components all play together to create a rich texture of sound. At the right moment the trumpets join in, and the cymbals are struck, or the cadence of the drums is added. Themes are introduced and re-echoed to produce a sense of coherence. The emotional coloring shifts and shimmers. The miraculous process of mental activity occurs, routinely, in all of us, all of the time, whether we are considered gifted or ordinary. Each of us—each individual mind/brain—not only plays a uniquely rich and complex symphony but also spontaneously composes its own score at the same time … and conducts it as well.
>
> —Nancy Andreason, 2001, pp. 85–86

Figure 2.2 shows how the conductor of this incredible "brain symphony" is the prefrontal cortex, center of executive function that enriches our lives by enabling us to wait before acting, ponder possible consequences, thoughtfully decide, think more of others than of self, remember and compare, and process abstract thought. To do all this, the brain must learn how to tune out irrelevant stimuli that can be left for later, or not respond at all. In a nutshell, the primary roles of executive function are *to enable the whole brain to wait* and *to guide the higher brain in deciding*. Waiting without impulse and deciding without distraction are the missing ingredients for individuals with ADHD or ADD.

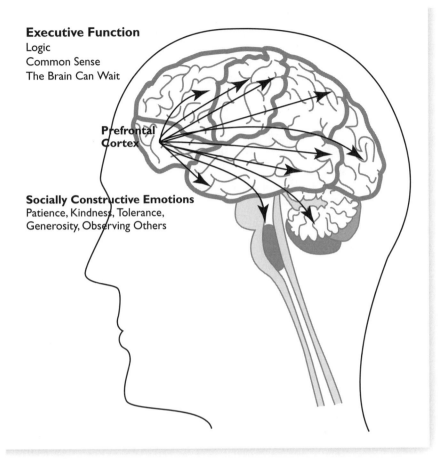

Executive Function
Logic
Common Sense
The Brain Can Wait

Prefrontal Cortex

Socially Constructive Emotions
Patience, Kindness, Tolerance,
Generosity, Observing Others

39

FIGURE 2.2. At about age 5 in most children, the left-brain prefrontal cortex begins
to take charge of the whole brain, the way an executive takes charge of an organization.
From age 5 to about age 22, the frontal cortex gradually exerts increasing control through
logic, commonsense reasoning, and socially constructive emotions that are essential for
social success. The primary task of the prefrontal cortex is to enable the brain to wait before acting while the person thinks about the consequences.

The Emotional Brain

> Without emotions to guide us, we would be incapable of either deci-
> sions or plans.
>
> —Richard Restak, 2002, p. 112

One of the most profound results of recent brain research is new understanding of the powerful role of emotions and feelings in human achievement. Antonio Damasio, Richard Restak, Daniel Schacter, and others have

documented the function of emotions and feelings in how the higher brain does its cognitive work of thinking, learning, and remembering. Chapter 1 reviewed Descartes's mistaken assumption that *the brain is a thinking machine that feels, but feelings must be left outside the work of thinking.* In fact, the brain is an *emotional machine that thinks, and emotions and feelings must be taken seriously as the brain thinks* (Andreason, 2001; Block et al., 1997; Damasio, 1994, 1999; Dennet, 1991; Jordan, 1998, 2000a, 2000b, 2002; McGinn, 1991; Ramachandran, 1993; Ratey & Johnson, 1997; Schacter, 1996; Searle, 1997; Sutherland, 1992; Ungerleider & Haxby, 1994). This point of view has profound implications for classroom curriculum design, mental health treatment, and early childhood development programs.

The Emotional Brain That Thinks

Before the brain has formed after conception, the very first neurological function of emerging neurons is to begin filtering and coping with primitive feelings. Figure 1.1 shows the neuron clusters that by day 28 of pregnancy are feeling sensations that touch the embryo. This is the beginning of the *visceral somatosensory system,* which is the lifelong entryway for all new data approaching the brain. Because the brain is locked safely inside the thick bone box called the *cranium* or *skull,* all information must be translated from sensory impressions (feelings) into electrical codes that tell the brain what is happening outside the cranial box. The visceral somatosensory system monitors, filters, accepts, or rejects every bit of outside data on its way to the brain. By the 35th day of pregnancy, a second avenue of information for the brain begins to work. This is the bloodstream, called the *circulatory system.* As the visceral system processes new sensory data from the outside world, the bloodstream delivers chemical messages that tell the brain what is happening in every cell inside the body. Before the higher brain thinks a thought, these visceral and circulatory systems test new sensations with the feeling-centered question: "Is this safe?" From the moment of birth, feelings are expressed as emotions that show what is happening internally. For the rest of each person's life, feelings and emotions come first as the brain does its work.

Dual Centers of Emotion

Figures 2.1 and 2.2 show the two centers of emotion that determine the quality of mental health throughout our lives. By the ninth month of fetal development, a complex network has formed within the limbic system, as Figure 2.3 shows. This network governs and filters the spectrum of basal feelings and emotions before the higher brain becomes involved. This limbic network controls the fight-or-flight reflex. As executive function gains control over whole-brain functions, a balance emerges between midbrain feelings and higher brain emotions. This is called *homeostasis*. The goal of the midbrain network shown in Figure 2.3 and executive function is to produce a balance of feelings and emotions that permits the individual to cope with challenges without becoming overwhelmed. When a child grows up with the positive nurture of praise, love, and language stimulation, the prefrontal cortex is shaped by neuron pruning to guide the person's life through constructive social emotions and feelings. Youngsters within a nurturing lifestyle learn to wait their turn, notice the needs of others, extend kindness, and practice generosity. By age 7, these children are building strong enough self-esteem to cope with challenges without fear or harm.

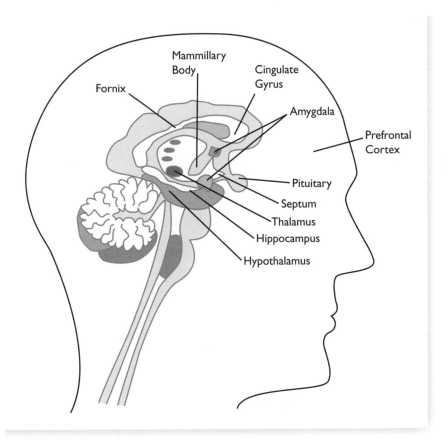

FIGURE 2.3. The amygdala is the primary source of basal emotions. As the midbrain matures, the amygdala becomes linked with the other regions of the limbic system shown above. This midbrain network incorporates feelings and emotions into all functions of the limbic system.

Executive Function and Executive Dysfunction

Their personalities become well balanced between healthy self-confidence and momentary challenges of failure or embarrassment.

The Risk of Stress in ADHD

Children who are ADHD are at high risk for imbalanced feelings and emotions. ADHD keeps these children in conflict with others because of inattention, poor organization, and lack of self-control (inhibition). This lifestyle is filled with stress that overwhelms them with fear, dread, and the shame of failure. This negative, high-stress lifestyle shapes the midbrain emotional control center in a way that sabotages emotional homeostasis. A remarkable psychiatrist, James Gilligan, calls this emotional imbalance *death of self-esteem* (Gilligan, 1996). In his work with violent men serving prison sentences, Gilligan has shown that the root of violence (antisocial behavior) usually is deeply embedded shame that causes death of self-esteem. When a child's emotions and feelings are shaped by the toxic shame of more failure than success, that individual loses the self-confidence and self-esteem that are vital for achieving or maintaining executive function. When a child experiences too many unsafe emotions with no safe place for protection or shelter, the brain is shaped toward executive dysfunction that is described later in this chapter. The executive dysfunction of ADHD places youngsters at high risk for becoming so filled by shame of failure that they cannot develop constructive social emotions and feelings.

Many recent studies of brain development have centered on the role of stress in how neurons are pruned and brain regions are shaped. Research of the effects of stress hormones, especially *cortisol,* have shown that unrelieved stress during early brain development has potentially catastrophic consequences for midbrain and higher brain formation (Andreason, 2001; Eliot, 1999; Haber, 2003; Hartmann, 2003; Pearce, 2002; Restak, 2002, 2003). When a child grows up in an atmosphere of constant stress, the balance of emotions and feelings is lost. The overstimulation of cortisol constantly energizing the limbic system creates a toxic environment for developing constructive feelings and emotions.

How the Brain Remembers

The Brain's Inner Voice

To understand the role of executive function, first we must understand how the brain builds and retains memory. Andreason (2001), Damasio (1994, 1999), Ratey & Johnson (1997), Restak (2002, 2003), Schacter (1996), and others have explored the mystery of how the brain remembers. During the first trimester of fetal development, the basal brain begins the lifelong process of constructing memory codes of every experience of one's life. During early childhood, the brain develops an active *inner voice* that permits a type of inside-the-brain communication. Through this inner voice, the brain regions talk with each other. In 1977 Jacob Branowski developed an intriguing model of how this "brain language" separates human beings from animals. Bronowski believed that before the brain sends action signals to the rest of the body, various brain regions hold a "mental language conference" that forces a pause between impulse and action. During this pause for mental conversation, regions of the brain that do logical reasoning confer with other brain regions that control emotion and feeling. According to Bronowski's model, a mature brain with a good balance between logic and emotion quickly comes to reasonable, commonsense conclusions that take into account the consequences of any action. This brain network conversation asks: "If we do this, what will be the consequences? If we don't do this, then what will be the consequences?" In milliseconds the brain decides on the safest, most reasonable course of action. Signals then are sent to activate the body to carry out that internal decision, or to refrain from doing so. Attention deficit disorder is caused when the brain cannot carry on these inner voice dialogues. When this mental voice deficit is mild or moderate, attention deficit disorders occur. When the inner voice deficit is extreme, oppositional-defiant behavior and conduct disorders arise.

The Noisy Brain

In their book *Shadow Syndromes*, John Ratey and Catherine Johnson (1997) described the *noisy brain*, which chatters on and on and cannot be still. Brain imaging research has developed a "snapshot" of the noisy brain, as shown in Figure 2.4. When the brain cannot stop talking to itself, the individual is handicapped by a lifelong inability to pay full attention to the outside world. Ratey and Johnson demonstrated how the noisy brain is the cause of a variety of dysfunctions, including obsessive-compulsive disorder, intense self-focus that may evolve into narcissism, or even chronic depression, which causes the person to withdraw into a self-contained private world of noisy emotional misery. Chapter 7 describes how medication and diet control can help rid the brain of excess noise so that the inner voice can function without distraction.

Emotional Memory

The brain's inner voice plays a major role in how the central nervous system recalls knowledge and builds memory images. When old information must

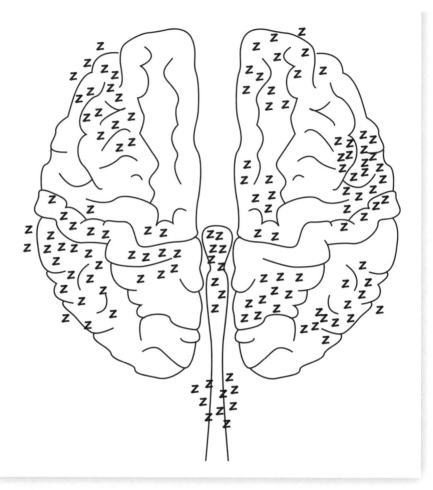

FIGURE 2.4. Brain imaging science has revealed the "noise" that fills the brain when executive function loses control of the basal emotions. This noise is much like static that interrupts radio and television during electrical storms. This "brain noise" is triggered when too much stress hormone (cortisol) is present in the bloodstream.

be recalled, the frontal lobes search their databases and locate part of that knowledge. At the same time, other regions throughout the brain conduct their own search for data that is related to the information the frontal lobe is activating. However, the brain never simply calls up facts or figures as a computer does. Commands for memory material also activate emotions and feelings that were present when that original event occurred, or when that old information was first encountered.

In his book *Searching for Memory*, Daniel Schacter (1996) documented the impact that emotions and feelings have on the memory images activated by memory searches throughout the brain. As new information enters the brain, that data is coded and stored in neuron clusters that Schacter calls *engrams*. These engrams are like computer memory chips that hold analog or binary codes for future use. Every bit of information the brain receives is encoded in a series of interconnected engrams that are scattered throughout the higher brain. When the brain needs to activate any stored information, a locator signal is broadcast in waves throughout the brain. Those engrams holding portions of that particular data become active, forming a neurological network that brings that mental image alive. If the original event related to the awakening memory was peaceful, the brain produces a peaceful mental image. If the original event was traumatic or unsafe, then the brain brings up an image that is colored by strong emotions and urgent feelings that trigger the fight-or-flight reflex (Damasio, 1994, 1999; Schacter, 1996).

Changes in Memory

Contrary to popular belief about the accuracy of human memory, the brain never re-creates the same memory image twice. Each time the brain develops memory images of knowledge or experience, the new image differs somewhat from other times when that event or set of facts was recalled. Andreason (2001), Damasio (1994, 1999), Restak (2002, 2003), Schacter (1996), and others have described how strong emotions, which are governed by the limbic system (amygdala, thalamus, hypothalamus), and higher emotions, which are governed by the prefrontal cortex, change in time. As persons mature and become wiser, or as individuals fail to mature or become neurotic, emotions and feelings that are linked to early experiences change. Memory images evoked at age 14 often are quite different from memories of those same events when one is age 40 or 55 or 72. There is much evidence that memory cannot be held to fully logical or factually correct standards. As we call up memory images of the past events, those recollections may be no more historically or factually accurate than the symbolic images of a dream.

Memory and Attention Deficit

This new understanding of how the brain learns and remembers greatly enhances our understanding of the impact of attention deficit disorders, learning disabilities, obsessive-compulsive behavior, autism, and other types of socially disruptive lifestyles. As later chapters describe, difficulties in learning and remembering become strongly emotional events for struggling learners, classmates, teachers, and families. The more negative the first learning event was, the more unsettling and unreliable each future memory of that event will be. In the book *Overcoming Dyslexia in Children, Adolescents, and Adults,* I described patterns of school phobias, panic attack, and chronic anxiety that many struggling learners display when asked to do schoolwork (Jordan, 2002). When unsafe emotional memories are triggered by tasks the person cannot do, the limbic system triggers the fight-or-flight reflex that causes tightness of the chest, contraction of the digestive tract, faster heartbeat, shortness of breath, and a strong urge to flee the threatening situation.

How the Brain Pays Full Attention

Executive function has the responsibility for enabling the brain to pay full attention from start to finish of each task. Brain imaging research in the 1990s revealed a composite brain map that showed how many regions of the brain are engaged in the process of paying attention. Figure 2.5 shows what is required of the whole brain for a person to maintain full attention. ADHD and ADD rob the brain of this ability.

The Profile of Executive Function

Executive function has three faces by which we recognize this critical lifestyle as children grow up: *Attention* (habits by which a person pays attention), *Organization* (habits by which a person organizes and regulates his or her life), and *Inhibition* (the degree of self-control over impulses). As the adolescent brain becomes "hardwired" for executive function, a distinctive lifestyle emerges with specific habits and patterns of constructive behavior. Mature executive function blesses individuals with the foundation for happiness, lifelong contentment, strength to cope with stress, and skills for solving problems as they occur.

The Lifestyle of Paying Attention

The individual with good attention:

- *Keeps attention focused on tasks* without darting off on mental rabbit trails or drifting off into daydreams
- *Tunes out or ignores* what goes on nearby in order to finish tasks
- *Keeps on listening* until the flow of oral information is finished
- *Understands new information without interrupting* with "What?" or "Huh?" or "What do you mean?"

Three-Step Brain Sequence in Paying Full Attention

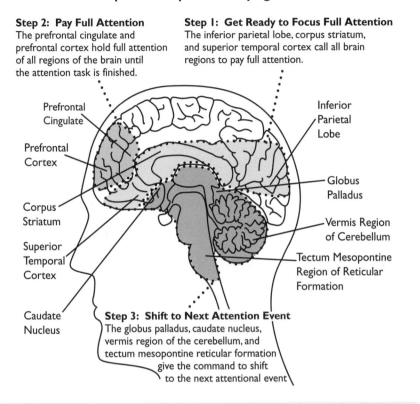

Step 2: Pay Full Attention
The prefrontal cingulate and prefrontal cortex hold full attention of all regions of the brain until the attention task is finished.

Step 1: Get Ready to Focus Full Attention
The inferior parietal lobe, corpus striatum, and superior temporal cortex call all brain regions to pay full attention.

Prefrontal Cingulate

Prefrontal Cortex

Corpus Striatum

Superior Temporal Cortex

Caudate Nucleus

Inferior Parietal Lobe

Globus Palladus

Vermis Region of Cerebellum

Tectum Mesopontine Region of Reticular Formation

Step 3: Shift to Next Attention Event
The globus palladus, caudate nucleus, vermis region of the cerebellum, and tectum mesopontine reticular formation give the command to shift to the next attentional event

47

FIGURE 2.5. All of these regions of the brain must work together so the person can keep on paying attention from start to finish of a task. If any of these brain regions fails to stay engaged during an attentional event, the brain loses the mental image and attention goes elsewhere.

- *Finishes tasks* before starting something new
- *Completes necessary tasks* without being reminded or supervised
- *Is a cooperative team member* from start to finish in group activities
- *Follows rules and regulations* without being reminded or supervised
- *Has long-term memory of what to do* without being reminded or supervised
- *Has long-term memory* for messages, instructions, and essential information
- *Keeps personal space tidy* without being reminded or supervised
- *Does routine chores* without being reminded or supervised

Executive Function and Executive Dysfunction

- *Keeps on paying attention* to movies, television shows, sermons, and lectures without becoming restless or distracted
- *Notices how others respond* to his or her behavior
- *Picks up cues* about how personal behavior should be adjusted to help or show respect for others
- *Notices details* without being reminded
- *Notices where things are* so as not to bump or knock them over
- *Notices how materials are organized* (how lines are numbered, where written responses should go, how details are arranged and spaced)
- *Participates in conversations* without interrupting or changing the subject too soon

The Lifestyle of Being Organized

The organized person:

- *Keeps track of things* without losing or misplacing them
- *Gathers up and returns things* without being reminded or supervised
- *Keeps personal space clean and orderly* without being reminded or supervised
- *Follows through on instructions and directions* without being supervised or reminded
- *Returns tools, toys, and equipment to proper places* without being reminded or supervised
- *Spaces written work* evenly and neatly
- *Budgets time and plans ahead* without being supervised or reminded
- *Has realistic, accurate sense of time* without being reminded
- *Budgets and manages own money* without supervision
- *Plans ahead for special occasions* (birthdays, anniversaries, holidays)
- *Notices and follows sequence patterns* in how things should be arranged
- *Groups things together* (books on shelves, papers for school or work, shoes in pairs, tools in sets, silverware in correct places)
- *Keeps school or work material organized* in notebooks, files, or folders
- *Works and plays by the rules* without being reminded
- *Does tasks in order* from start to finish without skipping around

The Lifestyle of Inhibition (Self-Control)

The individual who exercises inhibition:

- *Thinks of consequences* before doing what comes to mind
- *Postpones pleasure* until necessary work is finished

Overcoming Attention Deficit Disorders in Children, Adolescents, and Adults

- *Follows own sense of right and wrong* instead of being influenced by others
- *Puts the needs and welfare of others* ahead of personal wishes and desires
- *Willingly says "no" to impulses* when responsibilities must be carried out
- *Makes an effort to grow up* instead of remaining immature/impulsive
- *Tries to change mannerisms and habits* that bother or offend others
- *Learns from experience*
- *Lives by rules or spiritual principles* instead of by whim or impulse
- *Accepts responsibility* instead of blaming others or making excuses
- *Asks for and responds to advice* instead of being stubborn
- *Apologizes or asks forgiveness* when personal behavior has hurt or offended others
- *Is recognized by others* as being mature, unselfish, dependable, teachable, cooperative
- *Stops inappropriate impulses* before they emerge so that others will not be bothered or offended
- *Sticks to promises and agreements* without supervision
- *Goes extra miles for others* without complaining or feeling self-pity
- *Sets long-term goals* and works toward them without reminding or being supervised
- *Absorbs teasing or rudeness* without flaring or becoming defensive
- *Practices kindness* toward others by avoiding sarcasm or hateful, put-down comments
- *Resists urges* to take things apart, damage things from rough handling, pick at things with fingers
- *Is flexible and creative* instead of being ritualized and rigid

49

The Impact of Emerging Executive Function

What if an individual had all of these positive, constructive qualities? Would such a person be too good to be true? Appendix A (*Jordan Executive Function Index for Children*) and Appendix B (*Jordan Executive Function Index for Adults*) present two inventories that show how close individuals are to achieving these lifestyle goals. These inventories reveal where persons are in their developmental journey toward becoming mature, thoughtful, sensitive members of society. As time goes by, it is easy to map progress toward rewarding lifestyles by watching how individuals achieve higher-ranking levels on these executive function characteristics. There is reason for hope when Luis or Jacob, whom we met in the Introduction, move up from Never to Sometimes on the checklist. There is reason to rejoice when, in their adolescent years, they move up from Sometimes to Usually. By their late teens, their checklist profiles will gain several "always" responses, compared with Never or Sometimes five years earlier.

Rapid Emergence of Executive Function During Adolescence

During the spring of 2004, my family rejoiced at the splendid emergence of executive function in our wonderful granddaughter Alex and our remarkable grandson William. Alex and William were born six years apart. Both were high-need infants and toddlers. Each of them faced major challenges learning to read and write, and both struggled with impulsivity and acute emotional sensitivity that required special educational support for several years. Alex and William were extremely active, with the inwardly driven attention surplus patterns Thom Hartmann describes as "Edison-gene hunter" children. Eventually Alex was diagnosed as ADHD and began taking cortical stimulant medication to reduce her emotional stress and impulsivity. William was diagnosed as being dyslexic but never was medicated for attention control.

These grandchildren were born as my wife and I entered middle age. By their teen years, we had become "early old age" grandparents as their parents crossed the threshold into middle age. All of the deep love within our family for these amazing kids did not keep us from becoming exhausted after being with them for a while. Throughout their childhood years, both Alex and William had insatiable "go-go-go" needs long after we adults had reached the point of needing to "sit-sit-sit." Alex thrived within a public school special education program that was tailored for students with her kinds of special needs. Until age 11, William was homeschooled to shelter him from overwhelming stress he could not tolerate in a classroom setting. Alex was a late bloomer who needed several extra years to reach the "hardwiring" brain maturity of late adolescence. William was an early bloomer who entered adolescence ahead of schedule. Our family had the experience of witnessing both grandchildren reach executive function maturity at the same time.

At age 16, with puberty under way, Alex entered a richly supportive high school program designed to prepare her life skills and job skills for early adulthood. At age 11, and well into puberty, William enrolled in a private school for dyslexic learners. That year we saw amazing changes in Alex and William as each of them began to thrive in social skills at the same time that their academic skills increased. In each grandchild, new levels of attention emerged. Each year of hardwiring progress brought forth growing maturity in organization without so much supervision. New levels of self-control over impulses (inhibition) blossomed overnight. By age 19, Alex was a charming, thoughtful young adult with remarkable new manifestations of executive function. At age 19, she no longer needed medication for attention control. Before his 14th birthday, William was six feet tall and unusually talented at golf. Through computer keyboarding, both of them gained literacy skills that were beyond their reach a few years earlier.

In the fall of 2003, 20-year-old Alex was earning part-time income while attending community college part time. A few years before, no one predicted that she ever would achieve that level of success. As the family held its breath, William entered ninth grade in a large high school, his first experience with public school education. Would this dyslexic adolescent, who had struggled so hard his first 14 years, find ways to cope and succeed in this stressful new environment? In the spring of 2004, Alex approached her 21st birthday and William turned 15. Alex was radiant with workplace success and the joy of being an adult student at the community college level. She still needed help managing money, staying on time schedules, and making major decisions. But she had become a thoughtful, generous, self-confident young adult with greatly increased attention, organization, and inhibition habits that brought tears of joy to her grandparents' eyes. The week he turned 15, William won a place on the high school golf team, beating out several senior students with his superior golf skills. He attained honor roll status by making all A grades his freshman year in high school.

Our family has been richly blessed by the emergence of executive function, which changed the lives of Alex and William forever. By the time Alex is 25 and William is 19, both of our grandchildren will have completed most of the hardwiring passage into their executive function lifestyles, which will continue to be fine-tuned and refined into their 30s. Our family is amazed at the hope and blessings that have come through emerging executive function.

The Impact of
Residual Executive Dysfunction

Many research studies have reported the tendency for a majority of ADHD and ADD youngsters to overcome most of their difficulties by their late teens or early 20s (Barkley, 1990, 1995; Hallowell & Ratey, 1994a, 1994b; Hartmann, 2000, 2003; Jordan, 1998, 2000a, 2002; Restak, 2002, 2003; Taylor, 1994; Weiss, 1992, 1996; Wender, 2000). Most of us agree that when ADHD or ADD children receive positive support, encouragement, and assurance during their formative years, their brains become wired away from habits and tendencies for inattention, disorganization, and poor impulse control. Approximately 8 out of 10 ADHD youngsters achieve executive function that brings them into adulthood mostly free from childhood challenges with attention, organization, and inhibition.

Unfortunately, 2 out of 10 of these individuals do not. Residual ADHD or ADD follows 20 percent of these inattentive, impulsive, and poorly organized youngsters into adulthood. This residual ADHD, called *executive dysfunction*, creates the disruptive, counterproductive lifestyles seen in the following profile.

The Lifestyle of Inattention

The individual with attention problems:

- *Does not keep attention focused* on tasks or activities
- *Does not tune out or ignore distractions* in the classroom, on the job, or in relationships
- *Does not keep on listening* at work, in the classroom, or in relationships
- *Interrupts the flow of oral information* by blurting out "What?" or "Huh?" or "What do you mean?"
- *Does not finish tasks* without being reminded or supervised
- *Cannot function as a team member* at work, at school, or in relationships
- *Cannot follow rules or regulations* without supervision and reminding
- *Cannot remember what needs to be done* after leaving work or school
- *Cannot remember phone messages* unless they are written down immediately
- *Cannot keep personal space tidy* without supervision and reminding
- *Cannot do necessary chores* without supervision and reminding
- *Cannot keep attention focused* on movies, television shows, sermons, lectures, textbook reading, assignments or projects
- *Does not notice how others respond* to his or her habits, mannerisms, and behavior
- *Does not notice details* in his or her environment without being reminded
- *Does not notice where things are* to avoid bumping/knocking things over
- *Does not notice how materials are organized* at work or at school
- *Cannot participate in conversations* without interrupting, changing the subject, misunderstanding what others say

The Lifestyle of Poor Organization

The poorly organized person:

- *Cannot keep track of personal things* without reminding or supervision
- *Does not return things to where they belong* without reminding or supervision
- *Cannot keep track of work or school materials* without reminding or supervision
- *Does not keep personal space or work space* tidy and organized
- *Does not keep clothes and personal things* organized without supervision or reminding
- *Does not follow instructions* in an orderly, sequential way
- *Does not keep tools or materials organized*
- *Creates a messy clutter* doing jobs and projects
- *Cannot keep handwriting projects neat and legible*
- *Does not budget time realistically* without reminding or supervision
- *Cannot budget or manage own money* without supervision
- *Does not plan ahead for special occasions* (birthdays, anniversaries, holidays)
- *Cannot carry out plans for activities* without help and reminding
- *Does not notice how things should be arranged* without help or reminding
- *Cannot keep things together in appropriate groups* without reminding or supervision (shoes in pairs, books on shelves, tools in sets, work or school papers in order)
- *Forgets the rules during games* and must be reminded
- *Does not follow an orderly sequence* in doing work or school tasks

The Lifestyle of Poor Inhibition (Lack of Self-Control)

The individual with poor inhibition:

- *Does not think of consequences* before doing what comes to mind
- *Does not postpone pleasure* in order to finish necessary work
- *Follows own sense of right and wrong* instead of heeding advice of others
- *Puts own desires, needs, or wishes first*
- *Seldom says "no" to impulses* when responsibilities must be carried out
- *Seldom makes a conscious effort to "grow up"* and become more mature
- *Seldom tries to change habits or mannerisms* that bother or offend others

- *Seldom learns from experience*
- *Seldom practices rules or spiritual principles* instead of following own whims and impulses
- *Seldom accepts responsibility* without blaming others or making excuses
- *Seldom asks for or accepts advice* instead of being stubborn
- *Seldom apologizes or asks forgiveness* when personal behavior has hurt or offended others
- *Is regarded by leaders* as being self-centered, immature, unteachable, undependable, uncooperative
- *Does not go the extra mile* without complaining or feeling self-pity
- *Does not set long-term goals* or work toward them without reminding and supervision
- *Seldom absorbs teasing or rudeness* without flaring or becoming defensive
- *Is usually sarcastic or uses putdown remarks* when speaking of others
- *Rarely refrains from urges* to take things apart, damage things from rough handling, pick at things with fingers
- *Clings to self-focused rituals and habits* while refusing to try new ideas or do something differently

The Social Gift of Executive Function

54

Perhaps the most beneficial gift the human brain offers is the hope of executive function. This incredible characteristic of the higher brain makes it possible for us to live at peace in comfortable, safe relationships, no matter where we might be. When executive function is in charge, we greet others with generosity, trust, and mutual goodwill. When the prefrontal cortex is in charge, individuals form creative bonds that build relationships of affection, friendship, and respect. Enormous loss occurs when executive dysfunction takes charge of human lives. The ultimate cost of lifelong ADHD is that such individuals never live a day that is free from conflict, disappointment, and frustration—outcomes over which they have virtually no control.

The Challenges of ADHD in the Classroom and Workplace

This chapter introduces the major problem we encountered in discussing Attention Deficit Disorder. Throughout the vast body of literature about this topic, authors disagree on what to call this difference in behavior. Is it ADHD? Or is it ADD? Both labels are used by specialists to define ADHD: Attention-deficit/hyperactive disorder (see *DSM–IV–TR*). This chapter is devoted to discussing ADHD, which is distinctly different from ADD, described in Chapter 4.

> Recently, several authors have argued that Attention Deficit Hyperactivity Disorder (ADHD) is a myth. Nothing could be further from the truth. It is a very real entity [that] has been called by many different names over the past fifty-five years. Perhaps as many as 15 percent of our children and adolescents are receiving medical treatment for ADHD, which can be severely devastating in the areas of learning, thinking, working, and social interaction. There is no question that the number of children diagnosed with the disorder is increasing.
>
> —Julian Stuart Haber, 2003, p. xiii

Is ADHD a Personality Difference or a Mental Health Disorder?

The Introduction of this book described the ongoing debate among professionals who work with people with attention deficits about whether ADHD and ADD are differences in personality structure, or whether they are types of mental health disorders. This question stands at the crossroads of how ADHD and ADD are defined and accommodated. In the Introduction, we met Luis, who fits Thom Hartmann's criteria for an "Edison-gene hunter," an individual who should not be labeled as having a mental health disorder. We met Jacob, who displays enough symptoms of ADHD to meet Russell Barkley's criteria for having a mental health disorder that requires medical treatment. We also met Anna, the daydreamer, whose challenges are described in Chapter 4. As we entered the 21st century, we did not have a universally accepted answer for the question of whether ADHD is a difference or a disorder. This chapter presents a survey of the many approaches to defining or diagnosing ADHD. If this challenge in classroom learning, job performance, and personal relationships is a personality difference, then it will be treated in a much different way than if it is classified as a mental health disorder.

What Is ADHD?

ADHD is heterogeneous, with multiple causes. While genetic susceptibility appears to account for approximately 50 percent of its occurrences, ADHD is also a known outcome of neurological injury or disease, prenatal exposure to toxic substances, and prenatal variables such as prematurity, low birth weight, and birth anoxia.... ADHD is a final "common symptom pathway" for a variety of causes ...
—Lucy Jo Palladino, in Hartmann, 2003, p. xiii

For more than 100 years, educators, neurologists, psychologists, psychiatrists, and pediatricians have tried to develop a universal definition of this attentional difference that frustrates so many individuals and disrupts families, classrooms, workplace situations, and personal relationships. Despite countless clinical studies, worldwide brain imaging research, and probing investigations of body chemistry and genetic patterns, we entered the 21st century still divided over what to call this persistent condition, which disrupts the lives of 10 to 15 percent of the human population (Haber, 2003; Jordan, 1998, 2000a, 2000b, 2002; Quinn, 2001) This dilemma is not helped when authors use contradictory terminology in describing attention deficit disorder. For example, the prolific author Thom Hartmann has published a series of works about attention deficit issues with titles such as *Thom Hartmann's Complete Guide to ADHD* and *The Edison Gene: ADHD and the Gift of the Hunter Child* (2003). Yet throughout his texts, Hartmann uses the term ADD while describing hyperactive, impulsive, inattentive, risk-taking individuals. In a similar way, Daniel G. Amen's book *Healing ADD: The Breakthrough Program That Allows You to See and Heal the 6 Types of ADD* (2001) is mostly devoted to the hyperactive, impulsive, disruptive symptoms of ADHD. For many of us, ADD refers to nonhyperactive attention deficit disorder that is distinctly different from ADHD, as Chapter 4 explains. Before we explore current attempts to define ADHD, we must recognize the wide range of severity in attention deficit behaviors.

Range of Severity of ADHD Symptoms

Through the years, I've … met hundreds of Edison-trait children and adults who don't have ADHD. Because their problems with inattention, impulsivity, or hyperactivity do not interfere with their daily lives, they do not qualify for an ADHD diagnosis. In diagnostic terms, *interference with daily living* is the critical line that separates personality and pathology.

—Lucy Jo Palladino, in Hartmann, 2003, p. xiv

ADHD is many things, all of which can trigger disruptions in personal relationships, classroom learning, workplace performance, and social behavior. ADHD has many faces that are seen at different levels of severity. An ADHD symptom that appears in one situation might not emerge in different circumstances. The following severity scale shows the range of ADHD symptoms described later in this chapter.

1	2	3	4	5	6	7	8	9	10
	Mild			Moderate			Severe		

▶ **Mild ADHD**
This person displays some, but not all, of the faces of ADHD described in this chapter. Soon after starting a task, he or she becomes restless and bored. Body motion emerges and increases after a few minutes. This person often fails to comprehend what he or she hears. Reading comprehension usually is spotty and unpredictable. Often, the mildly ADHD individual must be reminded to stay on task or to finish what is started. With occasional supervision or reminding, this person can finish job tasks or make good grades in school. At this mild level, ADHD is more a nuisance than a problem. Mildly ADHD persons can develop self-reminder strategies for finishing tasks without always needing outside help.

► **Moderate ADHD**

This individual displays most of the faces of ADHD that are described in this chapter. He or she continually jumps track and fails to follow through on tasks without frequent reminding. A moderately ADHD person must have frequent supervision to succeed in the classroom or at work. With adequate supervision and guidance, this individual can succeed most of the time. This person continually triggers conflict in social relationships, in workplace performance, and in classroom learning. He or she lives more by feelings and emotions than by logic and commonsense thinking. Since early childhood, this person has been a difficult member of the family. Success is possible if others show enough patience and willingness to tolerate the lifestyle habits described later in this chapter.

► **Severe ADHD**

Individuals with severe ADHD face almost impossible challenges in social relationships, classroom performance, and workplace success. At the severe level, it is not unusual to find all of the faces of ADHD described in this chapter. Severely ADHD individuals are very difficult at home, at school, at work, and in the community. Their volatile emotions flare too easily when criticized or challenged. Severely ADHD persons are undependable, overly touchy and irritable, and generally irresponsible. In most instances, these individuals are social misfits because of aggressive, self-focused, immature, and inappropriate behavior. As time goes by, they do not learn from their mistakes or from the advice of others.

How ADHD Is Identified or Diagnosed

A major cause for different professional opinions about attention deficits is that there is no standard medical or neurological test for ADHD. In seeking to define this cluster of challenging behaviors, clinicians have three options for arriving at a diagnosis of ADHD: 1) an informal questionnaire that yields an anecdotal word picture that describes but does not diagnose ADHD behavior; 2) a semiformal questionnaire that produces a score-based profile that shows the probability that ADHD exists; or 3) a clinical diagnosis of the mental health disorder ADHD based upon criteria from the American Psychiatric Association *Diagnostic and Statistical Manual of Mental Disorders*. Often all three of these options are used before a final diagnosis is made.

Informal Evaluation of ADHD/ADD Behavior

A popular approach to identifying ADHD patterns is to use one of the many informal questionnaires that are available to teachers, counselors, physicians, and mental health providers. These questionnaires ask parents, teachers, and often inattentive persons themselves to check the symptoms frequently seen in the classroom, on the job, or in daily life. These questionnaires estimate where the individual fits along the mild/moderate/severe continuum of ADHD behaviors. These informal inventories do not diagnosis ADHD or ADD. Instead of yielding a diagnosis, they are designed to build a word picture of how the person functions when asked to pay attention, organize, and say "no" to impulses.

Semiformal Evaluation of ADHD/ADD Behavior

Numerous questionnaires yield score profiles to show the level of severity of ADHD or ADD symptoms. For example, Appendix B and Appendix C present three comprehensive semiformal questionnaires, the Jordan Executive Function Index for Children, the Jordan Executive Function Index for Adults, and the Jordan Attention Deficit Scale. These surveys of ADHD behavior yield an estimate of whether symptoms are mild, moderate, or severe. Neither the informal nor semiformal approach labels attention deficit patterns as a mental health disorder. These types of questionnaires are used to identify individuals whose differences can be accommodated without medication or mental health intervention. These questionnaires also identify persons whose symptoms are severe enough to need intervention through medication or talking therapy.

59

Clinical Diagnosis of ADHD

For physicians and psychologists who regard ADHD as a mental health disorder requiring medical intervention and/or talk therapy, the point of reference is the American Psychiatric Association *Diagnostic and Statistical Manual of Mental Disorders*, Fourth Edition, Text Revision 2000 (*DSM–IV–TR*). Figure 3.1 shows the categories of mental health disorders used to diagnose four subtypes of ADHD. This recently revised diagnostic guide classifies Attention-Deficit as a *Disruptive Behavior Disorder* that occurs in four variations:

314.01 Attention-Deficit/Hyperactivity Disorder, Combined Type
314.00 Attention-Deficit/Hyperactivity Disorder, Predominantly Inattentive Type

Attention-Deficit/Hyperactivity Disorder

A. Either (1) or (2):

    (1) six (or more) of the following symptoms of **inattention** have persisted for at least 6 months to a degree that is maladaptive and inconsistent with developmental level:

    Inattention

    (a) often fails to give close attention to details or makes careless mistakes in schoolwork, work, or other activity.

    (b) often has difficulty sustaining attention in tasks or play activities.

    (c) often does not seem to listen when spoken to directly.

    (d) often does not follow through on instructions and fails to finish schoolwork, chores, or duties in the workplace (not due to oppositional behavior or failure to understand instructions).

    (e) often has difficulty organizing tasks and activities.

    (f) often avoids, dislikes, or is reluctant to engage in tasks that require sustained mental effort (such as schoolwork or homework).

    (g) often loses things necessary for tasks or activities (e.g., toys, school assignments, pencils, books, or tools)

    (h) is often easily distracted by extraneous stimuli.

    (i) is often forgetful in daily activities.

    (2) six (or more) of the following symptoms of **hyperactivity-impulsivity** have persisted for at least 6 months to a degree that is maladaptive and inconsistent with developmental level.

    Hyperactivity

    (a) often fidgets with hands or feet or squirms in seat.

    (b) often leaves seat in classroom or other situations in which remaining seated is expected.

    (c) often runs about or climbs excessively in situations in which it is inappropriate (in adolescents or adults, may be limited to subjective feelings of restlessness).

    (d) often has difficulty playing or engaging in leisure activities quietly.

    (e) is often "on the go" or often acts as if "driven by a motor."

    Impulsivity

    (a) often blurts out answers before questions have been completed.

    (b) often has difficulty awaiting turn.

    (c) often interrupts or intrudes on others (e.g., butts into conversations or games).

B. Some hyperactive-impulsive or inattentive symptoms that caused impairment were present before age 7 years.

C. Some impairment from the symptoms is present in two or more settings (e.g., at school [or work] and at home).

(continues)

FIGURE 3.1. These are the diagnostic categories used by physicians and mental health providers to diagnose the four subtypes of ADHD. *Note.* From American Psychiatric Association (2000), *Diagnostic and Statistical Manual of Mental Disorders* (4th ed. TR). Washington, DC: Author. Copyright 2000 by the American Psychiatric Association. Reprinted with permission.

D. There must be clear evidence of clinically significant impairment in social, academic, or occupational functioning.

E. The symptoms do not occur exclusively during the course of a Pervasive Developmental Disorder, Schizophrenia, or other Psychotic Disorder and are not better accounted for by another mental disorder (e.g., Mood Disorder, Anxiety Disorder, Dissociative Disorder, or a Personality Disorder).

Code based on type:

314.01   Attention-Deficit/Hyperactivity Disorder, Combined Type: if both Criteria A1 and A2 are met for the past 6 months.

314.0   Attention-Deficit/Hyperactivity Disorder, Predominantly Inattentive Type: if Criterion A1 is met but Criterion A2 is not met for the past 6 months.

314.01   Attention-Deficit/Hyperactivity Disorder, Predominantly Hyperactive-Impulsive Type: if Criterion A2 is met but Criterion A1 is not met for the past 6 months.

Coding note: For individuals (especially adolescents and adults) who currently have symptoms that no longer meet full criteria, "In Partial Remission" should be specified.

314.9   Attention-Deficit/Hyperactivity Disorder Not Otherwise Specified: This category is for disorders with prominent symptoms of inattention or hyperactivity-impulsivity that do not meet criteria for Attention-Deficit/Hyperactivity Disorder. Examples include

1. Individuals whose symptoms and impairment meet the criteria for Attention-Deficit/Hyperactivity Disorder, Predominantly Inattentive Type but whose age at onset is 7 years or later.

2. Individuals with clinically significant impairment who present with inattention and whose symptom pattern does not meet the full criteria for the disorder but have a behavioral pattern marked by sluggishness, daydreaming, and hypoactivity.

61

FIGURE 3.1. *Continued.*

   314.01   Attention-Deficit/Hyperactivity Disorder, Predominantly Hyperactive-Impulsive Type

   314.9   Attention-Deficit/Hyperactivity Disorder, Not Otherwise Specified (NOS)

For more than 30 years, the American Psychiatric Association (APA) has labored to construct a universally accepted definition of attention deficit differences. Clinicians who depend upon the *Diagnostic and Statistical Manual* (DSM) often are frustrated and confused as, every few years, the standards for diagnosing ADHD change. Adults who were first diagnosed as ADHD during childhood in the 1970s have seen their attention deficit

ADHD in the Classroom and Workplace

syndrome redefined several times. With each revision, the DSM diagnostic language reflects the lack of agreement among psychiatrists and psychologists who set the diagnostic standards for mental health disorders in our culture.

Welcome changes in the *DSM–IV–TR* edition permit us to separate four subtypes of attention deficit more easily: 1) inattentive but not hyperactive; 2) inattentive and hyperactive; 3) inattentive/excessively hyperactive/impulsive; and 4) inattentive and hyperactive, but not ADHD. These criteria are followed by a significant Coding Note: "For individuals (especially adolescents and adults), who currently have symptoms that no longer meet full criteria, 'in Partial Remission' should be specified." This revision of DSM criteria acknowledges the fact that many ADHD or ADD individuals outgrow most of their symptoms during adolescent emergence of executive function, a process described in Chapter 2.

Without using the label ADD, this revised diagnostic guideline acknowledges the passive, nonhyperactive type of attention deficit described in Chapter 4. Classification 314.9, *Attention-Deficit/ Hyperactivity Disorder, Not Otherwise Specified,* includes this significant concession:

> This category is for disorders with prominent symptoms of inattention or hyperactivity-impulsivity that do not meet criteria for Attention-Deficit/Hyperactivity Disorder. Examples include … individuals with clinically significant impairment who present with inattention and whose symptom pattern does not meet the full criteria for the disorder but have a behavioral pattern marked by sluggishness, daydreaming, and hypoactivity.

However, it remains a mystery why the specialists who authorize these diagnostic standards cling to the nonsensical concept "hyperactive/ nonhyperactive disorder." Without conceding the obvious contradiction in this diagnostic format, without using Thom Hartmann's label "Edison-gene hunter" type, diagnosticians now may acknowledge this form of attention deficit without calling it a mental health disorder.

Alternative Clinical Diagnostic Methods for ADHD

For 35 years, the DSM has set the standard for diagnosis of ADHD. However, alternative methods for defining and diagnosing attention differences are emerging. For example, Daniel G. Amen, through extensive brain imaging research, has developed a much broader, more comprehensive view of this issue. Amen's research identifies six subtypes of attention deficit disorder

(Amen, 2001). Often his work is less than clear as he uses the label ADD to describe ADHD symptoms and behaviors:

1. Type 1 *Classic ADD:* Inattentive, distractible, disorganized, hyperactive, restless, and impulsive.
2. Type 2 *Inattentive ADD:* Easily distracted with a low attention span, but not hyperactive. Instead, often appears sluggish or apathetic.
3. Type 3 *Overfocused ADD:* Excessive worrying, argumentative, and compulsive; often gets locked in a spiral of negative thoughts.
4. Type 4 *Temporal Lobe ADD:* Quick temper and rage, periods of panic and fear, mildly paranoid.
5. Type 5 *Limbic ADD:* Moodiness, low energy. Socially isolated, chronic low-grade depression. Frequent feelings of hopelessness.
6. Type 6 *"Ring of Fire" ADD:* Angry, aggressive, sensitive to noise, light, clothes, and touch; often inflexible, experiencing periods of mean, unpredictable behavior, and grandiose thinking.

Amen's point of view is pressing traditional thinking about ADHD to expand and become more comprehensive. His regrouping of symptoms includes but does not name the tag-along syndromes Oppositional/Defiant Disorder, mood disorder, and autism, described in Chapter 5. This expanding attitude toward attention deficit disorders is reflected in the work of Nancy Andreason (2001), Julian Haber (2003), Thom Hartmann (2003), Diane Kennedy (2002), Joseph Chilton Pearce (2002), Patricia Quinn (2001), Richard Restak (2003), Paul Wender (2000), and others.

Recognizing the Many Faces of ADHD

ADHD Individuals Have Poor Self-Regulation

Since the early 1980s, Russell Barkley, a pioneer in defining ADHD, has insisted that the problem of ADHD is more than, or likely different from, lack of attention control. During the 1990s, Russell and his research colleagues developed a new model for understanding this form of disruptive behavior:

> ADHD probably is not primarily a disorder of paying attention but one of *self-regulation:* how the self comes to manage itself within the larger realm of social behavior. ADHD is … a disturbance in the [individual's] ability to use self-control with regard to the future … an inability to use a sense of time and of the past and future to guide … behavior. What is not developing properly … is the capacity to shift from focusing on the here and now to focusing on the future.
> —Russell Barkley, 1995, pp. vii–ix

This point of view recognizes the major difficulty that ADHD individuals have over time in coping with classroom expectations, workplace requirements, family responsibilities, personal relationships, and community standards for public behavior. If the individual is "time blind," he or she cannot see the past, present, and future as a logical sequence or unbroken continuum. Because of this chronic deficit in comprehending time, ADHD individuals cannot develop appropriate behavior to fit into society without being disruptive. Being "time blind" is much more challenging than simply not paying attention well enough.

ADHD Individuals Cannot Wait

Chapter 2 described a major problem with executive dysfunction when the person cannot wait. To be successful at school, in the workplace, in personal relationships, and in the community, individuals must have the ability to pause before acting, wait a moment before responding, and take extra time to be sure that this is appropriate before doing something. Waiting involves keeping impulses under control long enough to think about the consequences of personal action. Waiting—inviting others to go first while holding back the impulse to push ahead—is the heart of thoughtful behavior. Waiting to spend money is the key to managing one's own affairs, keeping bills paid on time, and following a budget of what one can afford. Inability to wait costs ADHD individuals friendships, job success, and classroom achievement.

ADHD Individuals Are Too Noisy

Chapter 2 presented John Ratey and Catherine Johnson's concept of *the noisy brain*. This model of ADHD is based on the fact that the ADHD brain is filled with "noise" much like static that overloads radio or television broadcasts. The noisy brain never is quiet or at peace. Chapter 1 described the brain's inner voice, which carries on an inner brain dialog, enabling all the brain regions to communicate. In the ADHD brain, this inner voice does not stay quiet long enough for the person to listen well. The overly verbal (*hyperlexic*) brain fails to pay attention to important new data that enter the basal brain and limbic system. The hyperlexic brain attends to bits and pieces of data instead of processing complete streams of new information. Without waiting to understand the full incoming message, the noisy brain jumps to conclusions before all the data are in. The overly verbal ADHD brain continually makes mistakes in judgment because the chattering inner voice interrupts frontral lobe executive function as it tries to think things through. The noisy brain becomes sidetracked by emotions and feelings that surge beyond normal levels. The voice of the ADHD brain clamors on and on, demanding immediate action instead of becoming quiet enough to think things through from start to finish. Cascades of emotions overwhelm logic, triggering impulsive behavior that does not pause to think of consequences. Decisions are based largely on feelings and emotions because the inner voice is talking too much to hear the rest of the story. The motor cortex sends premature signals that create inappropriate body activity. The ADHD brain talks too much, keeps the body in constant motion, and overreacts with stronger emotions and feelings than the situation demands.

ADHD Individuals Are Too Quickly Bored

Authors who describe ADHD agree that boredom is one of the most disruptive traits of attention deficit disorder. In the Introduction, we saw the impact of boredom as Luis, Jacob, and Anna disrupted Mrs. Jolly's classroom. Parents of bored ADHD youngsters struggle to keep these restless ones focused from start to finish on homework and household chores. Chapter 2 explains how executive function governs the length of time the whole brain can pay attention before boredom interrupts.

Cell Firing Rhythms

To understand how boredom takes charge of executive function, we must review the role of *cell firing rhythms* in paying attention. During the 1990s, a remarkable discovery was reported by Rodolfo Llinas and his colleagues at Massachusetts Institute of Technology (Llinas, 1993). That research measured the speed of cell firing in several regions of the brain. Llinas described the rhythmic cell firing throughout the brain as "fluid motion" that transmits data in steady, continuous streams from one brain region to another. Each area of the brain maintains a different rate of cell firing, and these firing rhythms change as a person's level of activity changes. For example, during deep sleep, cell firing within the cerebral cortex of the higher brain drops to 2 cycles per second. As the brain enters the REM (rapid eye movement) phase of sleep and starts to dream, cell firing increases to 10 cycles per second. When the brain is wide awake and fully alert, cerebral cell firing jumps to 40 cycles per second. This 40-cycles-per-second rhythm sweeps the whole brain from front to back the way that radar sweeps the atmosphere in weather forecasting. Llinas and his colleagues demonstrated how attention deficit disorders interrupt these brain wave cycles.

Arousal and Underarousal of the Brain

For more than 50 years, we have recognized cycles in being alert (fully focused) and becoming less alert (losing focus) in the way individuals pay attention. Llinas's research into cell firing rhythms answered an important question about inattention and distraction in ADHD and ADD. When the cerebral cortex cell firing rhythm is at 40 cycles per second, the higher brain is fully aroused, enabling the individual to pay full attention, listen well, read with good comprehension, and stay on task from start to finish. When cerebral cell firing rhythm drops below 40 cycles per second, the higher brain begins to lose attention and becomes distracted. This is called *underarousal*. Firing rhythm at 37 cycles per second produces mild ADD or ADHD inattention (underarousal) as boredom emerges. Firing rhythm at 35 cycles per second produces moderate ADD or ADHD with interfering boredom and restlessness. Firing rhythm at 32 cycles per second triggers severe underarousal with distractedness, inattention, major boredom, and disruptive restlessness.

Low Glucose Metabolism in the Brain

In 1990, Alan Zametkin and his colleagues discovered a major cause for underarousal in ADHD and ADD. Figure 3.2 shows Zametkin's map of brain regions where metabolism of glucose (brain sugar) drops below normal levels. As glucose metabolism decreases in these brain regions, executive function loses control over attention. Chapter 7 describes several reasons why ADHD and ADD individuals tend to have unstable glucose metabolism that triggers inattention, boredom, restlessness, and distraction.

Slow Blood Flow in the Brain

To maintain full arousal and long-term attention, the brain must receive a steady supply of oxygen to metabolize glucose and keep cerebral cell firing at 40 cycles per second. Daniel Amen (2001); Nancy Andreason (2001); Richard Restak (2002, 2003); Frank Wood (1991) and others have studied the impact of blood flow and brain functions. Below-normal blood flow often is seen in brain scan images of individuals with ADHD and ADD. When blood flow slows down or remains below normal, the decreased supply of oxygen causes the brain to slip into underarousal. As underarousal increases, the higher brain becomes drowsy, the way a sleepy driver feels behind the wheel or a sleepy student feels during a lecture.

The brain is designed to wake itself up when blood flow and glucose metabolism fall below normal levels. As a sleepy driver or drowsy listener starts to nap, the body jerks to wake up the sluggish brain. A similar "wakeup call" sweeps the underaroused ADHD brain, triggering the motor cortex to

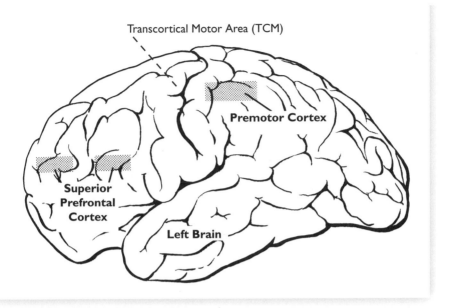

Transcortical Motor Area (TCM)

Premotor Cortex

Superior
Prefrontal
Cortex

Left Brain

FIGURE 3.2. Areas of the left brain where sugar usage (brain glucose metabolism) is lower in individuals who have ADHD than in those who do not have attention deficits. (Based on the model reported by Alan Zemetkin et al., 1990.)

fire muscle movement signals to make the body active. This "wakeup call" is sent over and over until the frontal cortex is wide awake. Hyperactive behavior in ADHD individuals often is the brain's way of making up for irregular, below-normal glucose metabolism and blood flow.

67

Underarousal and Boredom

A disruptive byproduct of underarousal in the left frontal lobe is quick boredom. The sluggish frontal lobe of the ADHD brain must have frequent stimulation to stay alert. As the frontal lobe loses interest, the brain searches for a more exciting, interesting, or faster-moving activity. This is why ADHD learners like Luis in Mrs. Jolly's classroom quickly become restless and fidgety doing paper-and-pencil activities. His understimulated brain needs more excitement, so Luis's attention shifts away from the assigned task, which for him has become too passive and boring. Without thinking about it, he scans his environment in search of something more active and stimulating. Through vision and hearing, Luis's brain spots more interesting events that draw him across the room as a magnet draws iron filings. This is why Mrs. Jolly never knows where Luis will go next. If he sits still even briefly and does passive pencil-and-paper work, his prefrontal cortex becomes underaroused, which triggers another seek-and-investigate cycle away from his workspace.

ADHD in the Classroom and Workplace

ADHD Individuals Are Aggressive

Often the most disruptive face of ADHD is aggressive behavior. Inner drives that push the ADHD person into hyperactivity can also cause the ADHD brain to ignore the privacy of others. As most individuals mature, they learn to look for boundaries that mark the privacy of others. In a society that is governed by rules of politeness, most young children begin to notice social signals that say they should stop and not press further into another person's private space. Individuals who are very private, even shy, must have a wide boundary zone that keeps others at a distance. Persons who need a lot of privacy give many signals that they want to be left alone, or that they must know ahead of time when someone plans to enter their private space. Outgoing people who talk a lot and want to be with others have much less need for privacy. Yet everyone sets limits on when outsiders are welcome to come into personal private space. Adults work hard to teach children how to recognize privacy signals that tell them when they are welcome to come closer, or when they should back away and leave others alone. During early childhood most youngsters learn to read body signals in the faces of adults and older siblings. A warm smile means "Come on in. You're welcome." A stern face, or a frown, means "Stay out of my space right now. You're not welcome." Body language sends clear signals that invite others in or warn others to stay outside private space. Arms crossed over the chest with the body standing stiffly or turned slightly away send the message, "Don't come near me right now." Arms open and relaxed, or the body standing in a relaxed posture, tell others that the gate is open and they are welcome to enter private territory. A stern, unemotional voice sends the signal to stay away. A warm, affectionate voice welcomes outsiders to come in.

When the ADHD brain is driven by churning emotions and hyperactive mental images, the individual does not read privacy signals from others. Impulsive ADHD individuals bound through closed gates, intruding into private space with no regard for the nonverbal signals to stay out. Individuals with ADHD are aggressive and intrusive. The ADHD brain does not learn the nonverbal language of reading social signals. This aggressive tendency quickly irritates and offends others who wish to be left alone and triggers resentment toward the hyperactive intruder, setting off a cascade of negative emotions and feelings that turns encounters into confrontations. Teachers, employers, friends, and relatives of ADHD persons must deal continually with disruptions caused by aggressive, thoughtless disregard for the privacy of others. This social blindness, or inability to read the signals that guide polite relationships, is often referred to as "social dyslexia."

ADHD Individuals Are Too Easily Distracted

It is impossible for the ADHD brain to ignore what goes on nearby. Instead of staying focused on any task, the individual's attention darts to nearby movement to see what is happening. An ADHD person's attention continually is drawn toward every new sound. Any unusual odor is an irresistible attraction that must be investigated. Visceral signals that air temperature has changed capture the brain's attention, tugging it away from the task before finishing. Pressure of clothing on the thighs or buttocks triggers squirming and tugging that cannot be postponed. An itch starts somewhere on the skin and must be scratched. The eyes glimpse something on the edge of the field of vision, and the head turns to examine that new visual image. An ear picks up a sound that draws the brain's attention to that new event. Feelings emerge inside the body as gas bubbles work through the digestive tract or a belch erupts. These visceral feelings cannot be ignored. Anything new or different in the ADHD person's environment calls for immediate investigation. The ADHD brain cannot ignore interesting or exciting temptations to abandon tasks that have become boring.

ADHD Individuals Are Poor Listeners

Individuals with ADHD cannot stay on track when listening. When flows of new oral information come their way, they cannot absorb the full meaning. Only bits and pieces of what the ADHD person hears move from the midbrain hippocampus, where long-term memory begins, into higher brain regions where permanent memory is established. When a listening experience is over, the ADHD person clamors, "What? What did you say? Tell me again." Later he or she claims "You didn't tell me that!" or "I didn't hear you say that." As a rule, the ADHD brain absorbs and retains less than 30 percent of oral information the first time it comes through listening (Jordan, 2000a, 2000b, 2002).

69

ADHD Individuals Cannot Finish What They Start

An earmark of ADHD is the trail of unfinished tasks and projects that are continually left behind and scattered around. ADHD individuals seldom finish what they start unless they are supervised and repeatedly reminded to do so. Classroom assignments are started but seldom finished. Household chores are begun but left uncompleted. Job tasks are started but not finished unless the ADHD worker is reminded and supervised. The first

ADHD in the Classroom and Workplace

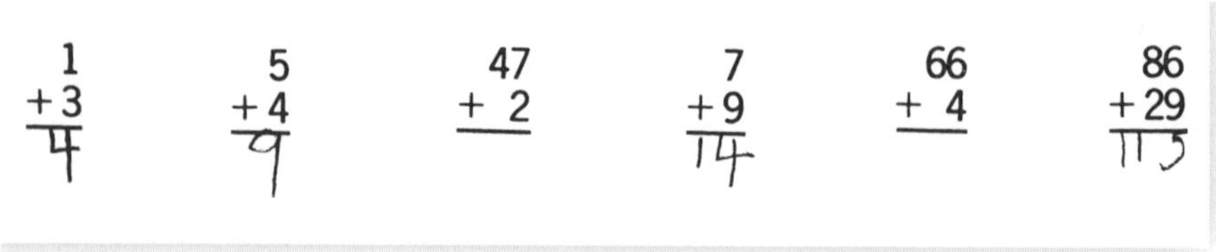

$$\begin{array}{r}1\\+3\\\hline 4\end{array} \qquad \begin{array}{r}5\\+4\\\hline 9\end{array} \qquad \begin{array}{r}47\\+\ 2\\\hline \end{array} \qquad \begin{array}{r}7\\+9\\\hline 14\end{array} \qquad \begin{array}{r}66\\+\ 4\\\hline \end{array} \qquad \begin{array}{r}86\\+29\\\hline 113\end{array}$$

FIGURE 3.3. Math assignment of a 9-year-old boy who has ADHD. He intended to come back to finish the problems he skipped, but he became distracted and failed to do so. He turned in his paper thinking that he had finished this assignment.

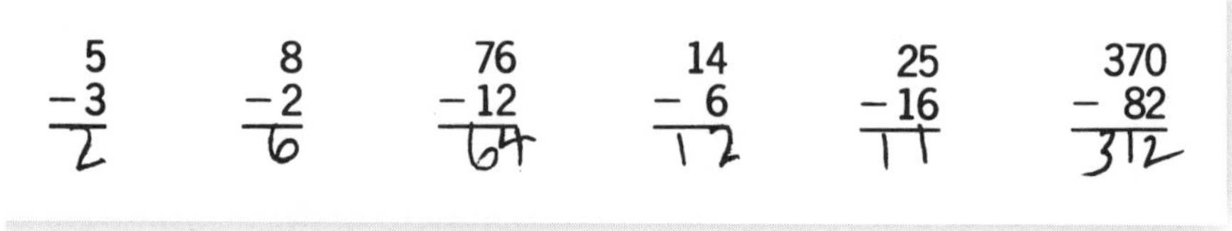

$$\begin{array}{r}5\\-3\\\hline 2\end{array} \qquad \begin{array}{r}8\\-2\\\hline 6\end{array} \qquad \begin{array}{r}76\\-12\\\hline 64\end{array} \qquad \begin{array}{r}14\\-\ 6\\\hline 12\end{array} \qquad \begin{array}{r}25\\-16\\\hline 11\end{array} \qquad \begin{array}{r}370\\-\ 82\\\hline 312\end{array}$$

FIGURE 3.4. Math assignment of a 10-year-old girl who has ADHD. She began to subtract, then became distracted. When she returned to her work, she did not notice the subtraction signs. By this time, she was too confused and disorganized to think clearly. To fill the answer spaces, she partly added and partly subtracted the remaining problems.

line of math problems may be worked accurately while the rest of the page is left unfinished. The first two or three lines on a worksheet are done well, but the rest of the page is left blank. Yet ADHD individuals believe that they have finished their work. Many arguments erupt when adults ask why work was not finished, and the ADHD person responds: "I did too finish. You always blame me for not finishing. I did all of it!" Figures 3.3 and 3.4 show examples of how ADHD interrupts math assignments. Students with ADHD seldom are aware when their attention leaves a task. The stimulation of jumping to a new track erases the short-term memory of laying aside an old task that has become too boring and uninteresting.

ADHD Individuals Are Impulsive

One of the major tasks of the higher brain is to control impulses that are generated by regions of the limbic system. The brain stem, amygdala, medulla, and basal ganglia are the first brain regions to deal with high-energy issues that demand immediate satisfaction. As new, unfiltered visceral or environmental information enters the basal brain, a lot of stimulating, exciting possibilities clamor for the higher brain's attention. Odors that signal something new, whether it is pleasant or unpleasant, call out for immediate response. New sounds that promise interesting relief from now-boring tasks demand investigation. A nearyby comment is so enticing that the listener simply must reply, often by butting in and triggering conflict. An invitation from friends to go do something exciting cannot be postponed, regardless of the consequences of leaving a task or chore undone. As these calls for action enter the higher brain, executive function from the prefrontal cortex has the responsibility to say no. The prefrontal cortex is the higher brain's logical adult to the limbic system's emotional child. In its logical way, executive function must maintain control over the midbrain's whims and impulses if the person is to live a self-regulated life.

In the ADHD brain, the prefrontal cortex cannot stay in charge of the emotions and feelings from the limbic system. As executive function loses these internal arguments, feelings and emotions take control of the ADHD person's behavior. He or she does not think of consequences as tasks are abandoned and the individual's attention darts off to a more interesting or exciting venture.

ADHD Individuals Are Poorly Organized

In their popular books *Driven to Distraction* and *Answers to Distraction,* Edward Hallowell and John Ratey (1994a, 1994b) tell many stories of how poor organization disrupts relationships, job performance, school achievement, and family life in people with ADHD. The ADHD brain does not develop a comprehensive sense of when things are organized or when they remain disorganized. Individuals with ADHD do not notice when things are out of order or in the wrong place. The individual parts of situations do not fit together into organized, complete mental images. An ADHD child does not see when his or her room is jumbled and overly cluttered. Most ADHD adults drive messy vehicles that are littered with trash the driver rarely tidies up. An ADHD employee works in a messy space with job stuff scattered around or loosely piled in overflowing stacks. An ADHD student is unaware that his or her locker or desk are crammed with old papers, lunch wrappers, and clothing from last season. The ADHD brain does not see a mess. Persons with ADHD perceive only one or two individual items at a time. They do not form a complete mental image that signals the brain when workspace, living area, or vehicle interior is cluttered and untidy. These individuals are bewildered when their unorganized lifestyle frustrates and irritates others. Being untidy seems normal to most ADHD persons, who see no problem with being poorly organized. They do not understand why their scattered lifestyle drives parents, teachers, bosses, lovers, and friends to distraction.

ADHD Individuals Are Too Emotional

Chapter 2 describes the link between strong emotions and attention deficits. Figure 2.1 shows the midbrain structures that regulate the rise and flow of strong emotions and feelings. In young children who do not have ADHD, the emotional centers of the limbic system begin to mature at the same time the prefrontal cortex takes charge of constructive emotions that govern social behavior (see Figure 2.2). By age 4 most children have begun to say no to strong feelings and yes to gentler emotions that make society pleasant and safe.

As children become fluent in oral language, and as they learn to read, they usually learn to stop urges to be angry, to cry over little bumps and bruises, or to crowd aggressively in front of others to be first in line. This development of social skills and self-control of emotional aggression lags behind schedule in youngsters with ADHD. These youngsters continue to have emotional eruptions that are no longer appropriate for their age. They disrupt group activities with tantrums when they fail to get their own way. They clamor for more when treats are given by adults. They aggressively "want what they want when they want it" without having a sense of politeness or of waiting one's turn. ADHD children, adolescents, and adults deal with life on a strongly emotional level rather than staying calm and thinking things through. The prefrontal cortex lags behind in executive function that reminds the limbic system to stop surges of socially destructive feelings and emotions.

ADHD Individuals Are Insatiable

One of the important signs of social maturity is the ability to be satisfied. The ADHD brain seldom is satisfied. Research by Nancy Andreason (2001), Lise Eliot (1999), and Richard Restak (2002, 2003) has mapped the reward pathway that links several pleasure centers in the limbic system, shown in Figure 3.5. Youngsters without ADHD reach reward pathway maturity on a predictable developmental schedule. They learn to be satisfied with one serving, a smaller helping, or just a taste of something delicious. They discover the social joy of sharing and being partners in having a good time.

Youngsters with ADHD do not. They lag behind in limbic system maturity, so that the reward pathway does not signal when they have had enough. Appetites are not curbed when enough has been eaten or drunk or experienced. When logical, commonsense reasoning of executive function says, "That's enough for now," hungry feelings and emotions from the limbic system yearn for more. Many ADHD individuals clamor, "He got more

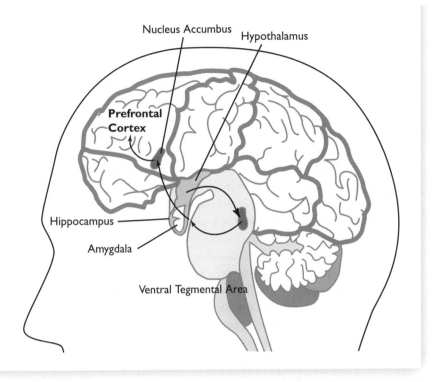

FIGURE 3.5. The arrows show the "reward pathway" within the limbic system. When these regions of the midbrain mature on schedule, the prefrontal cortex receives the signal "that's enough," and the person knows it is time to stop that activity. When neurons within the "reward pathway" do not mature on schedule, the prefrontal cortex does not send the "that's enough" signal. This causes the appetite or desire to continue. (Based on research reported by R. M. Restak, 2002.)

than I did" or "I never get my fair share." An ADHD adolescent shouts at his parents: "You always give my sister more than you give me!" as he starts the vehicle his parents gave him for his 16th birthday. He ignores the fact that his sister had to wait until age 18 for her first car. "I'm going to quit this dumb job!" an ADHD adult grumbles. "I can't ever please the boss. He always treats everyone else better than me." Jealousy is an active part of being insatiable. Envy eats away the heart of relationships as the insatiable ADHD person holds grudges against others. Insatiable ADHD individuals practice a lifestyle of grumbling, complaining, and accusing others of receiving more. "Life's not fair!" could be the motto of ADHD individuals. The aggressive habit of being insatiable disrupts family life, classroom environments, workplace cooperation, and personal relationships between friends and lovers.

ADHD Individuals Are Overly Sensitive

As children mature, they normally learn to welcome guidance and constructive criticism that enables them to win praise and higher achievement. Part of growing up should be to learn from one's mistakes and from the advice offered by wiser, older persons. One of the most disruptive characteristics of ADHD is being overly sensitive to criticism. Children, adolescents, and adults with ADHD cannot accept criticism without reacting aggressively in self-defense. Instead of listening to advice on how to do a task better next time, the ADHD person erupts in an overly emotional protest that is designed to stop the flow of criticism. Without thinking of consequences, the ADHD brain leaps to self-defense that involves argument, denial, and blaming someone else. "There you go criticizing me again!" the ADHD person blurts out. "I can't ever please you. No matter how hard I try, you always tell me I'm wrong. You never pick on anybody else. It's not my fault!" In the workplace, the ADHD employee blames equipment for ruining that piece of work. Or it is the custodian's fault for not cleaning the work area last night. Or it is the foreman's fault for changing the rules and not telling the worker. At home, parents are bombarded by aggressive verbal tirades about how the ADHD child always is the victim of another person's carelessness. In the community, the ADHD adult rails at the police officer who is issuing a speeding ticket. "It's not my fault I was going 70 miles an hour through that school zone. Someone took down the speed limit sign. Besides, you cops just pick on guys driving four-wheel-drive trucks." In a dating relationship, the ADHD partner has a tantrumn when a suggestion is made that he or she figure out a system to be on time for dates and appointments. "There you go again blaming me!" yells the ADHD partner. "It's not my fault I'm late. You just can't make up your mind when we're supposed to meet." Of all the faces of ADHD, being overly sensitive to constructive criticism is one of the most disruptive and costly traits of poor socialization skills.

ADHD Individuals Jump Mental Tracks

Chapter 2 described how the brain activates old memories and integrates new knowledge with what has been learned. From the moment new data enters the basal brain for safety checking, to the moment new information arrives at higher brain regions, an enormous amount of mental activity has taken place. Executive function from the prefrontal cortex governs this complex process of learning, remembering, and thinking. In order for the brain to think from start to finish, attention must remain fixed on specific idea tracks. Figure 2.8 in Chapter 2 shows the many brain regions that must work together to pay full attention. The ADHD brain cannot stay fixed on an idea track longer than a few seconds without becoming distracted. Without warning, the ADHD listener's attention jumps to a different track, leaving the original thought pattern unfinished. This is similar to surfing channels on a television set. Many ADHD individuals jump track when their brains pick up a new signal from a word that is heard or something that is seen. For example, an ADHD person might be listening to a conversation in which the speaker mentions "four-wheel-drive trucks." Without warning, the ADHD listener jumps from listening to the rest of the conversation to thinking about four-wheel-drive vehicles. The ADHD brain now is fixed on rapid images of high-energy vehicles instead of continuing to listen to the original idea track. Sometimes the ADHD listener sees something out the corner of the eyes or whiffs a new aroma. Suddenly the brain jumps track to that visual or olfactory event. It is not unusual for an ADHD person to begin a mental cascade of images that trigger a new idea track, then leap to still another track, then jump again to still a different track in a rapid mental sequence. Within seconds, the ADHD brain has leapfrogged far from the original mental activity, and none of the new mental processes is finished. Inside the ADHD brain, countless interrupted idea tracks are started but never completed.

ADHD Individuals Have Active Fantasies

When the ADHD brain jumps away from the reality of task performance, regions of the right and left brain that host imagination take over the person's thinking. Suddenly thoughts are off into the world of fantasy or make-believe. "What if I had a four-wheel-drive truck? Especially that red one with the chrome roll bars I saw last night. I would put in the biggest boom box in town. I would paint flame stripes down the sides. I would get mag wheel covers and put in purple shag upholstery. I would jack it up with the highest struts in town. Everybody would be pea-green jealous and want to ride with me. All the girls would be nice to me for a change." This kind of high-energy magical thinking is normal for persons with ADHD. Over time, a great deal of mental energy goes into fantastical make-believe instead of into the realities of life. Magical thinking or active fantasy is a highly desirable part of early childhood. Make-believe play is the first work of growing up. However, when fantasy continues to preoccupy the thoughts of older children, adolescents, and adults, the result is lost productivity and separation from the rest of society.

ADHD Individuals Are Immature

Individuals who have ADHD are noticeably less mature than others their age. As a rule, intelligence is far ahead of emotional development. Most persons with ADHD are quite bright, but that intelligence is not available for consistent use in the classroom, on the job, or in making mature lifestyle decisions. In an important way, ADHD individuals are upside down in their emotional maturity. The following maturity profile for a 14-year-old ADHD boy illustrates this frustrating imbalance between ability and behavior. The first column shows certain areas of behavior or skill development. The second column shows the age at which that skill would be measured. The third column shows what grade level this behavior or skill would fit.

Oral vocabulary age (ability to make conversation, use words correctly)	18	Adult level
Mental age (ability to do problem solving and logical thinking when the brain is fully focused)	17	12th grade
Reading age (ability to glean the full meaning of printed material)	17	12th grade
Spelling age (ability to spell words correctly from memory or dictation)	16	11th grade
Chronological age	14	9th grade
Math age (skills in arithmetic computation and number problem solving)	13	8th grade
Attention span age (how long attention can remain fully focused without jumping to another track)	8	3rd grade
Emotional maturity age (has tantrums, is self-centered, has no patience, is thoughtless, is impulsive and overly emotional)	7	2nd grade

ADHD individuals with this kind of difference between verbal skills, intelligence, and control of basal emotions are disruptive in most situations. Having the oral skills of a young adult while behaving like a spoiled child sabotages relationships and fosters a lifestyle of failure.

ADHD Individuals' Plugs Keep Falling Out

As I prepared to retire from private practice in diagnosing and treating learning disorders, I spent a day with an 11-year-old girl with severe ADHD. Her maturity profile resembled the one above. Jennifer's hyperactive behavior had exhausted her parents, and her disruptive behavior kept the classroom in an uproar. Yet adults agreed that she seemed to be highly intelligent. My office was well equipped for Jennifer's aggressive ADHD behavior. Heavy carpet was supported by thick foam padding. Chairs were on rollers. The work table was made of solid oak lumber sturdy enough to support an elephant. An enormous fuzzy beanbag sat at one end of the room, ready to absorb the energy of belly flops and flying leaps. As Jennifer and I worked through the diagnostic tests, she rolled on the floor, dived onto the beanbag, scooted around in chairs, and lay on her back kicking the underside of the table. With this freedom to discharge excess energy, she did not miss a beat in listening and responding to test questions. At the end of the day she still was bursting with energy, but she had demonstrated oral language development far beyond her age. I could talk with her on a young adult level.

As I prepared to review the day's work with Jennifer's parents, I asked her to tell me what it is like to have ADHD. While performing acrobatic leaps and bounds around the office, she told me of an experience she and her brother had had the previous summer. Their grandmother had taken them to Silver Dollar City in Missouri. There the children had enjoyed reconstructions of life in the early 1900s. Jennifer's favorite historical display was the telephone office where a lady sat on a tall stool and plugged cords into the switchboard as she said, "Number please." Jennifer stopped bounding and leaping long enough to explain that having ADHD is like that old-fashioned telephone exchange. "I put in all my plugs," she said, "but my plugs keep falling out." I have never heard a better explanation of what it is like to have ADHD.

This lifestyle of mental plugs falling out explains many of the irregular patterns we see when ADHD individuals take certain kinds of tests. For example, Figure 3.6 shows the irregular, seesaw pattern of subscores on the *Wechsler Intelligence Test for Children* (WISC–III) that signals attention deficit disorder. The higher scores show where the plugs stayed in all the way through the subtest activities. The lower scores show where the student's plugs kept falling out, making it impossible for the ADHD individual to maintain full attention and give fully organized responses.

Is ADHD Ever Outgrown?

Opinions differ as to whether ADHD ever is outgrown. Mental health specialists who developed the most recent diagnostic criteria for the American

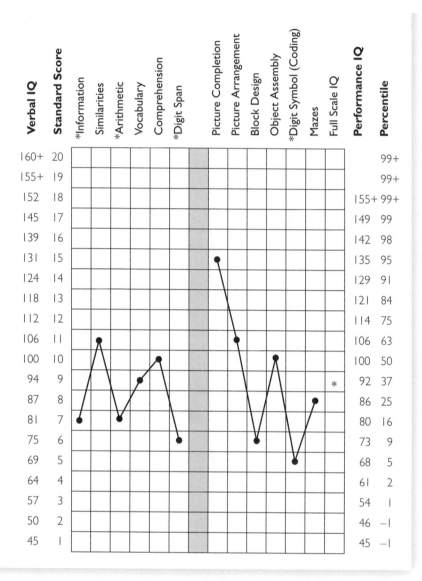

FIGURE 3.6. ADHD or ADD is indicated when we find wide differences between the highest and lowest scores on the WISC profile. This ADD boy is 12 years 8 months old in Grade 6.3. He struggles in all areas of classroom work when he must work alone. When he has a partner to help stay focused, he does outstanding work for brief periods of time. To do his best, he must whisper to himself as he touches his work. This multisensory technique enables his brain to compensate for underlying ADD tendencies.

Psychiatric Association *Diagnostic and Statistical Manual of Mental Disorders,* Fourth Edition, Text Revision 2000 (*DSM–IV–TR*) tucked a significant footnote inside the criteria for diagnosing Attention-Deficit/Hyperactivity Disorder (ADHD):

> Coding Note: For individuals, especially adolescents and adults who currently have symptoms that no longer meet full criteria, "In Partial Remission" should be specified.
>
> —Quick Reference to the Diagnostic Criteria
> from *DSM–IV–TR*, 2000, p. 67

For the first time since the DSM first established diagnostic codes for mental health disorders, this note acknowledges the fact that as ADHD youngsters pass through adolescence into early adulthood, many do outgrow enough of their childhood ADHD symptoms to be taken off the list of having an active mental health disorder.

In his book *Taking Charge of ADHD* (1995), Russell Barkley estimated that 70% of individuals with moderate or mild ADHD lose most of their childhood symptoms by early adult years. This reduction in ADHD symptoms permits these individuals to become well-educated and productive adults. During my 47 years of professional life, I have worked one-on-one with several thousand ADHD individuals. I have remained involved in many of their lives and have met children and grandchildren of the first ADHD youngsters I met. This multigenerational experience has allowed me to observe firsthand the developmental progress of three generations of struggling learners. On reflection, I estimate that 80% of all children with ADHD eventually outgrow most of their early attention deficit symptoms.

Sadly, the remaining 20% of this special population emerge into their adult years still handicapped by many faces of ADHD. As Chapter 7 describes, medication and diet control often reduce negative behavior and ADHD symptoms enough to let these residual-type adults earn a moderate living and enjoy some of the blessings of adulthood. Those who do not outgrow childhood ADHD struggle all their lives with the disruptive patterns described in this chapter.

Checklist of Executive Dysfunction Behaviors

This checklist provides a quick summary of the disruptive behaviors (executive dysfunction) seen by teachers, parents, employers, partners, or counselors. Each check has a value of 1. Subscore totals are found by counting the checks in each section. The total score is found by adding all of the subscores. Finally, the total score is entered in the appropriate section to show whether the individual exhibits mild, moderate, or severe ADHD behavior. Over time, this checklist is useful in showing progress as executive dysfunction behaviors decrease or disappear. For example, an initial total score would show a person's ADHD behavior at the start of a school year, or when medication, diet control, and/or counseling are begun. Then every three months or six months, this checklist would be done again and compared with the results of the original assessment. Everyone involved with this individual will be encouraged to see how much progress in executive function is being made.

Checklist of Executive Dysfunction Behaviors

Hyperactivity

_____ Excessive body activity

_____ Cannot ignore what goes on nearby

_____ Cannot say "no" to impulses

_____ Cannot leave others alone

_____ Cannot spend time alone without feeling nervous or left out

_____ Cannot keep still or stay quiet

Subscore Total _____

Short Attention Span

_____ Cannot keep thoughts concentrated longer than a short period of time

_____ Continually is off on mental rabbit trails

_____ Continually must be called back to the task

Subscore Total _____

Loose Thought Patterns

_____ Cannot maintain organized mental images

_____ Cannot do a series of things without starting to make mistakes

Subscore Total _____

Poor Organization

_____ Cannot keep life organized without help

_____ Cannot stay on schedule without supervision

_____ Lives and works in a cluttered space

_____ Cannot straighten up own space without help

_____ Cannot do homework or silent projects without supervision

Subscore Total _____

Change of First Impression

_____ First impressions do not stay the same

_____ Mental images immediately change

_____ Continually is surprised or startled as things seem different

Subscore Total _____

Poor Listening Comprehension

_____ Cannot get the full meaning of what others say the first time

_____ Continually says "What?" or "Huh?" or "What do you mean?"

_____ Cannot follow oral instructions without hearing again

_____ Does not keep on listening

_____ Attention darts or drifts away before speaker has finished talking

_____ Later insists "You didn't say that" or "I didn't hear you say that"

Subscore Total _____

Overly Sensitive

_____ Immediately has defensive reaction to criticism or correction

_____ Spends a great deal of emotional energy defending self and blaming others

_____ Flies into tantrum when criticized or corrected

_____ Jumps the gun; does not wait to receive all the information before becoming angry or defensive

_____ Leaders must spend a lot of time restoring calm and soothing hurt feelings

Subscore Total _____

Unfinished Tasks

_____ Does not finish tasks without supervision

_____ Leaves several unfinished tasks scattered around

_____ Thinks task is finished when it is not

_____ Does not realize when more is yet to be done to finish the task

Subscore Total _____

Trouble Fitting in Socially

_____ Cannot fit into group situations without conflict

_____ Whines and clamors for own way

_____ Fusses about rules not being fair

_____ Storms out of games when not winning

_____ Wants to quit and do something else before others are finished

_____ Tends to be abrupt, rude, impolite in expressing opinions

_____ Is overly critical of how social events are managed

_____ Keeps conflict going over unimportant issues

Overcoming Attention Deficit Disorders in Children, Adolescents, and Adults

_____ Displays self-centered attitude instead of noticing needs or wishes of others

_____ Is aggressive and domineering in order to get own way

Subscore Total _____

Easily Distracted

_____ Attention continually darts to whatever is going on nearby

_____ Cannot ignore nearby events

_____ Continually stops work to see what others are doing

_____ Is overly aware of nearby sounds, odors, movement

_____ Cannot ignore own body sensations

Subscore Total _____

Immaturity

_____ Behavior is obviously less mature than expected for this age

_____ Behaves like much younger person

_____ Cannot get along well with age-mates

_____ Prefers to play or be with younger persons

_____ Has the interests and thought patterns of much younger persons

_____ Does not make effort to "grow up"

_____ Refuses to accept responsibility

_____ Behavior is impulsive/compulsive

_____ Acts on spur of the moment instead of thinking things through

_____ Refuses long-term goals

_____ Insists on immediate satisfaction of wishes and desires

_____ Puts self ahead of others

_____ Blames others for own mistakes

_____ Triggers displeasure of companions

_____ Often is disliked by others

Subscore Total _____

Insatiability

_____ Desires are never satisfied

_____ Clamors for more

_____ Cannot leave others alone

_____ Demands attention

83

_____ Is quickly bored and wants something different

_____ Complains that others get larger share

_____ Blames parents and leaders for not being fair

_____ Drains emotions of those who must be involved in this person's life

_____ Triggers desire in others to push this person away

_____ Often is dreaded by others

_____ Becomes target of rejection by others

Subscore Total _____

Impulsivity

_____ Does not plan ahead

_____ Acts on spur of the moment

_____ Lacks common sense in making decisions

_____ Does not think of consequences

_____ Demands immediate satisfaction of wishes and desires

_____ Cannot put off desires or wishes

Subscore Total _____

Disruptiveness

_____ Is a disruptive influence in groups

_____ Keeps things stirred up

_____ Triggers conflict within group

_____ Disturbs neighbors during study time or work time

_____ Causes others to complain about how this person behaves

_____ Others are relieved when this person is absent

Subscore Total _____

Body Energy Overflow

_____ Some part of the body is in continual motion

_____ Cannot sit still

_____ Cannot be quiet

_____ Can hold body motions under brief control, but overflow starts again soon

Subscore Total _____

Overcoming Attention Deficit Disorders in Children, Adolescents, and Adults

Emotional Overflow

_____ Emotions always are near the surface

_____ Clamors in an emotional way

_____ Is easily triggered into a hysterical or overly emotional state

_____ Tantrums always are near the surface

Subscore Total _____

Lack of Continuity

_____ Lifestyle does not have continuity

_____ Lives life in unconnected events

_____ Must have supervision and guidance to stay with a course of action from start to finish

_____ Is continually surprised by each new task requirement, no matter how many times the routine has been done before

Subscore Total _____

TOTAL SCORE _____

Enter TOTAL SCORE in appropriate place below.

_____	Mild Executive Dysfunction 1–30	Requires occasional reminding and supervision to finish tasks, not disrupt, return from day-dreaming
_____	Low Moderate Executive Dysfunction 31–45	Requires frequent reminding and supervision to finish tasks, stay on track, not disrupt, return from daydreaming
_____	Moderate Executive Dysfunction 46–55	Requires continual reminding and supervision to finish tasks, stay on track, not disrupt, return from daydreaming. Must have help from teachers, job super-visors, partners to be successful.
_____	High Moderate Executive Dysfunction 56–69	Is disruptive, disorganized, dys-logical in making decisions, overly emotional, triggers conflict in groups, off on mental trails, hyperactive, inflicts high level of

stress on others. Needs medical intervention. Should eliminate trigger foods from diet. Must have supervision to succeed.

_____ Borderline Severe Executive Dysfunction 70–79

Cannot function without help, constant reminding and supervision. Cannot fit into groups. Hyperactive and impulsive. Cannot make logical/commonsense decisions without help. Is very untidy and disorganized. Must have medical intervention, diet control, and talk therapy.

_____ Severe Executive Dysfunction 80–89

Cannot function in a classroom, in the workplace, in a family, in personal relationships. Must have medical intervention, diet control, talk therapy. Must have alternative educational program.

_____ Acute Executive Dysfunction 90–99

Behavior is out of control. Must have medical intervention, diet control, and talk therapy. Cannot participate in educational or social programs until symptoms are reduced.

The Challenges of ADD in the Classroom and Workplace

Chapter

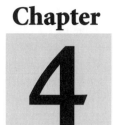

~~~~~~~~~~~~~~~~~~~~~~~~~~~~~~~~~~~~~~~

I start doing my work like the teacher says, but my brain just stops.
— how an 11-year-old girl described being ADD

The [child] with an attention deficit can pay attention. But it takes that [child] 100 percent motivation to do what a normal [child] can do with 55 percent motivation.... If you follow these [children] around throughout an ordinary day, the number of "nos" and "stops" and "don'ts" they hear is astronomical.
— Allan Phillips, Department of Psychiatry,
University of California at Los Angeles
(quoted in Ratey & Johnson, 1997, p. 158)

What Is ADD?

I began my career of teaching and diagnosing struggling learners in 1957, when the disruptive behaviors now called ADHD were labeled MBDS (Minimal Brain Damage Syndrome) and HID (Hyperkinetic Impulse Disorder). During the 1960s my generation largely accepted the newer label MBD (Minimal Brain Dysfunction). During the 1980s we changed to using the new labels ADD+H (Attention Deficit Disorder with Hyperactivity) and ADD−H (Attention Deficit Disorder without Hyperactivity). To the dismay of most diagnosticians, 1987 brought still another shift to the single label ADHD (Attention-Deficit/Hyperactivity Disorder). In 1994, diagnostic specialists were asked to switch to yet another set of diagnostic labels that stipulated hyperactivity while permitting nonhyperactive forms of ADHD. Again in 2000, *DSM–IV–TR* restated the diagnostic criteria for ADHD. The arguments for labeling all forms of attention deficit as ADHD are largely academic. Supporters of this point of view usually are scientists who accept only what can be measured by standard technology as being true attention deficit disorder. This rigid diagnostic model often fails to include quietly disruptive behaviors that fall through the cracks of standard evaluation for attention deficit disorders.

The Existence of ADD Without Hyperactivity

As a hands-on teacher, diagnostician, and counselor of struggling learners for almost 50 years, I came face to face with the fact that not all persons who have attention deficits are hyperactive. In fact, my experience with several thousand struggling learners from around the world convinced me that fewer than half of all attention deficit individuals are hyperactive. If hyperactivity is required for diagnosis of attention deficit disorder, then Russell Barkley and others are correct when they estimate that 5% of the population are ADHD (Barkley, 1995). This means than only 5 individuals out of 100 display the faces of ADHD described in Chapter 3. However, if nonhyperactive ADD is included as a form of attention deficit disorder, then 13% (Jordan, 1998, 2002) to 15% (Haber, 2003) of the human population have attentional disorders. This chapter explores the many faces of ADD (Attention-Deficit Disorder without Hyperactivity), which quietly disrupts families, classrooms, personal relationships, and the workplace around the world.

88

ADD Individuals Are Passive

Lack of Body Motion
In sharp contrast to hyperactive ADHD, persons with ADD exhibit no unusual movement, other than slow eye movement toward the ceiling or subtle head turning away from the task. There is no squirming, bouncing, or moving about to attract attention. Individuals with ADD often sit quietly for long periods of time with no display of excess energy. Nothing on the surface reveals the internal loss of attention that interferes with the ADD person's interaction with his or her environment. ADHD individuals make a lot of noise and get right up in the face of others. ADD individuals drift through life making very little noise and experiencing infrequent confrontations. This passive exterior causes many parents, teachers, diagnosticians, and job supervisors to miss the subtle signs of underlying loss of attention.

Passive/Aggressive Personality Style

It is possible to provoke ADD individuals to the point of triggering a strong emotional response. Passive individuals absorb great amounts of pressure and stress without responding openly. In fact, before the mid-1970s, passive/aggressive tendencies were regarded as a type of emotional disorder. Mental health specialists thought that holding in one's strong emotions and feelings was a sign of emotional disturbance. In reality, being able to absorb insult and stress without becoming angry usually is a positive trait. The world's peacemakers and diplomats usually are passive individuals who automatically absorb insult without handing it back through confrontation. For the ADD brain, the lifestyle habit of absorbing criticism, rejection, or unfair discipline without response can become a problem.

The quiet, passive exterior of ADD often misleads aggressive persons into thinking that it is fine to push ADD strugglers who do not push back. At a certain point of stress, the ADD limbic system erupts with a shout that means "Enough!" Without warning, a storm of aggressive emotions boils out of the ADD individual. These delayed, infrequent reactions to stress always shock parents, teachers, and employers, who did not see the aggressive storm coming. When passive/aggressive ADD individuals reach their limit of accepting stress, they react in one of two ways. Either the exasperated person blasts the environment with explosions of temper, hostility, and revenge for old grievances, or the explosion is kept inside, sending the insulted individual into very active magical thinking that unplugs executive function from control of strong basal emotions. Inside this private, almost invisible battlefield of make-believe, the angry ADD person broods, sulks, and role-plays how to get revenge. Many ADD individuals who explode internally start a crusade of hidden vengeance to get even with the person who triggered the aggressive blast. It is not unusual to see such ADD aggression destroy things that belong to the enemy, or sabotage the enemy's vehicle, or send anonymous mail designed to damage the other person's reputation. Aggression that is held inside comes out in quietly destructive ways that outsiders did not suspect could happen. In some instances, murders have occurred when the totally aggrieved ADD individual decided to remove his or her adversary from the face of the earth.

ADD Individuals Are Quietly Confused

Internally, the ADD brain is as filled with noise as the ADHD brain. Plugs quietly drop out of thought patterns, in contrast to the commotion created when ADHD plugs fall out. Continual "short circuits" occur as the prefrontal cortex tries to communicate common sense and logic to the limbic system and brain stem. The ADD brain fails to absorb or comprehend much of the new information that reaches the higher brain. Individuals with ADD rarely follow streams of oral or visual information from start to finish. Too many bits of data fail to register, causing the ADD brain to give up trying to stay involved with what goes on nearby. When ADD individuals describe their mental images, they reveal constant confusion. "I don't get it," the ADD brain says. "What do you mean?" Then the ADD person gives up trying to comprehend and drifts away into a world of invisible but active make-believe.

ADD Individuals Are Slow in Processing

The ADHD brain races ahead, darts off on side trails, and jumps to conclusions. Body movement follows these sudden changes in where the brain is focused. ADHD moves too fast with too much distraction. In contrast, ADD moves forward too slowly in thinking things through and deciding what to do next. Many ADD individuals need two or three times longer than their neighbors to do the same amount of mental work. Making decisions is a slow, frustrating, often confusing process. If outsiders apply pressure to make the ADD brain work faster, the slow-processing person loses mental images and comes to a standstill. As an 11-year-old ADD student explained to me, "My brain stops." If the plugs stay in, ADD individuals must back up and start the thought process again. If plugs fall out under pressure to hurry, the ADD person gives up in silent confusion and stops trying. Yet the body does not signal this breakdown in mental processing. Careful observers see the eyes of the ADD person slowly shift away to "star gaze" toward the ceiling or out the window. The ADD brain cannot speed up enough to stay on schedules set by faster thinkers.

ADD Individuals Are Forgetful

Parents, teachers, partners, and job supervisors of ADD individuals tell many stories of their frustrations in keeping track of all the things ADD persons forget. The ADD brain does not keep mental lists of objects to be transported, schedules to be kept, projects to be started or finished, or commitments to be honored. Outsiders must monitor ADD individuals to make sure they remember. Children and adolescents with ADD leave trails of lost clothing, school supplies, sports equipment, and tools. The ADD brain does not keep track of where things were last seen or set down. Later the ADD youngster cannot remember what happened to a jacket, pair of shoes, Dad's tools from the garage, schoolbooks needed for homework, or homework to be turned in next day. Adults with ADD are forever losing car keys, wallets or purses, workplace items, shopping lists, and even their vehicle that was parked somewhere in the parking lot. Money management often is impossible because ADD persons forget to record checks written, or they lose important receipts for purchases. This chronic forgetfulness triggers conflict and frustration in those who must share space or life with one who is ADD.

ADD Individuals Are Poor Organizers

The ADD brain does not keep track of time, nor does it keep track of sequence. Internally there is no "clock" that tells the ADD brain how much time has passed or how much time remains before the next event begins. ADD individuals do not think in start-to-finish segments. Those who have ADD deal with one issue at a time, slowly thinking about it until attention drifts away to a new idea. As the ADD brain leaves an unfinished thought and moves to another, the individual is unaware of any sequence. Mental images occur without connection to what went before or what is to follow. Consequently the ADD person's lifestyle is disorganized. Personal space becomes cluttered with forgotten items scattered about. Conversations are left unfinished. Tasks are partly done. Reponsibilities are only partly carried out. Formal learning is spotty and filled with gaps in knowledge. Skill development is incomplete. The ADD brain wanders here and there, leaving an untidy trail of unorganized business. Memory for detail is full of holes, often called "Swiss cheese memory." The ADD person often is poorly groomed because he or she does not comprehend the time or sequences required for combed hair, brushed teeth, matched clothes, and timely bathing. From early childhood to old age, ADD individuals are out of step with a culture that values good organization.

ADD Individuals Are Often Late

Persons with ADD rarely are on time. Their lifestyle is that of being late for meetings and appointments. My grandmother, who had no knowledge of ADD, would say in exasperation: "He is always late. He'll be late to his own funeral!" Because the ADD brain has no internal clock that keeps track of time, these individuals are known for being tardy to class, late for scheduled appointments, not there on time for dates, and running behind in job completion. Teaching tardy ADD learners often challenges an instructor's patience to the breaking point. Supervising ADD workers on the job brings conflicting time standards into confrontation. Yet the passive surface behavior of ADD individuals does not reveal their internal confusion over time. Being on time is as foreign a concept for ADD as sitting still is foreign to ADHD.

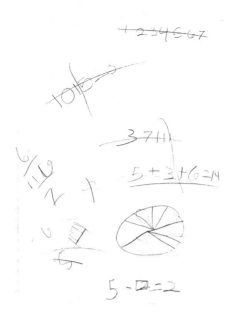

A   (*continues*)

FIGURE 4.1. Math work of a 14-year-old boy who has ADD. He cannot maintain organized mental images to work math problems. He tries to keep track by jotting "counting marks" on his paper or drawing shapes (A). Soon he becomes confused as he counts the marks and practices on scratch paper (B). Then he gives up in frustration and does not finish the assignment.

ADD Individuals Are Loose

Success in the classroom and the workplace depends on individuals having tight, concise mental images that stay clearly focused over periods of time. The ADD brain is too loose to achieve this kind of success. Mental images that begin with clear focus soon melt away into fuzzy, poorly formed thought patterns. What the ADD person knows is not stored as precise, well-organized memories. Chapter 1 reviewed how the brain stores permanent memories in engrams, and how those engrams are activated to call up knowledge in organized images. The ADD brain stem and midbrain are too loose to filter out irrelevant information, then pass on to the parietal lobes what the higher brain needs to know. ADD individuals pick up bits and pieces of new knowledge but not well-sequenced whole concepts. Memory for details is spotty. Later when engrams are activated to recall specific data, the ADD brain produces partial images and incomplete information. Thought patterns and memories are loose instead of sharply fo-

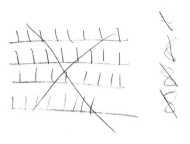

B

FIGURE 4.1. *Continued.*

cused. Learning new skills is unsatisfactory because the ADD brain fails to comprehend all of the skill steps in sequence. As the ADD person responds to questions, he or she stumbles over words and delivers only part of the information that is expected. Loose thought patterns cause the ADD brain to stumble every step of the way in learning and remembering.

Loose thought patterns are easily seen in paper-and-pencil assignments about which ADD learners are confused. In spite of drill and practice with basic skills, these students continue to struggle with simple assignments. Figure 4.1 shows how ADD interferes with arithmetic problem solving. The ADD brain often cannot keep track of the many variables that are involved in doing homework, especially math assignments.

ADD Individuals Cannot Listen

Listening well requires maturely developed self-discipline. For listening to be successful, the frontal lobes, temporal lobes, and parietal lobes must maintain clear communication between each other and the mibrain. The listener must tune out distractions in order to pay full attention to the flow of oral information. The ADD brain cannot do so. Very soon after the ADD individual starts to listen, his or her plugs quietly fall out and attention drifts elsewhere. As a rule, individuals with ADD retain less than 30% of what they hear, unless the oral information is repeated several times. Part of good listening for most persons is eye contact, except when cultural standards forbid looking directly at others. The ADD listener does not maintain eye contact. Soon after listening begins, the eyes drift away and attentional focus is lost. ADD individuals are known as "star gazers" because of this tendency for the eyes to drift away from the speaker. If an ADD individual is to listen successfully, he or she must be supervised. The ADD brain must be called back frequently to continue to hear. Without supervision and reminding, ADD persons soon drift beyond the voice of the speaker and do not come back.

ADD Individuals Are Too Easily Distracted

Paying full attention is a learned behavior. A major goal of wise parents is to teach preschool children how to pay attention. As certain developmental milestones are reached in playing together, sharing with others, and learning to take responsibility, children also are expected to turn attention away from themselves and pay attention to others. A critical part of this developmental sequence is learning how not to pay attention to certain things. Through a lot of practice over time, children are taught how to tune out and ignore irrelevant events nearby. Parents and teachers spend much time coaching youngsters: "Everyone look here, please. Don't let your eyes look away. Is everyone ready? Fold your hands in your lap. Don't let your eyes or hands get busy doing something else. Pay attention now." By age 6 most children learn how to attend to others well enough to fit into a classroom successfully.

The ADD brain does not follow this developmental sequence in paying attention. Loose thought patterns, plugs that fall out too easily, trouble thinking in sequence, and poor listening ability make it impossible for ADD individuals to ignore nearby events. What happens nearby leaks through the midbrain filter into higher brain pathways. On their own, ADD persons do not distinguish between what is necessary and what is irrelevant. This poor midbrain filtering creates a state of constant distraction.

ADD Individuals Live in a Make-Believe World

Where does the ADD person's attention go when the plugs fall out and he or she is no longer connected to what is happening? Chapter 3 described the high-energy magical thinking of an ADHD adolescent daydreaming about owning a fancy truck. When a person with ADHD daydreams, it is noisy and often openly disruptive. As ADD attention is lost, the person silently slips into a private world of make-believe. This world of magical thinking is much like writing a play or creating a musical show. Once it disconnects from the outside world, the ADD brain imagines a vividly colorful active scene filled with wished-for objects, pleasant sounds and colors, and the person's favorite music. On center stage of this magical world is the ADD individual doing whatever he or she dreams secretly of doing well. During childhood, girls often dream of being a skilled dancer on a stage, or riding a special horse, or being a famous movie or television star. Boys often imagine being the champion at martial arts, or flying space ships, or beating everyone else in roller blade hockey or basketball. Sometimes the body begins to display the content of the daydream as pretend dance steps are done or karate chops are delivered. Mostly, however, ADD make-believe remains hidden from the outside world. Individuals who engage in this make-believe are shy or even fearful of revealing where they spend their mental time. It takes a kind, patient adult to establish enough trust with the ADD dreamer to start him or her talking about this private world of make-believe.

ADD Individuals Are Too Quickly Bored

Fight-or-Flight Reflex
Chapter 3 described the rapid boredom of ADHD that is triggered by underarousal of the prefrontal cortex. The boredom experienced by an individual with ADD comes from a somewhat different source. As the ADD brain becomes overwhelmed by confused mental images, the brain stem and limbic system receive danger signals to prepare for fight-or-flight response. Some overly sensitive ADD individuals feel too easily threatened by failure or shame as their mental images fall apart. In the basal brain, the medulla, pons, and basal ganglia are triggered by the amygdala to stand by for possible flight from danger. If the brain decides that this overwhelming situation poses too much danger, the basal emotions trigger surges of anxiety that may reach the catastrophic level of panic attack or phobia. In most instances, the ADD brain learns in early childhood simply to enter the safety of make-believe. There the mind builds magical scenes in which the ADD person feels safe. If an ADD child is the victim of repeated abuse, he or she may create a negative fantasy world in which the victim takes revenge on persecutors. In this private world of magical thinking, the hurt child may spend a great deal of time getting even or plotting revenge. Whether the ADD brain chooses to create a pleasant world that surrounds the dreamer with success, or a dreadful world in which the hurt person fashions revenge, the private world of make-believe is the refuge for ADD individuals when they cannot cope with the realities of their lives.

Escape Through Doodling

Often it is possible to watch the ADD brain engage in make-believe. Many ADD individuals develop the habit of doodling when their plugs fall out and they embark on daydreaming or magical thinking. Figure 4.2 shows how a 10-year-old boy escapes from overwhelming confusion as he does math assignments. Since kindergarten his teachers have been irritated by this habit of doodling on his work pages while leaving the assignment unfinished. Figures 4.3 and 4.4 were produced by graduate students I taught in a doctoral-level seminar on learning disabilities. Both of those adults came to realize that they were ADD. These doodles opened the door for new understanding of themselves and focused their motivation to become specialists in treating ADHD and ADD.

ADD Individuals Are Immature

Compared with others their age, ADD individuals display immature interests and habits. Many ADD persons create inventive private games to entertain themselves when boredom overwhelms executive function. However, these games are similar to those of younger children, such as rolling a pencil up and down the desktop, making paper airplanes, drawing stick

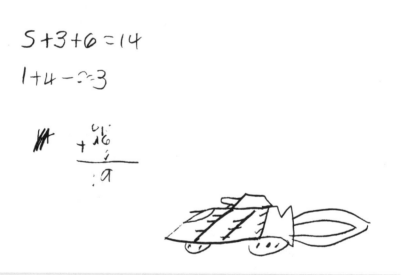

FIGURE 4.2. Math assignment of a 10-year-old boy who has ADD. After working two problems correctly, his plugs fell out and he was engulfed by confusion. After struggling with the third problem unsuccessfully, he drifted into his private world of make-believe and started to doodle. By this time he was unaware of what the rest of his class was doing.

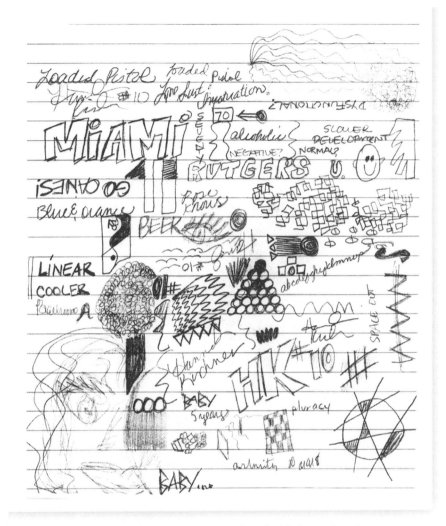

FIGURE 4.3. During a graduate seminar I conducted with doctoral students, an outstanding student produced this elaborate doodle as he followed every word I spoke in describing attention deficit disorders. Later he made the highest score in the class on an exam over that day's work.

figure cartoons, or counting buttons on their clothes. When given a choice, ADD individuals tend to choose television programs and movies with shallow themes, silly antics, and a lot of artificial laughter. If an ADD person must view an educational program or drama, he or she soon becomes bored and restless. ADD adults often prefer popular magazines that feature gossipy information about famous people. It is not unusual for ADD adults to develop an obssessive interest in mail-order catalogs, or spend many

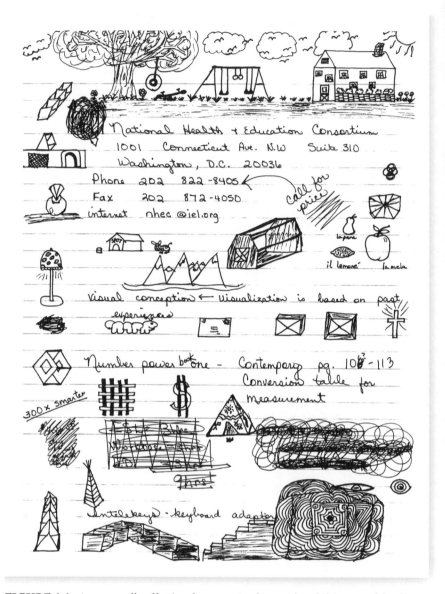

FIGURE 4.4. An unusually effective classroom teacher produced this page of doodles during a staff training seminar I conducted at her school. That year she was voted Teacher of the Year by her colleagues. During the seminar, she realized for the first time why she always has doodled while listening to lectures and sermons. Gripping a pen or pencil and creating intricate fine motor doodles enables her higher brain to concentrate for long periods of time without distraction.

hours on Internet channels that offer things for sale or auction. This kind of activity triggers active make-believe thinking: "Oh, what if I could have that? Oh, this would really look good in the bedroom." Lifestyle habits of ADD persons often include rituals and ingrained habits that seem "weird" to others. All of these less mature behaviors are linked to topics of magical thinking and make-believe that occupy so much of the ADD individual's time and energy.

ADD Individuals Are Often Depressed

Dark Thoughts of Make-Believe

Active make-believe can be a strongly positive attribute. However, in emotionally sensitive persons with ADD, drifting away from reality into the world of make-believe often involves depression. Hidden beneath the surface of slow processing, stargazing, and underachievement is the tendency for brooding and imagining dark possibilities. If the ADD individual is a victim of abuse or overly strict punishment, magical thinking moves toward thoughts of dying. "I would be better off dead," depression whispers. "I wish I could die and get away from all this pain." When the ADD brain sinks into depression, the sorrowful person cannot cheer up. Yet he or she rarely tells others of the heavy emotions and feelings that have blanketed the mind and heart. ADD persons in depression begin to brood and cry in private. They withdraw from talking with others, playing games, or attending meetings. They stop eating normally, lose interest in sexual expression, and often become "emotional zombies" with virtually no interaction with others.

ADD children with depression hide from others and find excuses not to join in group activities. They stop eating but refuse to tell why. Nightmares increase and minor fears become active phobias. ADD adolescents who are depressed often stop caring about personal hygiene and grooming. They withdraw from friends and break off social contacts. Frequently they write morbid poetry or draw black images with heavy strokes. Figure 4.5 was discovered by Jane's history teacher who had noticed the girl not paying attention day after day. When the kind teacher quietly asked Jane if something was wrong, the girl burst into tears and ran from the room. An exceptionally comforting counselor gained Jane's trust, and soon she was pouring out her sorrow and dark fears. That intervention helped Jane to recover hope and self-confidence. Later she told her counselor that she had come very close to trying to take her own life.

Figure 4.6 was done by a 15-year-old boy who became overwhelmed by the algebra class he was required to take. By the third week of fall semester,

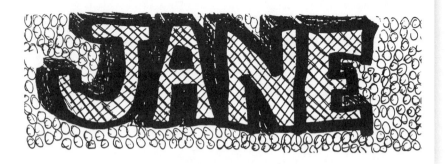

FIGURE 4.5. The 15-year-old girl who created this heavy doodle had become severely depressed as she entered adolescence. She hid her emotions and feelings and did not confide her mental anguish to anyone. When this doodle fell out of Jane's book as she left history class, her intuitive teacher started the counseling process that led Jane and her family to find the help the girl needed to regain emotional balance.

he was so far behind he had no idea what the teacher was talking about, and he was overwhelmed by the shame of failure described in Chapter 2. One day this doodle fell out of his notebook as he left the classroom. His wise teacher showed the sketch to the high school art instructor who was ADD and had struggled with math. As the teachers and parents talked about the boy's school struggles, they realized that his behavior fit the symptoms of depression. The art teacher volunteered to let the boy come to his studio instead of attending algebra class. As they did art projects together, the teacher recognized ADD symptoms in the student's behavior, and soon a diagnosis of ADD was made. The boy agreed to try cortical stimulant medication (described in Chapter 7) to help his thoughts stay focused. Also, he began working one-on-one with a patient math tutor. Together they discovered his hidden talent for math, once he understood the concepts in correct sequence. As Gilligan's research reported (see Figure 5.1) this ADD student's crushed self-esteem was resurrected through new hope, unexpected affection, and support. Soon his depression was transformed into positive hope and success.

Risk of Suicide

During the 1990s, many studies documented the increased risk of suicide among ADD children and adolescents (Barkley, 1995; Hallowel & Ratey, 1994a; Jordan, 1998, 2000a; Ratey & Johnson, 1997; Weiss & Hechtmann, 1993). Chapters 2 and 3 present the severity scale from 1 to 10 showing mild, moderate, and severe levels of attention deficit disorder. If ADD

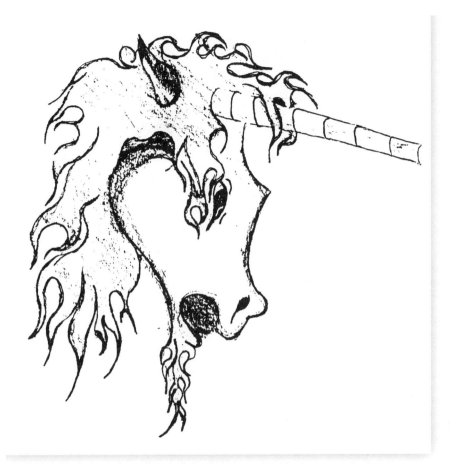

FIGURE 4.6. This doodle was done by a 16-year-old boy who had stopped participating in class or doing homework assignments. He had slipped into deep silent depression and no longer talked with adults. The high school art instructor became the boy's mentor. Through appropriate medication and art therapy, he became a talented artist and successful student.

is mild, symptoms of depression come and go with no real problems resulting. If ADD is moderate, cycles of depression are more frequent and intense, causing a drop in school grades, withdrawal from social contact, increasingly poor hygiene, and refusal to talk to family members or friends. If ADD is severe, onset of depression is so frightening that the individual is likely to try to die. For individuals of all ages with severe ADD, dying becomes more appealing than continuing to live under the dark clouds of failure, shame, and acute sadness.

Religious Belief

Religious belief plays a major role in how ADD individuals react to depression. Those who believe in a better life after death, where pain and sorrow do not exist, are in fact drawn more closely to dying. "After all," their emotions say, "wouldn't I be better off in heaven? Wouldn't my family be better off without having to put up with me?" Younger ADD individuals caught in depression begin to think: "I wish I was in heaven with Grandad. He always loved me and I miss him so much!" This "what if" thinking leads the sorrowing person into visions of heavenly peace. On the other hand, individuals who believe that human life ends with death often come to prefer vanishing from the universe through death rather than continuing to live like this. Many ADD persons with depression are afraid to try to die because of fear that they would go to hell. Yet they cannot go on living in a state of torment caused by their depression. When ADD symptoms are above Level 5 on the severity scale, the risk of suicide becomes a major concern for parents and companions.

Checklist of ADD Behaviors

Passive Behavior

_____ Has below-normal level of body activity

_____ Is reluctant to become involved with group activity

_____ Tries not to be involved in group discussion

_____ Avoids answering questions or giving oral responses

_____ Does not volunteer information

_____ Prefers to be alone in play situations and social activities

_____ Avoids being included in games and parties

_____ Spends long periods of time off in own private world of thought and imagination

_____ Uses fewest words possible when required to talk

Short Attention Span

_____ Cannot keep thoughts focused longer than brief periods of time

_____ Continually is off on mental side trails

_____ Continually must be called back to finish tasks

_____ Drifts away from tasks before finishing

Loose Thought Patterns

_____ Cannot maintain organized mental images

_____ Continually loses important details

_____ Cannot do a series of things without starting to make mistakes

_____ Cannot remember a series of events, facts, or details without being prompted or reminded

_____ Must have help to tell what has happened

_____ Cannot remember a series of instructions

_____ Cannot remember assignments over time

_____ Cannot remember game rules or game routines

_____ Keeps forgetting names of people, things, places, events

Poor Organization

_____ Must have help to keep life organized

_____ Continually loses things

_____ Must have supervision to stay on schedules

ADHD in the Classroom and Workplace

_____ Does not remember simple routines from day to day
_____ Lives and works in a cluttered space
_____ Cannot straighten up room or work space without help
_____ Vehicle is littered with trash
_____ Must have supervision to do homework

Change of First Impression
_____ Continually erases and changes as writing is done
_____ Has the impression that others are "playing tricks" because things seem to shift and change
_____ Word patterns, spelling patterns, math problems seem to change

Poor Listening Comprehension
_____ Rarely gets the full meaning of what others say
_____ Must have oral instructions repeated and explained again
_____ Sits without doing anything instead of asking for information to be repeated
_____ Does not keep on listening
_____ Attention drifts away before speaker has finished
_____ Cannot remember later what speaker said

Time Lag
_____ Pauses for long intervals before responding
_____ Does not start tasks without being pushed or guided to start
_____ Spends long periods of time doing nothing
_____ Spends long periods of time searching memory for information
_____ Whispers softly to self while searching memory or doing written assignments
_____ Continually lags behind schedules set by parents, teachers, or job supervisors

Unfinished Tasks
_____ Leaves tasks unfinished unless closely supervised
_____ Leaves several unfinished tasks scattered around
_____ Thinks tasks are finished when they are not
_____ Does not realize when more is yet to be done to finish a task

Overcoming Attention Deficit Disorders in Children, Adolescents, and Adults

Daydreaming

_____ Spends much time off in a private world of daydreams and make-believe

_____ Drifts into make-believe to escape stress of learning or performing tasks

_____ Doodles and draws pictures while daydreaming

_____ Refuses to talk about it when asked about daydreams

Boredom

_____ Becomes bored immediately after starting to do tasks

_____ Begins to play quietly with things instead of working as boredom sets in

_____ Eyes drift away as star gazing replaces boring tasks

_____ Slumps in seat and appears sluggish as boredom starts

_____ Begins to sigh and yawn deeply as boredom sets in

Easily Distracted

_____ Attention drifts to whatever is happening nearby

_____ Cannot ignore nearby events

_____ Stops work to watch what others are doing

_____ Begins quietly to tug at clothes, pick at lint or threads, fiddle with buttons, buckles, or shoelaces

Immaturity

_____ Role-plays imaginary situations like much younger individuals

_____ Does not pay attention to informational programs or drama in movies or television

_____ Chooses shallow or "silly" things to do when others that age choose more serious activities

_____ Sense of humor is like that of much younger individuals

_____ Spends time with comic books, mail-order catalogs, surfing the Internet, or other picture-related activities instead of reading books

_____ Does not fit in socially with others of same age

_____ Is bored with what others of same age like to do

_____ Cannot carry on small talk at social events

_____ Wanders off alone at social events

Depression

_____ Withdraws into private world of sad make-believe

_____ Stops eating an adequate diet, but refuses to explain why

_____ Stops brushing teeth, combing hair, taking a shower, wearing clean clothes

_____ Hides from others in out-of-the-way places

_____ Becomes irritable or tearful when questioned or pressed to talk

_____ Explodes suddenly in aggressive anger when pressed too hard to share private thoughts

_____ Cries when alone, but refuses to tell why

_____ Writes morbid poetry or draws dark pictures with morbid themes

_____ Becomes obsessed by themes of death or dying

_____ Expresses wish to die, or writes private notes about dying

How ADHD and ADD Challenge One's Personal Life

↗ ↗

Chapter 5

I often wonder if people without ADHD have any real idea of the amount of energy one with ADHD expends in just keeping above the tidal flood of their minds. When one's thoughts change faster than the stock market. The work of just writing a letter that begins to make sense. Of sitting down and trying to study and learn. People without ADHD think they have it hard. Let them trade places with me for a week. They couldn't handle it for a day, let alone a week.

—letter from Calvin, a 42-year-old ADHD man after he attempted suicide

I am so glad I am ADD! Are you surprised? You might be, if you have always associated ADD with problems, with limits, and with difficulties. But that's not the way I look at it. The way I see it, I possess special skills and strengths because of ADD, and with those skills I have been able to experience life in Technicolor. I've known diversity, drama, creativity, and sensitivity—all as a result of my ADD. I've had lots of experiences because of it, learned many lessons, and led a rich life.

—Lynn Weiss, a therapist who specializes in helping individuals overcome ADHD/ADD challenges, 1996, p. 1

For 25 years, the American Psychiatric Association has classified attention deficits as types of mental health disorder under the heading *Attention-Deficit and Disruptive Behavior Disorders* (*DSM–IV–TR*, p. 65). According to this point of view, ADHD and ADD are unhealthy, undesirable human characteristics that need to be fixed through medical/psychiatric intervention so that society will not be disrupted. Sadly, this approach to meeting the challenges of ADHD/ADD has not saved Calvin and countless others from lifelong failure and loss of hope.

Alongside this rather pessimistic point of view have been the cheerful, optimistic, hope-filled careers of Lynn Weiss, Edward Hallowell, John Ratey, Thom Hartmann, Dale Jordan, and many others who show ADHD and ADD individuals how to overcome the challenges of attention deficits. This chapter presents frank discussions of the classroom, family, and workplace challenges of ADHD and ADD when symptoms approach the severe level (see Chapter 2). Those of us who have conquered our challenges often have needed medical help and wise counseling. Not everyone has the internal strength to turn pessimistic defeat into optimistic victory. We who work with prison populations, troubled adolescents who are adjudicated delinquent, individuals enslaved by chronic addictions, and homeless individuals who are mentally ill live with the sad reality that certain individuals cannot overcome genetically linked differences that disable their lives. For them, we mourn our helplessness to relieve such awful loss. However, in the remarkable spirit expressed by Lynn Weiss, we roll up our sleeves in readiness to help those with the inborn potential to overcome lifelong challenges. This chapter explores the many challenges that ADHD and ADD bring to the classroom, family life, personal relationships, and the workplace. Chapter 8 presents a range of positive, encouraging, helpful strategies that enable most ADHD and ADD individuals to emulate Lynn Weiss's remarkable success.

ADHD and ADD in the Classroom

In the Introduction to this book, we visited Mrs. Jolly's classroom and watched her efforts to maintain order as three students continually disrupted the class in different ways. Luis, the ADHD "Edison-gene hunter" was all over the room, following his exuberant curiosity by scanning his environment and reacting to every new event inside and outside of the classroom. It never occurred to Luis that his hyperfocused roaming behavior was a disruptive nuisance in that environment. We watched Jacob's emotional reaction to stress that triggered a tantrum with destructive behavior. We saw examples of his struggle with the overlapping layers of ADHD, dyslexia, and dysgraphia. Also, we observed quiet, passive Anna off in her ADD daydream world, unplugged from what was happening around her. With no teacher's aide to help, Mrs. Jolly did her best to meet these disruptive challenges so that the other students could have an orderly place to learn.

Social-Behavioral Challenges

Self-Centeredness

Most individuals with ADHD or ADD are likable in brief, one-on-one relationships. When they are alone for a while with a friend, playmate, or instructor, a good relationship usually occurs. As Luis demonstrated, these individuals often are quite sensitive. They feel the same emotions others experience. They care deeply for pets. They grieve over sorrows that come into the lives of family and friends. They laugh, make jokes, and have lots of fun when they are free to set their own pace in working out mental images. Being hyperactive with a good sense of humor can be an endearing trait for a while. Being quiet, "loose as a goose," and forgetful can awaken affection and extra concern in classmates, partners, and teachers.

When ADHD or ADD individuals enter a group, a critical difference emerges. When these persons must interact with several others for an extended period of time, the successful interaction they achieve in one-on-one relationships breaks down. Individuals with ADHD or ADD spend most of their time dealing with themselves. Inattention usually makes it impossible for them to focus on the needs of others or to put their own needs aside in order to see the needs of others. However, these persons are not necessarily selfish. Many ADHD and ADD individuals are generous to a fault in letting others share their things. The problem is that the ADHD or ADD brain is preoccupied by personal needs, moments of fear and uncertainty, episodes of magical thinking, figuring out what others are saying, and handling all the impulses that spring from the limbic system. In the classroom, the ADHD or ADD brain is preoccupied with itself, usually in some form of make-believe.

As we reviewed in Chapter 4, ADD individuals like Anna spend many hours off on private rabbit trails, mentally acting out stories or situations they invent. These quiet ones spend long periods of time drifting through imaginary adventures that would make remarkable movies or stage plays. The body usually is still with no outward sign of activity, while the mind is busy creating complicated fanciful scenes. We watched Jacob's ADHD make-believe spill out through humming and foot action against the table leg. ADHD becomes disruptive as these individuals begin to act out their inner stories by rocking their chairs, "marching" or "dancing" with feet drumming the floor or bumping furniture, humming or singing the music of their daydreams, or mumbling the dialogue of their make-believe adventure. Within these private fantasy episodes, Jacob and Anna are the stars of their invisible shows. During these make-believe moments, they are aware only of themselves. As this self-centered creativity spills out into the real world, the teacher or supervisor must stop other tasks to deal with these disruptions that cause classmates to grumble about losing time and being distracted. As we have seen in previous chapters, during adolescence most youngsters with moderate ADHD and ADD outgrow most of their childhood hyperactivity and daydreaming. As her executive function matures, much of Anna's daydreaming will disappear, and she will become a more successful group participant. During adolescence, most of Jacob's ADHD tendencies will melt away, leaving dyslexia as his major challenge. However, during the first several years of formal education, self-centered behaviors are disruptive barriers between children with ADHD or ADD and others in the classroom.

Self-Gratification

During the self-centered years of ADHD and ADD, these children spend most of their mental energy on self-gratification. When do we go to lunch? How much more do I have to do? When can I go home? Did you see my new jeans? I got new roller blades from my granddad. I can't find my pencil. I have to go to the restroom. I don't want to play this game anymore. When can we go outside? You know what I saw last night? These are the concerns of self-centered, less mature individuals who have attention deficits. Whether hyperactive or passive, these kinds of self-centered thoughts occupy most of their time. Formal group learning in the classroom does not penetrate this thicket of self-concern. We watched Mrs. Jolly's extraordinary efforts to break through the self-preoccupation of ADHD and ADD students to implant new academic knowledge and skills. The self-centered ADHD or ADD student often is beyond the reach of others except in one-on-one relationships where tight structure can be maintained by the adult.

Boredom

In Chapters 2 and 3 we reviewed the concept of underarousal that triggers boredom in the prefrontal cortex of ADHD and ADD individuals. When these students are pressed into group learning, a strong sense of isolation occurs. The ADHD or ADD brain cannot stay plugged into the variety of events happening in the classroom. Loose thought patterns do not develop an organized sense of what the group is doing. Too many loose ends keep the attention deficit individual from following conversations and discussions well enough to be a responsive group member. Children and adults with attention deficits cannot deal effectively with a group environment. We saw how quickly Luis, Jacob, and Anna became isolated from the streams of interaction taking place all around them. Whether hyperactive or passive, ADHD and ADD individuals cannot enter into the spirit of the group as new skills are practiced. Because youngsters with ADHD or ADD cannot compete successfully, they quickly become outsiders in competitive group tasks. Alone on his or her island in the stream of learning, the attention deficit person has nothing meaningful to do. Copying from the White Board or working a page of math problems is too risky and boring for Jacob. Caught in an activity that gives him no immediate rewards or pleasure sends Luis off to find stimulation someplace else. Within 90 seconds or less, Anna's brain becomes so bored she escapes into her wonderfully fulfilling world of make-believe. Inside the brains of these three ADHD/ADD youngsters, the prefrontal cortex begs for a jolt of excitement. Bored eyes and ears scan the room for something interesting going on. Memory drifts or darts away to an experience that was lots of fun. Desires and wishes for something that has not happened yet carry the mind away from a boring assignment into a more exciting, pleasure-filled fantasy adventure. As boredom sets in, assigned work stops. Soon the bored child is in conflict with the teacher for not following instructions, and with classmates for disrupting their concentration.

Restlessness

Bored ADHD bodies soon become restless. Chapter 3 explained how the midbrain triggers body action to stimulate the underaroused prefrontal cortex through squirming, handling things, tapping a foot, bumping against furniture, making vocal sounds, rattling pencils, and whispering to neighbors. A visitor to Mrs. Jolly's classroom would see that with nothing meaningful to do, Luis's brain triggers his body to start doing something. He stands up, walks across the room, looks out the window, checks the aquarium, sees how Zeke is doing, inspects the growth of the seedlings, investigates the noise outside, sees what is making noise in the hall, double checks messages on the White Board, and answers Mrs. Jolly's question to her reading group. This restless cycle quickly intrudes on the concentration of Luis's classmates, who begin to complain to the teacher, which stops the group process in its tracks. Jacob's restlessness turns to anger toward the writing assignment he cannot do, and he destroys the worksheet that shames him with failure. Soon he turns inward to make-believe that overflows in humming and restless foot action that annoys his neighbors. Anna's restlessness immediately "goes there" inside her daydream world so that no outward activity is involved. Within a few minutes everyone in the room is distracted and begins to complain. Mrs. Jolly finds herself in the middle of a restless classroom that must be brought back to order. She has no choice but to leave her group to take Luis back to his seat, call Anna back to reality, calm Jacob's erupting emotions, and get everyone back on track. Chapters 2 and 3 describe the "noisy brain" that is a major factor in ADHD and ADD. Restlessness in the classroom reflects the intensity of the noisy brains that disrupt the classroom many times each day.

ADHD and ADD in One's Personal Life

Emotional Sensitivity

Students with ADHD and ADD live on the edge of failure. No classroom task is free from the hovering threat of shame and failure. Loose thought patterns, gaps in knowledge and skills, and plugs that keep falling out are like goblins dancing around the learner's desk, threatening to cause mistakes at any moment. ADHD and ADD persons who live under this never-ending shadow of defeat are understandably sensitive. From their earliest days in school, they have been criticized for "not trying harder." Teachers have said many times: "You didn't follow my instructions. Don't you ever listen when I explain?" Parents have said since early childhood: "I've told you a dozen times. Don't you ever hear what I say?" Since kindergarten, adults and classmates have made comments and jokes about how forgetful the ADHD or ADD student is. The statement "He would lose his head if it weren't fastened on" stopped being funny years ago to the youngster who has attention deficits. Being labeled "lazy" or "careless" is painful and embarrassing. Before the child with attention deficits has been in school very long, he or she has become quite emotional about these accusations, which seem very unfair.

Self-Defensive and Bullying Behavior

Most students with ADHD learn to defend themselves against teasing or bullying. Some do not. Those with passive ADD take the pain deep inside instead of showing it outwardly. Aggressive ADHD individuals tend to lash out at those who criticize them. They often start fights to avenge their honor. They develop habits of getting even with classmates who tease or make sarcastic remarks. Many schoolbus, playground, and lunchroom scuffles are triggered when ADHD persons fight back. A great deal of attention has become focused on the disruptive problem of bullying that often targets ADD individuals who do not think quickly enough to cope with aggressive behavior. In 2001 Susan Swearer and her colleagues at the University of Nebraska-Lincoln reported the first in-depth analysis of how depression and anxiety shape the destructive relationships between school-age bullies and their victims (Swearer & Doll, 2001). In 1997 G. M. Batsche reported that 15% to 20% of students in elementary, middle school, and high school experience bullying, defined as "the physical or psychological abuse of an individual by one or a group of students" (in Olweus, 1994). Ironically, Swearer and her colleagues concluded that a majority of bullies and their victims suffer from undiagnosed/untreated anxiety and depression that triggers aggressive action from some students and passive acceptance of aggression by others who are ADD.

The pioneering work of psychiatrist James Gilligan with violent prison inmates has defined the powerful role of shame and accompanying severe depression in violent criminal behavior (Gilligan, 1996). Figure 5.1 shows

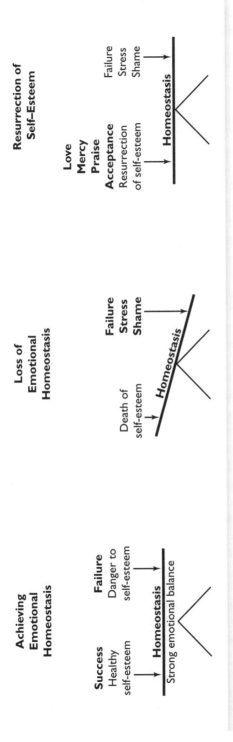

FIGURE 5.1. This model of emotional homeostasis shows how too much failure, stress, and shame crush a child's self-image and self-confidence in what Gilligan calls "the death of self-esteem." However, if such a person begins to receive continual love, mercy, affection, praise, and acceptance, he or she experiences "resurrection of self-esteem" as emotional homeostasis is restored.

113

ADHD and ADD in One's Personal Life

Gilligan's model of "death of self-esteem" that can occur when individuals grow up under the crushing stress of chronic failure, which overwhelms them with feelings of shame. Gilligan's research with men serving prison sentences for violent crime shows that when lifelong shame is replaced by new hope and success, individuals who have spent their lives in aggressive, bullying behavior experience "resurrection of self-esteem," which replaces shame and depression with new self-respect and self-confidence. Gilligan has documented how this resurrection of self-esteem transforms often violent bullies into hopeful, respectful citizens by releasing their feelings and emotions from the bondage of shame.

Quiet students with ADD seldom storm out overtly in self-defense. Instead, they build emotional fortresses where they silently retreat by turning inward and tuning out sources of conflict. For ADD, the most common defense is a silent decision to pull out all the plugs and become detached. If these overly sensitive students do not hear what others say about them, they will not be hurt by critical words. In choosing this deeply passive retreat into magical thinking, ADD individuals cut themselves off from classroom and peer group participation. Formal learning stops while overly sensitive feelings are protected. It is possible for ADD learners to build such thick walls of passive self-protection that it becomes impossible for adults to reach through the emotional barriers.

Misunderstanding

The lives of ADHD and ADD persons are clouded by misunderstanding. These individuals continually misunderstand what others say or mean. Meanwhile, parents, teachers, siblings, and friends misunderstand ADHD or ADD behavior. Well-organized adults who have no difficulty with their own thought patterns cannot believe that these healthy, bright individuals cannot do better. Far too often, teachers, parents, and job supervisors interpret attention deficit behavior as disobedience, laziness, or lack of effort. Adults often try to force disorganized youngsters to function more efficiently. However, no amount of discipline changes the patterns of ADHD and ADD. If one adult gives too much one-on-one attention to help the child function, another adult may say that too much coddling is going on: "Jacob has to learn to accept responsibility on his own." If adults back away and place all responsibility on the attention deficit child, nothing improves. In fact, when ADHD and ADD students are left alone to carry out responsibility, they are helpless.

Misunderstanding multiplies rapidly in the classroom. Instructions continually are misunderstood and not carried out by ADHD and ADD learners. Friendly comments by classmates often are misinterpreted and blown out of proportion by overly sensitive attention deficit children. Classmates misunderstand the stumbling speech of the ADHD or ADD person who has lost his or her words while trying to tell a story. Diagnosticians who evaluate these strugglers often misunderstand their answers to questions and thus do not see the full extent of attentional problems. ADD and ADHD individuals are among the most seriously misunderstood persons in our culture. They live most of their developmental years being misunderstood and failing to understand the world around them.

Insatiability

Chapter 3 describes the problem of insatiability in many persons who are ADHD. Insatiable individuals never get enough. In the classroom, insatiable needs for personal attention and constant approval become disruptive. An insatiable person does not leave others alone. This individual cannot study silently or alone. The need for feedback from others is overwhelming. The insatiable student clamors for the teacher's attention regardless of how much time already has been spent in one-on-one contact. Children with insatiable habits cannot stay in a designated space without having someone to share that space. The insatiable individual cannot leave classmates alone during independent study time. He or she must have continual contact through touching, speaking, and being spoken to. This person is overly sensitive, even phobic, about being alone. When frustrated classmates and teachers reach the point of firmly saying: "Stay in your own seat and leave me alone," his or her feelings are hurt. Insatiable individuals burst into emotional pleading, or they blame others for being selfish or not caring. Sometimes the insatiable student retreats into a pout, brooding about how unfair everyone is. The insatiable person is extremely immature and cannot deal with life issues realistically.

The need for constant company overpowers other needs of the insatiable person. He or she runs surprising risks to gain the attention of others. These individuals expose themselves to the risk of rejection or ridicule in order not to be isolated. An insatiable student's disruptive behavior places heavy pressure on the emotions of the group. An insatiable person in the classroom demands more than others can give. This individual has no concept of privacy or appreciation of territorial rights of others. Inner hunger for response from others overwhelms other considerations as these individuals clamor to be satisfied.

Impact of Failure on Self-Esteem

A potentially devastating result of ADHD or ADD is loss of self-esteem through repeated failure. As children progress through their developmental years, the normal growth process is to accumulate good stories to tell about personal success, prizes won, awards received, and praise earned. For the most part, persons with ADHD or ADD are left out of this nurturing developmental experience. They seldom win prizes for good work. Their papers rarely are displayed on the bulletin board. Their progress reports seldom earn praise. In fact, most teacher comments to an ADHD or ADD child are negative: "Luis, you didn't follow my instructions again." "Anna, you forgot to put you name on your paper again." "Jacob, this is the fourth time I've had to repeat my instructions. Don't you ever listen?" "Anna, you forgot to give me your homework again." "Jacob, your handwriting must be neater." "Luis, I'm tired of telling you to sit down and mind your own business." This litany of criticisms and complaints never ends for those with ADHD or ADD. From their earliest years, these struggling youngsters build memories of adults saying negative things about them. Luis, Jacob, and Anna have no permanent memories of adults praising their work, complimenting their achievement, or congratulating them for jobs well done. Students with attention deficits have few positive stories to tell. When they do tell stories, they usually resort to make-believe to compensate for their history of failure. Then they are accused of telling lies.

Having no good stories to tell leaves deep scars on a youngster's self-esteem. If everyone else has good stories to tell, but the ADHD or ADD child does not, his or her impression of self becomes negative and inferior. If everyone else wins praise, but the attention deficit individual hears mostly blame and criticism, the impression of self becomes "I'm not good." All our lives, we who have overcome early challenges of ADHD or ADD to become happy and creative continue to flash back to the shame of failure and low self-esteem that darkened our developmental years. Despite adult success and achievement, remnants of childhood shame from failure hover over our memories. Being unable to satisfy adult expectations during developmental childhood years implants deeply rooted impressions that the self is bad, inadequate, and of low value. The feeling of low self-worth is an unfortunate legacy when ADHD and ADD are not recognized early so that constructive help can be given.

Problems with Academic Learning

Poor Listening Comprehension
Misunderstanding New Information. Understanding a stream of oral information is a major challenge for ADHD and ADD individuals like Luis, Jacob, and Anna. As a rule, the level of comprehension through listening is seldom higher than 30% (Jordan, 2000a, 2000b, 2002). This means that the ADHD or ADD listener fully understands and retains only one third of what he or she hears in the course of a school day. This deficit in auditory perception has nothing to with the ability to hear. These struggling listeners usually hear well enough. Chapter 1 explains how the midbrain is designed to filter and organize incoming oral data. When ADD or ADHD exist, this

midbrain oral language filtering is inadequate. Incomplete pruning of neuron pathways within the brain stem and midbrain causes the higher brain to receive bits and pieces of new oral data, not complete streams of what the individual hears others say. Often ADHD and ADD listeners try to keep up by interrupting the speaker with "What?" or "Huh?" or "What do you mean?" Frequently, however, they give no signal that they have not heard everything correctly. When slow thought processing is a factor, the ADHD or ADD student cannot develop full mental images fast enough to respond to what he or she just heard. Poor listening is a major challenge for Luis, Jacob, and Anna in their classroom performance.

Trouble Participating In Discussions. Students with listening deficits find it difficult to participate in class discussions. Streams of oral information that are shared rapidly by several classmates, or between Mrs. Jolly and her students, do not connect into meaningful mental images for Anna, Jacob, and Luis. For them, what Juan said to his reading group does not connect with what Mia replied. Again, these students with ADHD and ADD are alone on their islands within the stream of flowing talk and discussion. This sense of isolation increases rapidly as group discussion continues. Within a short time these attention deficit listeners are lost and overwhelmed by boredom. Soon boredom triggers Luis into restless traveling about the room. Boredom sends Anna deep into daydreaming, while Jacob drifts away to make-believe about his own private issues. Conflict disrupts the group as Mrs. Jolly is forced to bring Luis back to his seat, waken Anna from her daydream, and refocus Jacob on tasks made difficult by dyslexia. Again and again these disruptive cycles repeat during the school day.

Trouble Following Oral Instructions. Mrs. Jolly works very hard to make new information clear to her ADHD and ADD students. They do not follow as she explains, gives instructions, and teaches new skills. Things are somewhat better when she takes the time to display printed information on the White Board, but even then, she must devote extra time to reminding Luis, Jacob, and Anna to refer to the White Board guidelines. As Mrs. Jolly finishes explaining or giving instructions, she asks: "Does everyone understand?" Luis sometimes does, but then he wants to tell a lot more about the topic than others want to hear. This tendency to talk too much (*hyperlexia*) would be welcome in a one-on-one situation when others were not involved. However, when 19 classmates are waiting to start their work, Luis's verbal outpouring quickly irritates others who clamor: "Make him hush, Mrs. Jolly! Make him stop talking all the time!" When calm has been restored and the class is ready to get to work, Jacob's hand goes up: "What are we supposed to do?" If Mrs. Jolly loses patience and says, "I just told you what to do," Jacob responds with defensive emotions: "No you didn't! You never tell me what to do!" Sometimes he says "I didn't hear you say that." Through all this disruption, Mrs. Jolly notices that Anna is in another world, unaware of this discussion or this conflict. With a sigh, the teacher realizes that somehow she must spend enough one-on-one time with Anna to get the girl started on this assignment. These disruptive scenes are played again and again, hour after hour, day after day. Mrs. Jolly knows that no amount of scolding or fussing will change these listening challenges for Luis, Jacob, and Anna. She is coming to understand that ADHD and ADD midbrains cannot keep up with filtering and organizing new oral data on schedule.

Unpredictable Response

One of the most frustrating characteristics of ADHD and ADD is the tendency to do the first steps of a task rather well, then begin to make mistakes on later steps in the same task. In the Introduction, Figure I.1 shows how this breakdown in attention disrupts Luis's math processing. In one-on-one work sessions with a tutor, he demonstrates advanced knowledge of math and arithmetic skills. When he must work alone, his ADHD habits sabotage his ability to stay on task from start to finish. During the cycles when her plugs stay in, Anna also shows mastery of third-grade math skills. However, like Luis, she cannot stay on task long enough to finish assignments unless she is supervised and reminded frequently.

ADHD and ADD students who are not dyslexic display short attention cycles as they do spelling and writing activities. Figure 5.2 shows the creative work of an 11-year-old student who is ADD. In the classroom, he rarely finishes a task. Alone with his tutor who guided him with immediate feedback, he demonstrated superior language skills with this creative writing assignment. One day in his sixth-grade classroom, this student was asked to do a rapid writing assignment that pressed him to hurry. Figure 5.3 shows his struggle to work alone in a hurry. He began the task well with no mistakes. Then he began to lose control of writing skills as errors emerged. After finishing this task, he said: "I should have used capital letters," revealing the strength of his memory when he has plenty of time without pressure to hurry.

These kinds of short-circuit patterns are not caused by carelessness or laziness. As an attention deficit student works through an assignment, memory becomes spotty and unpredictable. Mental images that were clear one moment become cluttered and confused the next. Students with these short-circuit patterns seldom maintain fully clear mental images longer than 90 seconds. They are at constant disadvantage doing assignments that require clearly focused thinking for 10 minutes or longer. No matter how often ADHD or ADD learners promise to do better, incomplete neuron development trips them up. Promising to be more careful next time does

ceremonial   dignity   impression

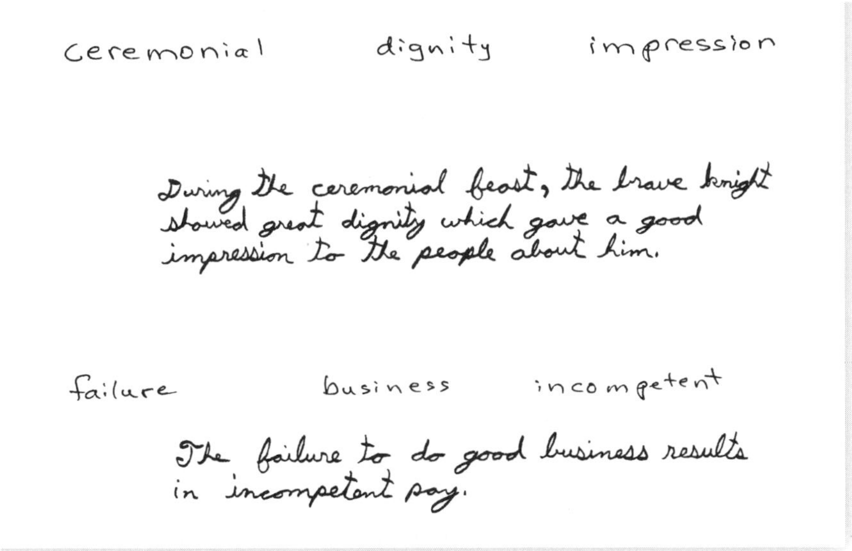

During the ceremonial feast, the brave knight showed great dignity which gave a good impression to the people about him.

failure   business   incompetent

The failure to do good business results in incompetent pay.

FIGURE 5.2. This 11-year-old boy has ADD. In classroom activities that require him to work alone, he rarely functions successfully and seldom finishes assignments. Working one-to-one with a tutor, he produced this excellent writing on a sentence-building activity. He made no mistakes in capitalization, punctuation, or spelling. This work was done in a quiet, private place where he had all the time he needed with no distractions.

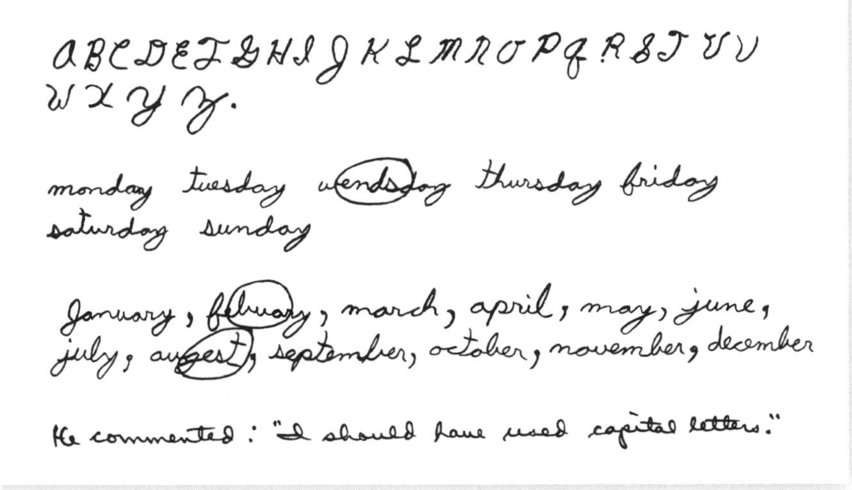

ABCDEFGHIJKLMNOPQRSTUV WXYZ.

monday tuesday wednesday thursday friday saturday sunday

January, february, march, april, may, june, july, august, september, october, november, december

He commented: "I should have used capital letters."

FIGURE 5.3. As part of a rapid memory activity in the classroom, the same 11-year-old boy was asked to write the alphabet, days of the week, and months of the year. He started the task with perfect recall of the alphabet, remembering how to write capital letters. Stress from having to hurry interrupted his memory as he wrote the days and months. Later he said to his teacher, "I should have used capital letters."

not change the underlying neurological differences that foster ADHD and ADD.

This unpredictability in memory tasks also is seen in oral responses that Jacob and Anna are asked to make. Luis's ADHD hyperlexic speech permits him to say much more than the situation requires or accepts. Jacob and Anna are challenged by too-slow speech (*hypolexia*). They cannot find their words quickly enough to give fluent oral responses or join in fast-flowing conversations successfully. In telling what they know, Anna and Jacob continually lose their words. For example, no matter how many times he has practiced naming geometric shapes, Jacob stumbles when Mrs. Jolly calls on him to name a triangle, rectangle, square, or "greater than" and "lesser than" math signs. This stumbling over the names of things triggers giggling and teasing from his classmates, which sparks Jacob's temper in self-defense. When Anna is asked to name shapes or signs, she quietly shakes her head and refuses to speak. She would rather appear not to know than to have classmates make fun of her effort to find her words.

These oral naming challenges of ADHD and ADD are deeply humiliating for Jacob and Anna. They are bright enough to realize that something is wrong as they watch their classmates do these tasks quickly and accurately enough to win praise. Beneath Anna's quiet surface and Jacob's angry self-defense, both of these attention deficit children believe that they are "dumb" or "stupid." These harsh adjectives often shock adults, who rush in to say: "Oh, Anna, you're not dumb! You're very smart!" or to assure Jacob by saying: "You're one of the smartest boys in the class." But being ADHD and ADD inside the left-brain linear box does not comfort Anna or Jacob. Secretly, each is convinced that "I'm dumb. If I weren't dumb, I could do it like everybody else."

As Mrs. Jolly does her best to help Jacob and Anna thrive in her classroom, she is not aware that the shadow of depression is darkening their emotions and feelings day after day. Depression often is described as anger turned inward. This is true for Anna, who is an intensely private, passive person by nature. What anger she feels over failure, being teased, or being left out of classroom praise turns inward and adds dark colors to her make-believe. In a different way, Jacob's anger bursts outward when stress reaches a certain level of discomfort. His tantrums actually are a healthy release that is more wholesome than bottling up dark feelings without expressing them. Chapter 4 describes the potentially destructive effects of depression. This erosion of self-image and self-esteem begins in early childhood for youngsters like Anna and Jacob and may continue throughout their years in school. Without patient, affectionate help, these ADHD and ADD individuals with unpredictable memory and hypolexia in expressing themselves do not develop positive self-image and self-esteem. Without help, they are prone to become discouraged adults like Calvin, whom we met at the beginning of this chapter. With good help and early encouragement, they have the potential to become a radiant, happy, victorious adult like Lynn Weiss.

Poor Organization

Lack of mental organization is a major source of friction in the classroom. The tools of learning are not seen by ADHD or ADD individuals as an organized, integrated whole. A book lying on the floor does not seem out of place to Jacob. A pencil left on the library table is not connected with the writing task that was interrupted when Luis went to check on Zeke and inspect the aquarium. The homework Anna forgot to bring to school does not connect in her thinking to Mrs. Jolly's irritation. As these loose, poorly organized students move through the day, they do not develop cumulative images of where things are or where they ought to be.

In a self-contained class where students stay all day, essential things are continually misplaced. When it is time for math, Anna's math book is missing and Jacob cannot find his writing paper. Luis is out of his seat helping both of them find their things while his own work remains unfinished. When it is time for reading, Luis cannot find his homework while Jacob grows angry looking for his book. Anna is off in a daydream and must be "awakened" to join the group. When it is time for art, none of these attention deficit youngsters can find their crayons. In a curriculum that requires classes to travel from room to room, ADHD and ADD students are at a serious disadvantage. If attention deficit individuals must go to their lockers between classes, they are forever tardy finding their books and papers. If they must catch the bus immediately after school, they cannot remember what to take for homework. Unless they are supervised the next morning, they forget to bring homework and books back to class. Scolding or punishment does not change these disorganized habits of forgetting, losing, and misplacing. Chapter 1 explained the neurological reasons why ADHD and ADD individuals cannot maintain organized, long-term memory for duties and responsibilities. If teachers or parents make lists for attention deficit students to follow, these "loose as a goose" youngsters often lose their lists.

Distractibility

When one is a member of a classroom group, progress depends upon being able to concentrate on the main activity while tuning out events that are not related to the task being done. Children with normal neurological processing ability soon learn to ignore anything that is not important at each moment. Youngsters like Luis and Jacob cannot. Little events, such as nearby sounds, unexpected activity across the room, movement glimpsed out of the corner of the eye, or a new odor, all clamor for the ADHD or ADD child's attention. He or she darts or drifts off on each new rabbit trail instead of saying "no" to new impulses. During reading, eyes glance away

ADHD and ADD in One's Personal Life

to see what is happening, and the reader loses the place on the page. While thinking through a math problem, the person's attention is attracted to something going on nearby, and the mental image of the task is lost. Being unable to ignore distractions leaves attention deficit students lost and wondering what to do after the distraction has been investigated.

Usually, it is impossible for these chronically distracted youngsters to finish a task. They continually leave jobs unfinished or assignments only partly done. They do not get all the way through a work page before attention goes elsewhere. Then they seldom manage to come back to finish their work. These restless ones skip portions of most assignments, thinking that all the work was done. Later, as adults scan the unfinished work, conflict is triggered as the student is accused of being careless or not paying attention. ADHD and ADD learners leave holes in their work, not realizing that everything has not been completed. They remember that they were doing tasks, but in their incomplete perception, they believe that they stopped because the whole assignment was finished. Persons with ADHD or ADD are not aware when their attention jumps track or drifts away.

Burnout

Most individuals with moderately severe attention deficits begin to lose their mental images within 60 to 90 seconds after starting a task. Those with mild ADHD or ADD may stay mentally focused for 3 to 5 minutes. After a certain length of time, a type of burnout occurs, causing mental images to fade away or disappear suddenly. This attention burnout happens in several ways. For some persons, the brain goes blank. As a bright ADD girl explained to me: "My brain stops." She described how she starts to do her work with clear images and well-organized information. After 2 or 3 minutes of steady thinking, her "brain stops" and her mind is blank. This always startles her. There is no feeling to warn her that her brain is about to stop.

In a different type of attention burnout, the brain does not go blank. Without warning, the brain jumps to a different thought, much like switching channels on a television set. An adult with ADHD described this to me as "blinking." He said: "I will be thinking clearly about one thing, then my brain blinks and I'm fully concentrated on a different thing. I never know when this will happen next." This blinking pattern starts after the man has been reading for 2 or 3 minutes. Once brain blinking begins, he must take a break to let his central nervous system settle down. "My brain really gets wound up if I keep on trying to read after blinking starts," he explained.

Still a different kind of mental burnout involves slow fading away of the original mental image, then a slow fading into focus of a different mental image. This fading cycle comes and goes slowly but steadily in many ADD individuals. Once started, this burnout cycle forces the person to leave the task until the brain has refocused. Changing from a passive task to something active recharges the brain, allowing individuals to return to the task until the next cycle of fading occurs.

For persons with ADHD or ADD, mental burnout occurs after a specific length of time in sustained thinking. To be successful, these individuals must develop work segments that allow them to accomplish what they can before the next burnout episode interrupts their thinking. After burnout is relieved by a short break, the person comes back to do a bit more before the next burnout cycle begins. Parents, teachers, and job supervisors can observe these burnout cycles rather clearly. Quality of work may have begun quite well with few errors, then a noticeable change occurs with mistakes popping up and accuracy deteriorating. Good spelling falls apart. Smooth left-to-right sequencing begins to scramble. Accurate math computation becomes filled with "careless" mistakes. Memory for a routine procedure suddenly is gone, leaving the person fumbling and groping for what to do next. Sentence structure falls apart, with fragments appearing instead of full sentences. Typing errors suddenly multiply in the middle of smooth keyboard writing. Essay writing falls apart after getting off to a good start. Students with these attention deficit patterns are bewildered, not realizing when burnout cycles start. Teachers often are puzzled, not understanding what causes such radical fluctuation in a student's performance. Parents who watch these burnout cycles often realize that the youngster is doing his or her best, yet the best efforts fall apart after a certain length of time. Neurological burnout is one of the common causes of disruption in the classroom, as irritated adults fuss at helpless students who have no control over these cycles of failure.

Messy Papers

Most attention deficit individuals have trouble writing neatly and producing attractive written work. As we saw in Chapter 1, the motor cortex and frontal lobes in the attention deficit brain cannot maintain well-organized thought patterns during the act of writing. In spite of having a clear mental image of the item to be copied or spelled, a breakdown occurs in the hand motion signals sent by the motor cortex. Without warning, the fingers make incomplete strokes, or the pencil moves the wrong way. Handwriting comes out messy and poorly done. Chapter 6 describes a subtype of dyslexia that interferes with handwriting. This lifelong encoding difficulty is called *dysgraphia*. The poor writing that accompanies attention deficit disorder usually is a different kind of tactile/kinesthetic challenge. It is the result of periodic burnout that interrupts fine motor signals during the act of writing. Figure 5.4 shows this periodic fine motor interruption in the copy work of a 13-year-old boy with ADD and moderate dysgraphia. Since kindergarten he has been criticized by adults who insist that he could learn good penmanship if he just tried harder. By the time he reached third

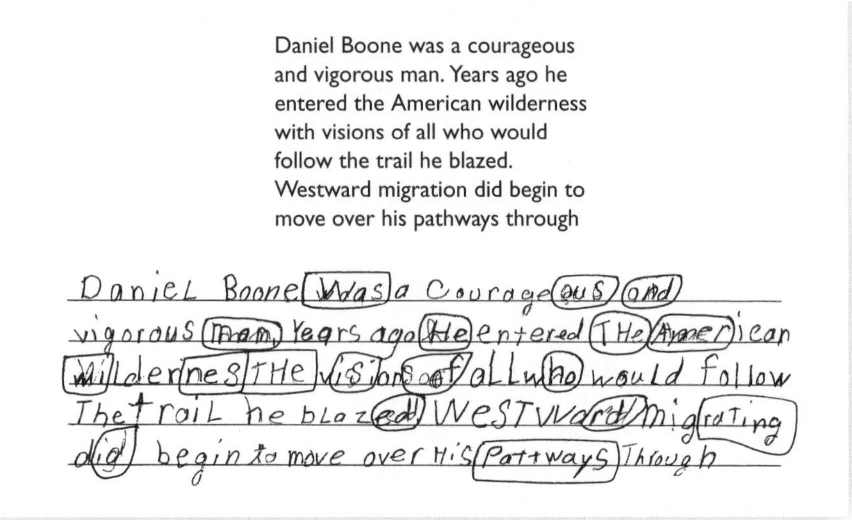

Daniel Boone was a courageous
and vigorous man. Years ago he
entered the American wilderness
with visions of all who would
follow the trail he blazed.
Westward migration did begin to
move over his pathways through

FIGURE 5.4. This copy task was done by a 13-year-old boy with overlapping ADD and moderate dysgraphia. He had all the time he needed in a quiet place to do this work. It took him 15 minutes to finish this assignment. His plugs kept falling out, he continually lost the place, and his tight pencil grip caused his fingers to ache. He described this kind of work as "very boring." *Note.* From *Specific Language Disability Test for Grades Six, Seven and Eight,* by N. Malcomesius, 1984, Cambridge, MA: Educators Publishing Service. Copyright 1984 by Educators Publishing Service. Reprinted with permission.

124

grade, he had become phobic about handwriting. He retreated into his private world of make-believe when penmanship tasks were presented.

Erratic Reading Comprehension

Most attention deficit individuals have adequate skills in phonics, word recognition, and reading comprehension. Unless they are also dyslexic, they do not have disability in learning and applying rules of phonics in decoding (reading) or encoding (spelling and writing). However, they tend to stumble over syllables within words, and they cannot always keep sound units in the right sequence. Yet they usually know how to blend sounds together and how to chunk (break words into sound units). Tests of phonics skills often show good knowledge of letter/sound relationships. However, reading comprehension tends to be well below grade level and unpredictable.

For example, if teachers study the reading patterns of students with ADHD and ADD, they often find wide fluctuations in what the reader comprehends from page to page. When the plugs are firmly in and the attention deficit reader is fresh, he or she may score 100% comprehension on the first page. As plugs fall out and burnout begins, the reader's comprehension may drop to 60% on the second page. If the reader takes a break, comprehension may rise to 80% on the third page. By this time the person has reached burnout, and the fourth page score may be 40% or lower. Jay's ADD score scatter in reading comprehension is reflected by the achievement test bar graphs shown in Figures 5.5 through 5.8. It is impossible for the ADHD or ADD brain to maintain full attention during sustained reading tasks.

This problem with reading comprehension is similar to irregularities in listening to oral information. As Luis, Jacob, and Anna listen to a stream of speech, they do not comprehend all they hear. Only bits and pieces of what an ADD or ADHD person hears are understood fully. The same pattern occurs as these individuals read. They may sound out or correctly

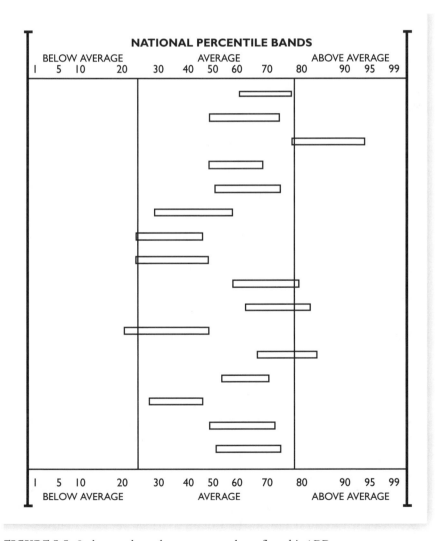

FIGURE 5.5. Jay's seventh-grade score scatter that reflects his ADD.

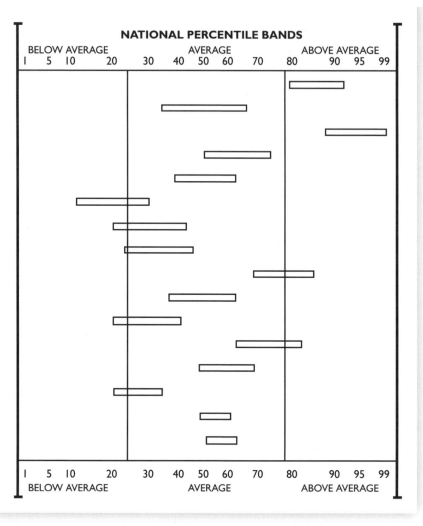

FIGURE 5.6. Jay's eighth-grade score scatter that reflects his continuing ADD.

recognize every word on the page, but only bits and pieces of the meaning are recorded by short-term or long-term memory. The reader with ADHD or ADD does not develop a cumulative, ongoing mental image of what the text says. Only some of the printed page is transformed into inner speech, so that the author's written message does not become fluent inner language for the attention deficit brain. The ADHD or ADD brain speaks the inner language of reading in the same broken, choppy way the student listens. This person leaves a reading task with partial images of what was on the page. Often it is impossible for the attention deficit person to answer follow-up questions successfully.

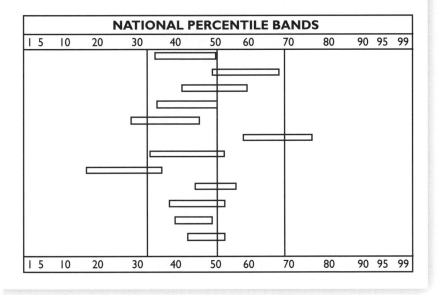

FIGURE 5.7. Jay's ninth-grade score scatter that shows continuing ADD.

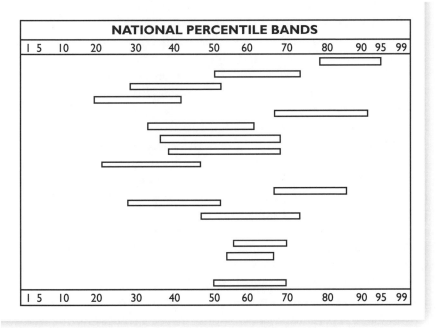

FIGURE 5.8. Jay's 10th-grade score scatter showing that he has not yet begun to out-grow ADD.

ADHD and ADD in One's Personal Life

The amount of material to be read is critically important for persons with attention deficits. Short attention and rapid burnout sabotage the task of reading large quantities of text material. Within a few minutes, the zigzag pattern of comprehension emerges, making it impossible for the reader to benefit from sustained reading tasks. However, these struggling individuals can be good readers if the assignment is divided into short segments that fit the cycles of burnout. It is not difficult for teachers to break reading tasks into short segments of 2, 3, or 5 minutes that permit the reader to take short breaks according to each person's burnout cycles.

Avoidance of Work

One of Mrs. Jolly's most difficult challenges is to keep Luis, Jacob, and Anna at their work. ADHD and ADD individuals have far more memories of classroom failure than moments of success. By the time attention deficit youngsters have entered second grade, they face schoolwork with great dread. If they are overly sensitive to criticism and teasing, they often develop phobias that erupt when a classroom task poses the likelihood of failure. In Chapter 1 we reviewed the issue of emotional memory. Recalling events or knowledge always awakens the emotions and feelings that occurred during the first moments of learning specific things. Many individuals with ADHD and ADD develop deeply ingrained habits of avoiding situations that threaten to confront them with failure or emotional pain. These overly sensitive learners cannot tolerate the normal pressure of academic work. They are too easily overwhelmed by emotional surges that accompany classroom failure. These attention deficit individuals spend a great deal of time and energy seeking ways to get out of assignments. They often complain of not feeling well. This complaint can indicate a source of real discomfort, such as eye strain or seasonal allergy attack. When poor vision or allergies exist, the person does indeed have frequent headaches or feels unwell. Chapter 7 describes immaturity of the digestive tract and intolerance for certain foods—conditions that cause authentic gastric misery. However, most students who make a habit of avoiding classroom tasks do not have these kinds of physical problems. Pleading to "go to the restroom" or "I need to call my mother" usually is an effort to avoid tasks that place too much stress on fragile skills.

Youngsters with ADHD actively avoid tasks any way they can. Pencil leads are broken every few minutes, requiring another trip to the pencil sharpener. It is easy to stretch a 45-second pencil sharpening chore into 2 or 3 minutes away from one's desk. Or the student may decide to look up a word in the dictionary across the room. This simple chore can be extended into a 15-minute adventure if the teacher is busy with a group. Or the ADHD student may have left an essential item in his or her locker and must ask the teacher for a hall pass. Once out of the room, it is easy to stretch a locker visit into half an hour. The fact that the procrastinator ends up in trouble does not stop the avoidance behavior. To him or her, avoiding threatening work is worth the consequence of being scolded.

Passive students like Jacob and Anna develop another type of avoidance. Instead of walking away from the task as Luis does, they drift away into daydreams. Sometimes these stargazers develop cover-up strategies of pretending to work when actually nothing is being accomplished on the assignment. These dreamers learn how to look busy from across the room while spending time adrift in a world of wishful make-believe. This is when a lot of doodling occurs. Later, daydreaming ADD youngsters must face the consequences of work not finished. Their passive mental drifting helps them pass the time without being involved in dreaded tasks. It is possible for these silent drifters to float for a year or longer before adults become aware that little or no skill development is taking place. If the student does just enough work to avoid failing the class, he or she might float for several years neither learning new material nor increasing important skills. The avoidance behavior of ADHD and ADD sometimes is beyond the reach of the teacher. If avoidance becomes too deep-seated, teachers may not be able to do anything effective to change the learner's negative response to schoolwork.

These are the main characteristics of attention deficits in the classroom. The student's surface behavior appears to be lazy, disinterested, unmotivated, and careless. Individuals with ADHD may drive everyone up the wall by roaming or clamoring, or they may silently drift away, intellectually apart from the mainstream learning taking place in the classroom. Scolding does not change the behavior. Forcing these students to work without help does no good. Poor organization, messy papers, and lost materials continue to frustrate parents, teachers, and students day after day. Punishment does not bring better performance. Unless the underlying neurologically based challenges are identified and helped, years of conflict and a lifestyle of chronic failure are set into motion with crushing effects on self-esteem.

ADHD and ADD at Home

As we consider how ADHD and ADD disrupt home life for parents, siblings, and other close relatives, we must keep in mind the severity scale we saw in Chapter 3.

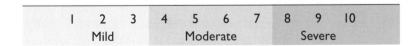

1	2	3	4	5	6	7	8	9	10
	Mild			Moderate			Severe		

The impact of ADHD or ADD on the family depends on the level of severity of symptoms and behavior. An aggressive child with ADHD at level 8, 9, or 10 creates much more disruption than a moderately ADHD child at level 5. A severely ADD child at level 8 creates a different kind of disruption that upsets family life. The clearest way to see the impact of ADHD and ADD on home life is to visit two families in which severe attention deficits disrupted their lives during each youngster's childhood and early adolescence.

James

I first met James when he was 8 years old. He is now 31 in a doctoral program in counseling psychology. His goal is to become a specialist in treating attention deficit disorders in children. James was born into a deeply religious family that tried hard to live according to biblical teachings. During the first trimester of her pregnancy with James, Mrs. King endured prolonged "morning sickness" that she had not experienced during her pregnancy with her daughter. During the third trimester of James's gestation, Mrs. King often said: "I think there's an entire soccer team playing inside me!" From the moment of his birth, James did not want to be cuddled or held firmly. He arched his back and screamed at anyone who tried to hold him longer than a brief time. In spite of this early resistance to being touched, Mr. and Mrs. King proudly took their son to church when he was 3 weeks old. Partway through the worship service, they were called to the nursery where their infant son was creating a crisis. His screams could be heard all over the church. At 3 weeks of age, he was fighting everyone who made physical contact with him. Thus began years of disruption for the King family's lifestyle as this newborn son brought his frustrations and tantrums into their home. James fought his parents, sister, and other relatives from the moment he came home from the hospital nursery. No one could reason with him. His demands were insatiable, and his temper was aggressive and often destructive.

As he learned to move about and handle things, the family lost the privacy that had been so important before his birth. Family members couldn't close a door, or a drawer, or take a break without having James invade their privacy. Before he could stand alone or walk, James climbed like a squirrel. In no time, he could be at the top of the bookshelves in the family room. When he was 11 months old, his father caught the tall bookcase as it was about to fall on top of the baby. After anchoring it to the wall, Mr. King packed away all of the pictures and crystal objects he and his wife had collected from vacation trips. By the time James was 12 months old, the house had been stripped of anything breakable that he could possibly reach. Before their son's first birthday, his parents knew that the next several years of their lives would be difficult. They had no idea how they had produced this angry little tiger who demanded everything, gave nothing in return, and seemed bent on destroying the home life that the Kings had worked so hard to establish.

As James grew older, he became the dreaded child of the neighborhood. He hurt several other children and was forbidden by their parents to play with them. He was so aggressive with pets that his parents were forced to give away their beloved cat and middle-aged dog. None of the grandparents or uncles and aunts could handle James's visits. He lived on the very edge of danger with no fear and no display of common sense. In fact, it appeared that he thrived on danger. James took incredible risks that no logical person would take. When he was 4 years old, he climbed to the top of the community water tower. Three firemen finally brought him down after chasing him several times around the catwalk 180 feet above the ground. Like a squirrel, he climbed the tall tree beside the house and leaped to the roof, then slid down the drainpipe to the ground, over and over. It was impossible to take him shopping unless he wore a harness with a leash tied to his father's wrist. If he were not restrained, he would dash off into the shopping mall and disappear.

Mr. and Mrs. King sought help from many sources. A child psychiatrist attempted psychotherapy with James and his parents. It was suggested that, as parents, the Kings were not doing their best with this child. If they paid more attention to him and less attention to themselves, surely their son would learn to behave normally. The Kings went through several years of guilt, believing that it was their failure that produced their son's disruptive behavior. They worked with two clinical psychologists who tried many kinds of management techniques, including biofeedback training to teach James's brain how to control muscle stress and reduce impulsivity. After making some improvement, he always returned to his aggressive ways. A series of pediatricians gave different opinions, none of which helped the Kings reduce the disruption in their home. Bedtime was a battle scene with both parents forcing James to take a shower, brush his teeth, get into his pajamas, and turn out the light. Evenings usually ended with his mother in tears, his father furious, and his sister hiding in her room. The only way bedtime was successful was when Mr. King showered with James, then lay down with the boy until he finally went to sleep. That procedure got everyone to bed, but it drove a wedge between husband and wife. James seemed to enjoy his power in keeping his parents apart at bedtime. Next morning he was up before sunrise racing about the house. He thrived on less than five hours of sleep. The rest of the family suffered from chronic exhaustion.

James was dismissed from three preschools in town. By the time he was 4 years old, no preschool would accept him. Every child care agency in the community had heard of this uncontrollable little boy. When he was 5, his

ADHD and ADD in One's Personal Life

parents found a private kindergarten that reluctantly agreed to let James attend for one week to see if their staff could work with him. After three days, he was told not to come back. By this time he had been labeled as emotionally disturbed, severely oppositional, and antisocial. By age 6 he was beyond the reach of the educational systems of his community.

Meanwhile, the King family was breaking apart. Mr. King moved out of the house one night after he and his wife had a verbal battle. Both had become so frustrated over James's incorrigible behavior that each blamed the other for his condition. Words became increasingly bitter. Their anger had been building for several years without being properly channeled or expressed. When it all exploded, the marriage came apart. That night James climbed into his mother's bed and went right to sleep. With his father gone, he had his mother all to himself. His bedtime tantrums stopped, and he began to act almost normally once he was in control. Mrs. King confided to a close friend, "I'm finding it very hard to love this child. When I look at my feelings honestly, I sometimes hate him. This child has cost us our marriage. We have not had a moment's peace since he was born. What am I going to do?"

The Kings were mature enough to patch things together so that the marriage survived, but the home was not a happy place. Finally, the grandparents put together enough money to enroll James in a special day school for emotionally disturbed children. Under the constant supervision of specialists in abnormal behavior, he learned to behave differently enough to remove some pressure from his home.

When he was 8 years old, James's parents brought him to me for an evaluation of his intelligence, learning patterns, and academic skills. My approach to evaluation was to duplicate the school day a child would have in his classroom. This all-day experience let me map the ups and downs in moods, energy levels, and cycles of inattention during regular school hours. I spent an entire day with this hyperactive boy who had been disruptive in every situation so far in his life. An amazing bonding occurred that day between James and me. Instead of forcing him to do tests in traditional fashion, I worked out ways for him to be himself as we did the assessment activities together. Sometimes he lay on the floor with feet bumping the underside of the work table as I asked questions and he answered. At times he rolled back and forth on the giant beanbag and chanted responses in rhymes he created on the spot. Sometimes he sat on my lap and snuggled against my chest. Then he lay flat on the carpet and pounded rhythms with his fists and feet. It was the first time in his life he had interacted with an adult in such a comfortable, safe, positive way. There were no pressures, threats, or fear of failure. In this relationship, he was free to use his right-brain novelty thinking to invent multisensory ways to communicate his knowledge and ideas. Twenty-three years later, James still talks about that day when he met an adult who did not fight his hyperactivity but accepted him as the intelligent, creative person he really was.

When we met, James was at Level 10 on the ADHD severity scale. His chronic aggression exerted enormous pressure on everyone involved in his life. He was totally disorganized and had no sense of how things should go or be arranged. He was insatiable, never receiving enough to satisfy his cravings for attention. He was completely self-focused, spending his energies on meeting his own needs and desires. He was angry, taking out his frustrations on anyone within reach. He was frightened and experienced awful nightmares that terrified him for days. He was phobic about many things that overloaded his emotions. For example, the sight of an inflated balloon sent him into hysterics. "It might pop!" he would wail, no matter where the family might be. They would have to leave the restaurant, party, or shopping mall where balloons were on display.

James often was vindictive, going out of his way to get even with anyone who offended him or made him angry. He had no friends, playmates, pets, or group of peers who would accept him. In all of this, he was bewildered. Why did other kids not like him? Why could he not spend a night at Grandma's house? Why did his family stop attending church services? Why did everyone always yell "No!" and "Stop that, James!" When he and I met, he was a lonely, frightened, stubborn, uneducated boy with underdeveloped social skills. Yet he had enormous potential that lay beyond our reach. What could we do to help this severely challenged child who showed all of the major signs of ADHD?

Mr. and Mrs. King were desperate for help with their son, yet they were afraid of the medications described in Chapter 7 that had been suggested by several pediatricians. The King family had been told by their church leaders that medications like Ritalin often turn hyperactive children into zombies with stunted growth. When I realized that it would not be possible to refer these parents to a physician for medication, I urged them to follow a controversial therapy of diet control. Something had to be done to help this desperate child and his battered family. In our city lived a psychiatrist who was regarded by the professional community as a maverick. For several years, he had practiced what he called "ecological psychiatry." This therapy method used diet control with extremely hyperactive, aggressive, impulsive individuals like James who did not respond to other treatments for emotional disturbance. I asked the King family to consider letting this psychiatrist try to help their son.

Because ecological psychiatry involved foods and beverages with no medications, Mr. and Mrs. King agreed to try. The approach was direct and simple. James became a guest in a private clinic for one week. He was treated like a very important person, and he was introduced to a computer that kept him busy. At the same time, he was systematically tested for food and beverage intolerance. The parents were asked not to see their son or call him for the first 4 days. Because of our strong bond, I visited James and spent time watching him work with his computer. For the first 3 days, he went through withdrawal symptoms as his body cried out for his old diet. He had tantrums and headaches, but he made it through that difficult time. An amazing difference greeted me when I visited him on the fourth day. James was relaxed and quiet. He was laughing over some jokes he had typed on the computer. He snuggled into my lap with deep affection, without any of his old game-playing tricks to take control. That morning his attention span was the longest I had ever seen. We began working with phonics skills he never had learned. The old disruptive James was out of the picture when his parents visited that day. Never before had they seen their son able to interact in normal ways that were filled with affection.

James and his family began to follow a careful diet that was developed as his intolerance for several foods were identified. He was severely reactive (cytotoxic) to wheat in any form. He could not tolerate milk, which he loved to drink by the quart. He had intolerance for several foods in the salicylate group (green pepper, peaches, apples, cucumbers, strawberries, tomatoes), and he could not tolerate caffeine. When these culprit foods and beverages were taken out of his diet, James became relatively calm and reachable, On this new diet, his ADHD symptoms came down to Level 6 on the ADHD severity scale. He still was antsy and easily bored, except with computer activities. He continued to lose his temper too easily, and he continued to balk and be stubborn when he was pressed too hard by adults. He continued to need a lot of supervision to keep things organized. Yet as long as he avoided trigger foods and beverages, he was a comfortable member of his family. He learned to function in academic work and eventually became a good student. I cherish the note of thanks I received from Mr. and Mrs. King a few weeks after they started the new diet control program: "We don't have the words to thank you enough, Dr. J. As the Bible says, through you God has restored to us 'the years that the locust hath eaten' (Joel 2:25). You have given us back our son we thought we had lost forever."

In his natural state, James's acutely severe ADHD symptoms placed so much stress on his environment, his family broke apart. Without dietary intervention, the King family home life could not have survived his aggression and hyperactivity.

Nate

I met Nate when he was 9 years old. After speaking to a parent group about attention deficit challenges, I was followed to my car by a woman who was crying. She had trouble talking through her sobs. "You have just described my son," she managed to tell me. "All these years I have tried to find out what his problem is. Tonight you have explained it. Everything you said about ADD without hyperactivity fits Nate to a tee." The more the mother talked about her son, the more I wanted to meet him. She was a single parent with two children. By working an extra job on weekends, she provided a modest living for her famly. She told me how no one in her family wanted anything to do with her son. "They call him weird," she explained. "His dad has nothing to do with him, and none of the grandparents pay any attention to him. Can you help me with my son?"

Soon after that I met 9-year-old Nate. Now he is 29 years old with a college degree in computer science. By his early 20s, he was regarded as a gifted computer programming specialist. Our first meeting was one of the strangest experiences of my life. Nate was unusually tall for his age. He was thin and awkward with poor motor coordination. He shuffled along in an awkward gait with his arms swinging in stiff jerks instead of being relaxed. I was greatly surprised to notice that he carried a Raggedy Andy doll. Nate introduced me to Roy, his doll. He placed Roy between us on the large round table where I worked with youngsters. He took a piece of gum from the candy dish and unwrapped it for Roy. He fussed with Roy's clothes and made all kinds of little sounds. Nate began speaking to Roy in a singsong voice (called *prosody*), and Roy answered in a high-pitched whining response. This conversation between Nate and his doll lasted several minutes. Finally I realized that Nate was telling Roy why they were in my office. He was assuring Roy that everything was fine. As I learned how to interpret this private language, I heard Nate explain: "Mommy thinks something is wrong with me and wants me to talk to this doctor. But nothing is wrong with me, is there, Roy? And nothing is wrong with you, either. This doctor just wants to ask me some questions, Roy. He isn't going to hurt me or give me any shots or any medicine. But it's OK, Roy. Don't be afraid. It's OK." This litany continued for more than 10 minutes while I listened with fascination. Here was a 9-year-old boy, as tall as most adolescents, speaking a private language to his doll, making sure that the doll was not afraid. No wonder Nate's relatives called him weird. I knew from the mother's information that Roy did not go to school with Nate. The moment the boy arrived home from after school care, he dashed into his room to be with Roy. They stayed behind the closed door until supper was ready. If Nate had his way, he would spend all of his time alone in his room talking things over with Roy in their private singsong speech.

As I worked with Nate over a period of time, we became close friends. However, it was six months before he came to me without bringing Roy. By working slowly and gently with Nate, I discovered that he had severe symptoms of ADD. Beneath his quiet, withdrawn surface was a cluster of attention deficits that blocked him in many ways. I finally determined that he was at Level 8 on the severity scale. No doubt he had been at Level 9 ADD when he first started attending school. Listening comprehension was very poor. Nate understood less than 30% of what he heard unless someone repeated for him. His thought patterns were extremely loose. He rarely went longer than 90 seconds without losing his mental image. He continually experienced the "blink" patterns described in Chapter 4. Without warning, the thought of the moment skipped to a different mental image. Along with this blink pattern were moments of going blank when he lost his thoughts altogether. As I worked with Nate, I remembered the comment of a bright 11-year-old girl who was ADD: "My brain just stops." So did Nate's brain. No matter how hard he tried to keep on listening, thinking, or doing his work, his brain "just stopped."

On the surface, we might wonder how a passive, intensely private boy who spent most of his time in make-believe with his doll could be disruptive within his family. The more I learned about Nate, the more easily I understood how disruptive his passive ADD patterns were for his mother, sister, and other relatives. Nate had almost no sense of time passing, and he had no sense of organization. His room was a mess, and he never attempted to clean it up. The small house in which the family lived was littered by things he absentmindedly left lying around. His clothing was scattered everywhere. He was extremely slow to start a task, then very slow doing it. He never went from start to finish without being supervised. He could not remember to get home with necessary school materials. After supper when his mother asked if he had any homework to do, Nate usually could not remember. On those days when he did get home with his stuff, he invariably forgot to take finished homework and books back to school the next day. Every morning began with his mother nagging him, Nate dawdling and procrastinating, and mother and son having a shouting match because time was running out. Visits with relatives were equally frustrating and discouraging for Nate's mother. He refused to go anywhere without his doll Roy. In spite of the snickers and teasing Nate received from relatives, he would not go without his make-believe partner. He sat in his grandmother's living room talking to Roy in their private singsong language even when adults showed irritation. Soon his grandparents, aunts, and uncles were making critical or sarcastic comments that caused Nate to burst into tears from hurt feelings. His mother could not remember a family visit that did not end with Nate crying, relatives criticizing her for not making him throw away that doll and grow up, and her yelling at Nate all the way home. The boy's immaturity, fears, ritualized behaviors, and deep-seated fantasies expressed through his doll were highly disruptive to this single-parent household where the mother exhausted herself earning a living, only to come home each night to this "weird" child who refused to grow up.

Two strategies built a bridge that a gifted tutor used to bring Nate from his world of make-believe into the world of reality. First, he was introduced to keyboard writing. Immediately he began to create fantastical stories that were filled with magical characters from his world of make-believe. Soon he had written his first illustrated book about Roy, a mighty warrior who saved his people from an invading tribe of barbarians. Through this medium we guided Nate into doing outstanding work in his language arts and reading programs at school. Second, the tutor introduced Nate to the magical worlds of the *Chronicles of Narnia* by C. S. Lewis and the hobbit tales by J. R. R. Tolkien. As he devoured these make-believe works, Nate's own imagination left behind the fearful immaturity I had seen at first. Soon he was self-confident enough to make some of the best grades in his classroom. By his 10th birthday, he no longer needed to use Roy as his surrogate self.

Nate remained a "slob" in his private life. He continued to litter his space with scattered stuff. He continued to be forgetful, forever losing books and clothing. He continued to dawdle and procrastinate at home. Yet the level of disruption within his family quickly dropped as his mother learned not to fret over ADD habits that Nate could not help doing. She agreed to stop taking him to family gatherings, and this removed a major source of heartache for her and her son. His mother learned to close the door to his room so that she did not see Nate's mess. He learned to keep his clutter out of the family living area of the home. Nate also learned to keep lists of his responsibilities and school assignments. Each day after school, an older student spent five minutes going over these lists with Nate to make sure he had all his things in his bookbag. Instead of engaging in arguments at home, he and his mother learned to review the lists, making sure Nate was ready for school each day. Part of this routine was the rule that if Nate became stubborn and refused to cooperate with his supervisors, he would face the consequences without making excuses. This stopped the nagging that had triggered so many morning arguments between mother and son.

As time went by, Nate gradually moved down the ADD severity scale. By age 13, his ADD symptoms were at Level 6. By age 16, his attention deficit was down to Level 5. By age 19, he was down to Level 4. Now at age 29, his ADD patterns are at Level 3. As ADD symptoms declined, another layer of challenge emerged more predominantly. Chapter 6 describes the tag-along *Asperger's syndrome* (very high functioning autism) that lived in the shadow of Nate's ADD. As an adult, he still is messy in his private space, has ritualized behavior, is forgetful enough to lose track of things, and is not yet ready for a romantic relationship because he remains self-focused and prefers time with his computer over time with friends. However, he has demonstrated extraordinary talent for computer science that does not require strong social skills for building a successful career.

ADHD and ADD on the Job

During the last two decades of the 20th century, dramatic changes occurred in the workplace. It became increasingly difficult for adults with attention deficits to earn a living. Restaurants were replaced by fast-food stores that demand rapid production and strict following of standard procedures. Self-service filling stations no longer needed human beings to clean the windshield, fill the tank, and check the tires. Auto mechanics must be expert at computer analysis of modern vehicles, which are run by computer chips. Working in a warehouse requires skills to interpret complex computer codes instead of relying on product names on shipping cartons. Loading trucks no longer is a simple matter of moving crates and boxes. Complex laws governing child care often make it impossible for women to earn extra income by supervising children in their homes. As our culture entered the 21st century, the workplace required computer skills, mature enough executive function to perform calmly under pressure, and enough education to qualify for licenses according to government regulations. Adults with residual ADHD or ADD find it difficult to earn a living. Several million young adults continue to live with their parents because they cannot earn enough to live on their own. Several million parents are caught in the "sandwich generation"—having to care for aging parents while still providing for adult children who cannot manage for themselves. Adults with residual ADHD or ADD swell the ranks of underemployed workers in our culture.

ADHD on the Job

For most of us, a psychological condition like [the noisy brain] ... threatens our effectiveness at work. Most jobs require that we know how to deal with people, and coping mechanisms like an escape into anger will almost inevitably get in the way. And of course, a decline in processing abilities will harm our ability to perform any work that involves abstract thinking or higher-level organizational skills.

The man or woman who is pulled to [sources of] stimulus is a person who may have tremendous difficulty formulating a plan and sticking to it. Goal-directed behavior, one of the bases of any kind of success in life and love, depends upon being able to organize one's thoughts and hopes, and act upon them in a direct and timely fashion. But the person who is pulled to [the source of] stimulus is constantly distracted—ambushed even—by the red spot [source of stimulus].

—John Ratey and Catherine Johnson, 1997, p. 62

Kim

I met hyperactive, impulsive Kim when she was 13 years old. I became her trusted friend and counselor, to whom she turned when her life got out of control. Twenth-nine years later, we are still good friends. Kim's parents held their marriage together in spite of the battering experience of rearing a daughter with severe ADHD. Until onset of puberty at age 12, Kim was at Level 9 in hyperactivity and executive dysfunction. The Springers survived those difficult years through the help of Ritalin (described in Chapter 7). This cortical stimulant medication brought Kim's hyperactivity and impulsivity down to Level 6 for a few hours each day when she was away from her parents. When the Springer family came together again for the evening, the parents endured emotional storms that were unleashed as Kim's pent-up energy and emotions rebounded because the cortical stimulant had disappeared from her brain. By dinner time each evening, she was climbing the walls and driving her parents crazy. Hormone development during puberty gradually reduced the force of her hyperactivity to Level 8, then to Level 7 by the time she entered ninth grade. With continued treatment through medication, Kim stayed in school with barely passing grades. Outbursts of impulsive, irrational behavior threatened school failure, but private tutoring and frequent counseling enabled her to graduate with her high school class. Mr. and Mrs. Springer wept with relief as they watched their difficult daughter receive her high school diploma. "Surely," they told themselves, "now we will get a break." After 18 traumatic years, they looked forward to the "empty nest" their friends described. Kim was their only child. They dared not have more children when the severity of her ADHD became clear.

On her 18th birthday, a few weeks before high school graduation, Kim stopped taking Ritalin. "I'm an adult now," she told her parents. "You can't make me take medication if I don't want to." Kim received several hundred dollars as graduation gifts. She talked about using that money to rent an apartment with a friend. The Springers encouraged this plan. They helped Kim and her friend look for an apartment they could afford and shop for household things. Three weeks after high school commencement, the Springers received a telephone call one evening. It was Kim telling them that she was at a summer resort with several friends. On the spur of the moment, they had decided to party because they were going separate ways in a few weeks. She would be home sometime. Then she hung up the phone without leaving her number or address. Kim was gone for 10 days. Late one night a call came from a sheriff's office in a neighboring state. "I'm in jail!" Kim said in her old angry voice. "This bunch of jerks arrested me for drunk driving. Come get me out of this crappy place!" Mr. Springer listened to several minutes of Kim's anger, then he talked with the sheriff's deputy. He learned that Kim and some friends had been stopped going 90 miles per hour in a 45-mph zone. Kim, who was driving, started to yell and resist the officer's effort to check things out. The deputy finally determined that she was driving without a license, and she registered .16 on the breath test for intoxication—twice the legal limit for blood alcohol in that state. Kim faced several hundred dollars in fines. She also needed an attorney to represent her in local court. That postgraduation party cost the Springers more than $3,000. All of Kim's gift money had been spent with nothing left for the apartment.

For several weeks following that upset, Kim lived in anger toward her parents. "We're back to the days when she was seven before we started Ritalin," Mrs. Springer sobbed one night. Relatives and church friends advised the Springers to practice "tough love" by forcing Kim to leave their home unless she obeyed their rules. Her parents could not bring themselves to take such a drastic step. By September, she began to calm down and become less angry. Her parents realized that Kim's anger actually was a smokescreen to cover intense anxiety. In reality, she was deeply afraid of stepping out on her own. Kim realized that she had no job skills to offer an employer. "I can't do anything right!" she sobbed one night to her mother. "All my life I've screwed everything up! I can't make it on my own without you and Dad. It makes me so mad at myself! I'm nothing but a failure!"

Kim swallowed her pride and agreed to talk things over with me. Finally she accepted my encouragement to apply for at least a part-time job. We worked out a list of jobs that would not press her too hard. Her ADHD patterns made it very hard for her to follow oral instructions, especially if there was background noise while she listened. Chapter 4 describes how the ADHD brain often "blinks" or "goes blank" instead of staying focused on a task. Lack of organization made it hard for Kim to keep a workspace tidy. Her poor sense of time meant that she must be reminded when and where to be. As we reviewed all of these issues, she made the decision to look for work. She was too bored and restless to stay at home and watch television all day. However, she refused to return to taking Ritalin. "I'm not going back on drugs," she declared. "I'm not a kid anymore."

I warned Kim that being turned down for jobs would be her most difficult challenge. "You're a very sensitive person," I reminded her. "Your first reaction will be to take it as a personal insult if you are turned down when you apply." That prediction proved to be correct. After being turned down three times following job interviews, Kim slipped into a state of depression for several days. Her old shame from failure returned heavily, and her lifelong battle with low self-esteem became acute. She cried, she was angry, and she began sleeping all day. Finally Mr. Springer asked a friend who owned several ice cream shops to give Kim a job to help build up her courage. The friend agreed, and Kim was to begin work at 3 P.M. the following Monday.

Kim was late to work that first day. As her parents left the house that morning, they reminded her to watch the clock. Mrs. Springer called at noon to remind her again, but this triggered an argument over the phone. "I'm not a baby!" Kim yelled at her mother. "Stay off my back!" Then she turned on the television and lost track of time. At 2:50 she saw the clock. She dashed to her car and raced off toward work. A few blocks from the house, she ran out of gas because she had forgotten to fill the tank when her father reminded her the day before. A neighbor brought gas from his garage and started her car. Then she discovered that she had left her purse and credit cards at home. Back to the house she raced, then rushed to work. She was 20 minutes late and out of breath.

Raul, the manager of the ice cream shop, was irritated by Kim's late arrival. He already was upset because a friend of the boss had gotten his daughter this job. An impressive young man had applied for the position, but Raul was told to hire Kim instead. The new job started on a negative note. Raul was impatient when it was clear that this new worker needed everything repeated. If the manager kept on explaining, Kim interrupted, "What do you mean?" Within a few minutes of on-the-job training, the manager was feeling hostile toward this new employee whom he had not wanted in the first place. Kim began to boil inside, as she always did when anyone in authority told her to listen and stop interrupting. Those words always triggered her anger because it made her feel "dumb" to be told to listen better. She tried to hold her temper under control, but as the work session continued, her old ADHD patterns emerged. Before she had been on the job two hours, Kim flared into a shouting match with her new manager. Raul reminded her who was boss. Those words were the last straw. "Well, you can take this rotten job and shove it!" she screamed as she stormed out of the shop.

During the next four months, Kim was hired, then fired, from seven jobs. Each time, she promised me and her parents that she would do better. Each time she started a new job, she fully intended to make this one a success. Each time, she soon reached the point of failure. Kim worked a few days selling tie-dyed T-shirts in a boutique. She made so many mistakes at the cash register that the boss finally let her go. She found a job making cinnamon pastries in a shopping mall, but that job required her to work in an open space where shoppers could stand and watch. She could not keep her attention focused on her work. After spoiling several batches of pastry dough, Kim was fired for being careless. Then she found part-time work that sounded exciting. She was to sell cosmetics by telephone. Like most of her friends, Kim loved talking on the phone. That job lasted half a day because she could not remember the sales message she was required to say. Besides, she began to feel angry when several people hung up as she

141

introduced herself by phone. Her love of telephone talking did not give her the right skills for this type of oral communication.

Finally Kim was hired to sell costume jewelry in a department store. All her life she had had a natural talent for fashion. She did well for the first two weeks and began to feel confident of her skills. One Friday evening during rush hour, three of her high school friends came by. As they laughed and talked about old times, customers stood in line. Several customers interrupted and asked Kim to help them with purchases. Her old habits of resenting authority flared, and she said sharply, "Just wait a minute! I'm busy!" Then she returned to gossiping with her friends. A customer complained to the floor manager, who came to see what the problem might be. When the manager told Kim's friends to leave and reminded her that customers were waiting, Kim's lifelong temper erupted. She walked off yet another job having a tantrum. Later she rationalized to me and her parents, "I hated that old job anyway. They make you work like a slave and they don't pay anything. I won't waste my time at a place like that!" Three more jobs came and went with similar stories.

As the Christmas season approached, the Springers realized with heavy hearts how handicapped their daughter was as a young adult with still-active ADHD behavior. They joined a parent support group called CHADD (see information in Appendix D). At CHADD meetings, they shared their sad story with other parents who also were trapped with adult children who had residual ADHD. To their dismay, the Springers learned that many families still support such children long after high school. These residual ADHD adults do not possess job skills that fit today's workplace needs, nor do they have the social skills to fit into the adult world successfully. They lack the emotional maturity to absorb normal social pressures without losing self-control. These young adults with ADHD are restless children in grown-up bodies. They still need the same type of supervision they required during childhood and adolescence, yet they are too proud, insecure, and self-focused to permit parents and other adults to supervise. These ADHD adults are demanding in the same selfish way that sabotaged relationships when they were young. They are too shallow to comprehend the principle that it is more blessed to give than to receive. They do not express gratitude to parents who are exhausted from many years of forgiving, providing, and carrying the burden with the family. These residual ADHD adults cannot establish separate lives. They cannot function successfully on jobs. They cannot stay in personal relationships that require give and take. They are locked into lifestyles that are immature, self-centered, and often destructive. And they tend to refuse the help offered by loved ones, friends, and the community. Parents like the Springers often search in vain for hope that things will soon improve as they confront the problems created by their adult children who still have ADHD.

In Chapters 3 and 4 we reviewed the question of whether individuals outgrow ADHD or ADD. We who work with these behavior challenges generally agree that during adolescence and early adult years, most individuals with mild or moderate ADHD and ADD do outgrow most of their childhood symptoms. During my career of working with individuals like Kim, I have seen an extremely late developmental cycle that seldom is reported by research. Among young adults with still-active ADHD, some begin to move down the severity scale as they near age 30. Many of the severely ADHD adolescents and young adults I have known began to mellow about age 28 and continued to mellow as they reached their early 30s.

Kim followed this extremely late blooming pattern. During her 20s, her life was a nightmare. At age 21 she became pregnant by an extremely immature ADHD man who paid for an abortion. Like most young adults with these behavior challenges, she began to use social drugs at parties and soon was habituated to cocaine and marijuana. This self-medication did relieve her churning emotions temporarily. Kim also became a heavy user of alcohol. She lived around the community with friends in low-rent apartments. Her parents were forced to install a security system to keep her from breaking into their home to steal things to sell for drug money. Every so often, Kim showed up at my office to talk with the only mature friend who had not rejected her.

When Kim reached her 27th birthday, I noticed a change in her attitude. She was using less cocaine and marijuana, and she stopped drinking alcohol altogether. She began staying on part-time jobs for 3 or 4 months instead of for only a few days. As she approached her 29th birthday, she came by one afternoon to introduce me to Pete, a new man in her life. He was well-groomed, well-educated, and appeared to be in love with Kim. That was the first time Kim had dated a mature man without destroying the relationship through her temper and sarcasm. Mr. and Mrs. Springer were able to let Kim come home for visits that no longer ended in tantrums and destructive words. On her 30th birthday, Kim and Pete told me that they were getting married. She had stayed successfully on a good job for more than a year. The Springers could hardly believe this good fortune. Between ages 27 and 30, Kim's ADHD patterns had gone down from Level 8 on the severity scale to Level 4. She was a true late bloomer, like many others I have known.

ADD on the Job

Although you can look like the most impressive job candidate to ever walk in the door—impressive degree from a well-respected university, a grade point average that anyone would envy, and a list of community service work a mile long—none of your credentials necessarily means you're equipped to be successful in the workplace if you have ADD.... Your education might have taught you how to produce an accurate profit-and-loss statement. However, chances are no one taught you how to deal with the frustration of trying to produce that statement in the middle of a noisy, chaotic office. Or how do you deal with a boss who looks over your shoulder twenty times a day? Or how do you deal with the distraction of the secretary's radio as it announces exactly when to call in for the next contest?"

—Lynn Weiss, 1996, p. 10

Robert came into my life when he was 9 years old, one of the most depressed children I had ever met. The first time we met, he quietly cried with his chin down on his chest. As we became acquainted that day, he surprised me by climbing into my lap. He wrapped his arms tightly around me and sobbed into my shoulder. From that moment, we were bonded for life. Soon I determined that Robert was at Level 8 ADD. That explanation helped his bewildered family come together as his strong support team. Since early childhood, he had been the most forgetful, absentminded person his family had ever seen. Through early childhood, kindergarten, and primary grades, Mr. and Mrs. Reyes tried every trick they could think of to help Robert remember. They covered the refrigerator with stick-on notes reminding him what to do after school, when to feed and water his dog, and where to be at certain times. Then they had to remind him to look at his notes. Every detail of Robert's young life had to be supervised, or else he forgot. After working at their jobs all day, Mr. and Mrs. Reyes faced the task of rounding up their son's schoolbooks for homework. They usually had to dash back to school to get something he had forgotten to bring home. They often had to drive to the bus barn to retrieve something Robert had left on the bus. Mr. and Mrs. Reyes lost track of how many new jackets, caps, gloves, and even socks their son lost during his years in school.

Without adult supervision, Robert could not finish anything he started. The attic was filled with half-finished models of all kinds. His room was littered with half-finished projects he abandoned. His school locker was stuffed with papers that represented half-finished homework never turned in. After dragging him through homework assignments at night, Mr. and Mrs. Reyes exhausted themselves reminding Robert to get all of his schoolwork into his book bag. He usually left something important behind as he ran to catch the bus. The orthodontist complained about Robert's failure to care for his teeth and braces. The optometrist could not believe how many times she replaced eyeglasses that Robert needed for school. After what seemed an eternity of constant supervision, the weary Reyes family watched their scatterbrained son receive his high school diploma. Their ray of hope was that Robert's ADD patterns had begun to decline during adolescence. At age 11, he was at Level 8 on the severity scale. By age 14, he was down to Level 7. At age 19, he was about Level 6. But he was still "loose as a goose," as his grandmother expressed it.

In every situation, Robert's good sense of humor saved the day. No one could stay angry with him very long. He never seemed upset. He was glad to see others, even when they scolded him for being so forgetful and inattentive. His kindness made quick friends everywhere he went. The fact that he was always rumpled and needed to comb his hair did not take away from his grin and friendly attitude. When Robert forgot to shower and use deodorant for several days, others overlooked his poor grooming. "That kid sure is ripe!" his Grandpa said every now and then. But Grandpa still bragged about this grandson to everyone who would listen.

Robert fully intended to go to college, but high school graduation was over and he had not gotten around to applying for college admission. He had forgotten to show up for the college admission test that was required by all of the state schools. He began looking for a job the week after graduation. Within 2 days, he was hired to deliver floral arrangements for a neighborhood shop. The owner of the floral shop was charmed by this young man's smile and friendly attitude. Part of Robert's responsibility was to take inventory of cut flowers and potted plants every Tuesday and Thursday afternoon. Keeping enough flowers on hand depended on those inventories. Robert could read well and had no trouble handling numbers, but as he hurried from work the first Tuesday to go fishing with his grandfather, he forgot to take the inventory. Two unexpected funerals occurred on Wednesday, and the shop ran out of flowers. The florist listened to Robert's apology. "Well, I'll forgive it this time," the manager said, "but don't let it happen again. We can't stay in business if we don't keep track of our inventory." Two weeks later Robert forgot again. This time the manager fired him. "You're one of the nicest boys I've ever had here," the florist said, "but, Robert, you've cost me five hundred dollars. I have to let you go."

It did not take long for Robert to find another job. This time he was hired as night-shift cashier in a self-service filling station. His job was to take money or credit cards before customers filled their tanks. He had to watch all the cars that pulled up to the 16 gasoline pumps. He was to stop any pump immediately if the driver tried to fill his tank before paying in advance at Robert's window or properly inserting a credit card at the pump. The third night on the job, a lull came in traffic. Ten minutes went by with no customers, so Robert started to read a book. Soon he was lost in the story and did not see two cars pull up to the pumps farthest from his booth. Those drivers knew how to activate the pumps without paying in advance. They filled their tanks, then slipped away without Robert seeing

145

ADHD and ADD in One's Personal Life

them. The next day, he was fired and had to pay the filling station owner for the stolen gas.

During the next 2 years, Robert was fired from more than 20 jobs. His mother kept a diary of her son's job history. "Someday when I write my book," she said many times, "people won't believe it." Robert lost jobs because he was late too many times. No matter how many alarm clocks went off beside his bed, he could not wake up without a struggle. He lost several more jobs because he forgot to do essential tasks. He was fired for wearing soiled uniforms after being warned to make sure he was fresh and clean. Twice he lost his job because he loaded merchandise on the wrong trucks. He had been watching something down the dock and did not notice what he was doing. Robert could not keep track of work schedules unless he was reminded. He lost several jobs because he failed to notice posted changes for his shift. Three times he was fined for losing important papers on the job. He was forever being nagged for having too much clutter in his workspace. Managers fussed at him for failing to put equipment away before leaving his shift. Yet every time he was fired, Robert was told, "You're one of the nicest guys we've ever had work here, but I have to let you go." This nice guy who had Level 6 ADD could not cope successfully with workplace expectations.

When Robert was 21 years old, he was still living at home with his parents, who continued to help him make car payments and pay his bills. Then he met a girl and fell in love. Mr. and Mrs. Reyes were delighted with Maria. "That girl has common sense," said Mr. Reyes, as they watched her reason with Robert. Maria was able to give advice in a way that did not offend or embarrass him. She began to help him notice that he needed to improve his appearance. On Saturdays they went shopping, where Maria taught Robert how to pay attention to clothes and styles. She suggested that he let her help him keep track of how he spent his money. Then she showed him how to keep track of time by using a pocket calendar and an electronic wristwatch. Maria coached Robert in watching clocks wherever he happened to be. She helped him understand why it is important not to start reading a book on the job or make personal phone calls at work. By the time Maria and Robert announced their engagement to be married, he was holding the first steady job he had had since high school. By letting Maria become his supervisor, Robert learned to compensate for residual ADD. As his mother eventually wrote in her book about rearing a son with ADD, "The key to success for anyone who has ADD is finding a supervisor. Children who have ADD need supervision. Teens must have supervision, although they rebel against it. Adults who still have ADD also need good supervisors. My son became a successful man when he had the good sense to marry the most wonderful supervisor in the world."

Chapter 6

Tag-Along Syndromes That Imitate ADHD and ADD

✦ ✦

The numbers are skyrocketing—and so is the confusion. Most parents—even many professionals—are perplexed by the overlapping syndromes, diagnostic categories, and classification schemes that are used to describe the rapidly growing population of behaviorally disordered children.

> —Bernard Rimland, November 2002,
> Autism Research Institute

Rarely does any type of learning difficulty (LD) exist alone. In most instances, several kinds of learning struggle overlap like layers of an onion. Seeing [dyslexia] clearly requires teachers and diagnosticians to peel away each layer of LD, give it an appropriate name, and define its characteristics. This process of separating the layers of LD brings into clear focus the overlapping factors that make classroom learning difficult. Before dyslexia can be defined correctly, it must be separated from other patterns that tend to hide in its shadow.

> —Dale Jordan, 2002, pp. 59–60

What Causes Socially Disruptive Behavior?

As far back in human history as the days of ancient Greece, physicians and philosophers have wondered about the disruptive behaviors of children, adolescents, and adults who are impulsive, hyperactive, emotionally volatile, subject to wide moods swings, and unable to live by the rules of society. Ancient Greek writers speculated that such behavior might be caused by "body humors" being out of balance. Those ancient scholars had no idea how close they were to understanding what causes such disruptive behaviors in many individuals.

During the 19th century, medical literature increasingly described behavior syndromes that disrupted personal and community lives through inattention, poor control of impulse, mood swings, explosive emotional patterns, and unexpected aggression and violence. Toward the end of the 1800s, William James became concerned about the socially disruptive presence of individuals who had poor moral control, did not control impulses, and could not maintain full attention long enough to finish what they started. James developed the theory that such behavior must come from an underlying neurological deficit (James, 1890).

The first clinical description of what we now call ADHD was offered in 1902 when George Still delivered a series of lectures at the Royal College of Physicians in London, England. Still expanded James's neurological theory as he described disruptive behaviors in children who were "aggressive, defiantly resistant to discipline, emotionally volatile, lawless, spiteful and cruel, dishonest, and apparently without inhibitory volition." In addition to being overly active, many of those disruptive children displayed chronic problems with maintaining attention. In the vocabulary of that day, Still reported that those youngsters had "a major deficit in moral control" (1901, pp. 1008–1009). In 1908 Alfred Tredgold elaborated on the work of James and Still by providing medical evidence that brain deficits contribute to disruptive behavior (Tredgold, 1908). Tredgold proposed a kind of special education for children who had impaired attention and inappropriate social behavior.

Defining Socially Disruptive Behavior

At the beginning of the 20th century, researchers believed that these socially disruptive behaviors arose from brain damage. If so, it was thought that such individuals always would be impaired in social functioning that sometimes could be modified through medication. Immediately following the close of World War I, an outbreak of encephalitis lethargica afflicted great numbers of children around the world. After recovering from that illness, many children displayed changed behavior that was hyperactive, impulsive, aggressive, inattentive, emotionally explosive, and socially inappropriate. During the 1920s, special residential treatment centers were established in the United States to care for these disruptive children. Eli Kahn and

Leonard Cohen (1934) concluded that this outbreak of disruptive behavioral changes was caused by encephalitic damage to the brain stem. Kahn and Cohen introduced the concept that this type of socially destructive behavior is "organically driven." This neurological model was confirmed by William Bradley's work (1937) with the new medication Benzedrine, which reduced disruptive behaviors in "organically driven" children. Benzedrine was the first application of the closely related chemical compounds dextroamphetamine and levoamphetamine (described in Chapter 7), which are used today to decrease inattention and hyperactivity.

From the 1930s to the mid-1950s, Arthur Strauss conducted studies to differentiate between brain-damaged and non-brain-damaged children who were thought to be mentally retarded. He described his brain-damaged population as having chronic problems with concept formation, language usage, emotional control, perception of new information and the world around them, and social behavior (Strauss & Kephart, 1955). Strauss further labeled these struggling children as *distractible* ("driven hither and yon by outside stimulation"), *impulsive* ("cannot master planful action"), *perseverative* ("perseveration obstructs the child's understanding of purposeful action"), and *hyperactive* ("motor disinhibition"). Stauss also documented the difficulty this special population had with cognitive learning. By 1940, research by Kahn and Cohen, Bradley, Strauss and others had produced the label *Minimal Brain Damage Syndrome* (MBDS). Until 1957, MBDS was the most widely used label for the cluster of behaviors that included hyperactivity, impulsivity, poor attention, mood swings, emotional volatility, and inappropriate social behavior.

Not everyone agreed with the MBDS "brain damage" label for struggling learners who were hyperactive. In 1942 Lauretta Bender proposed the concept of "maturational lag" to differentiate between disruptive behavior linked to brain disease or brain injury and hyperactive youngsters with delayed maturity of the central nervous system (Bender, 1942). Bender demonstrated that those "late bloomers" with no history of brain trauma tended to outgrow at least some of their inattentive, hyperactive symptoms as they passed through adolescence into early adulthood.

In 1957 Morris Laufer, Ernest Denhoff, and George Solomons introduced the concept *Hyperkinetic Impulse Disorder* (HID). HID syndrome labeled children who could not keep still. They were in some sort of constant motion, were always restless even in their sleep, and lived by impulse without thinking of the consequences. Laufer and his colleagues speculated that HID was caused by nerve pathway deficits in a portion of the limbic system called the *diencephlon* (Laufer, Denhoff, & Solomons, 1957). By 1960 many diagnosticians and counselors agreed that the models of Minimal Brain Damage Syndrome (MBDS) and Hyperkinetic Impulse Disorder (HID) were too narrow to continue to be useful as a diagnostic model. A broader point of view was proposed by Samuel Clements and John Peters at the Child Study Center in Little Rock, Arkansas. In 1962 they introduced the concept of *Minimal Brain Dysfunction* (MBD) with this statement:

> It is necessary to take into account the full spectrum of causality from the unique genetic combination that each individual is to his gestation and birth experiences, to his interaction with significant persons, and finally to the stresses and emotional traumata of later life, after his basic reaction patterns have been laid down.
>
> —Clements & Peters, 1962, p. 195

This model of MBD rapidly replaced the older labels MBDS and HID for impulsive, disruptive, underchieving youngsters. In 1968 the second edition of the *Diagnostic and Statistical Manual of Mental Disorders* (*DSM–II*, American Psychiatric Association, 1968) introduced the diagnostic category "Hyperkinetic Reaction of Childhood Disorder." During the 1970s, this classification largely replaced the earlier labels MBDS, HID, and MBD that had focused attention on underlying neurological causes for socially disruptive, inattentive, impulsive, disorganized behavior. In 1980 the third edition of the *Diagnostic and Statistical Manual of Mental Disorders* (*DSM–III*, American Psychiatric Association, 1980) introduced the concept of *Attention Deficit Disorder* ADD+H (with hyperactivity) and ADD–H (without hyperactivity). These new categories of attention deficits replaced all earlier labels for inattentive behavior. In 1987 the diagnostic labels ADD+H and ADD–H were replaced by the single label ADHD (*DSM–III–R*, American Psychiatric Association, 1987).

Separating the Layers of ADHD and ADD Syndromes

During the 1980s, Russell Barkley and his colleagues at the University of Massachussetts Medical Center undertook landmark research into the multiple layers of ADHD. In 1990 they published their conclusions that ADHD actually is a multilayered neurological condition usually consisting of several distinctive syndromes (Barkley, 1990). This research demonstrated that to understand attention deficit disorders, we must apply *principles of differential diagnosis to separate ADHD from other childhood and adolescent psychiatric disorders.* Barkley and his associates reported that 65% of those who are diagnosed with ADHD also present a lookalike syndrome called *Oppositional Defiant Disorder* (ODD), while 30% of ADHD individuals also display the highly disruptive syndrome called *Conduct Disorder* (CD). Furthermore, 5% of ADHD individuals present a distinctive struggle with language usage called *Multiplex Developmental Disorder* (MDD). In their book

Shadow Syndromes, John Ratey and Catherine Johnson separate ADHD and ADD from the comorbid syndromes of monopolar depression, hypomanic personality, rage disorders, mild autism, forms of addiction, anxiety, and attention hyperfocus disorder (Ratey & Johnson, 1997). During the 1990s, Dale Jordan began to document the frequent overlapping syndromes of ADHD, dyslexia, dysgraphia, and scotopic sensitivity syndrome (Jordan, 1996a, 1998, 2000a, 2000b, 2002). In 2002, Diane Kennedy demonstrated the many ways in which ADHD appears to be an extension of the autism spectrum (Kennedy, 2002). The 21st century began with growing emphasis upon *dual diagnosis* of comorbid syndromes as we seek to understand more clearly the nature of learning differences and how to overcome these challenges in children, adolescents, and adults.

In Chapter 5 we met James, the angry little ADHD tiger, whose often violent ODD and CD disorders were triggered by cytotoxic reactions to certain trigger foods and beverages. We met Kim, the extreme late bloomer, whose first 27 years were devasted by ADHD layered over ODD. Also, we met Nate whose ADD overlapped a type of very high functioning autism called *Asperger's syndrome.* Figure 6.1 shows how, like shingles on a roof, comorbid layers often obscure other types of disruptive disorders that hide behind each other to make positive identification of ADHD or ADD rather challenging.

Oppositional Defiant Disorder

Oppositional Defiant Disorder (ODD) is intensely disruptive without being violent or destructive. The surface of ODD presents many of the ADHD symptoms described in Chapter 3. However, hiding beneath the attentional deficit overlay is a lifestyle that is negative, hostile, and defiant of authority. No matter how much guidance and counseling parents or teachers might provide, the ADHD/ODD person cannot fit successfully into the family, a classroom, the workplace, or social groups. Yet this disruptive individual rarely meets the diagnostic criteria for such mental illness categories as Antisocial Personality Disorder or Psychotic or Mood Disorder. The following faces of ODD allow us to separate it from overlapping ADHD.

Temper Tantrums

The habitual temper tantrums of ODD go far beyond loss of temper that all persons experience from time to time. ODD tantrums are like thunderstorms that explode without warning and blow roofs off buildings or knock down power lines. Once the storm has released its aggressive energy, it quickly moves away. ODD tantrums follow a pattern that my grandmother

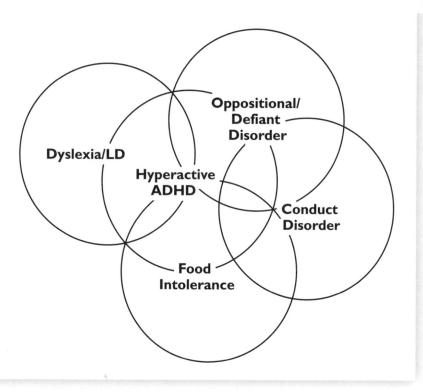

FIGURE 6.1. Usually when individuals struggle with classroom learning, we find two or more layers of difficulty that overlap like layers of an onion. It is not unusual to discover several layers of tag-along challenges that explain why certain individuals have difficulty in classroom performance.

explained: "She doesn't lose her temper. She uses her temper." I did not understand what she meant until I became a classroom teacher of ADHD/ODD youngsters. As their tantrums burst on classmates and adults, the exploding anger always had a purpose: to enable the self-focused child to get his or her own way. As soon as everyone gave in and the angry child got what he or she wanted, the tantrum stopped as suddenly as it had begun. As we saw in James's and Kim's behavior in Chapter 5, individuals with Oppositional Defiant Disorder do not just lose their temper. They use their anger to gain control over others in order to get their own way.

Arguing with Authority

A disruptive characteristic of ADHD is arguing over misunderstandings. However, when the misunderstanding has been corrected, persons with

ADHD stop arguing and begin to use the information they first misperceived. Arguing plays a different role in ODD behavior. Individuals with ODD "get up in the face" of whoever is in charge, daring that parent, teacher, coach, job supervisor, or police officer to enforce the rules. "You can't make me!" and "I don't have to!" are the battle cries of those with ODD. This hostile challenge toward authority comes as automatically as a sneeze. In Chapter 5 we met Kim, who defied authority all her life until her late-blooming epiphany after age 27. In one-to-one counseling relationships, frustrated individuals like Kim confess in pleading terms: "I don't know what makes me do this. I don't want to be this way. I just can't help it." Neuron development differences in the midbrain, as well as brain structure differences in the parietal lobes and prefrontal cortex, permit this runaway pattern of challenging authority. No matter how hard the ODD individual tries not to flare under authority, automatic "in your face" challenges occur.

Deliberately Annoying Others

Just as iron filings are attracted to a magnet, Oppositional Defiant persons are drawn to others. Being ODD means that the individual cannot leave others alone. It is important to separate normal childhood development from the pervasive patterns of ODD. It is normal for children of preschool age to pick on each other. This is partly to satisfy curiosity, partly to relieve boredom, and partly to exert individuality. Children with normal neurological development soon learn to stop picking on others. Oppositional Defiant youngsters do not.

An insatiable need to have the full attention of others is part of the disruptive package of ODD. Persons with ADHD/ODD not only are loose, poorly organized, and overly distracted, they also cannot leave others alone. These hyperfocused persons spend their time and energy scanning their environment to see what others are doing. Habitually they select a target and move into the private spaces of others, demanding to be part of that activity. If family members want to be quiet or alone for a while, the ODD individual does not. He or she begins to do things that force others to pay attention. For example, if a parent is reading quietly, the ODD person starts to make noises that he or she knows will irritate the reader. Soon the reader gives the desired attention by saying "Stop that!" or "Leave me alone!" Once the other person's attention is engaged, the ODD individual continues the intrusion by triggering still stronger emotions. Soon a battle of wills has begun, which was the ODD intention. In the classroom, if quiet work time has begun, the ODD child starts a subtle campaign to disrupt this group atmosphere. He or she begins by making small noises that are designed to attract attention. The ODD person may begin to flip bits of paper that hit a classmate's face or workpage. Or the ODD child may start foot games against a classmate's chair or table leg. Soon the quiet is broken, and the ODD individual has attracted the attention he or she craves—no matter that the attention received is negative or even harsh.

Blaming Others

Perhaps the most perplexing part of Oppositional Defiant behavior is the automatic reaction of blaming others. A dozen witnesses may have watched the ODD person commit a disruptive act, yet the automatic response when challenged is "I didn't do it!" or "He made me do it. It's not my fault." As ODD youngsters enter adolescence and then adulthood, this reflexive habit of blaming others brings them into confrontation with civil authority. We who work with adjudicated delinquents and convicted felons find this ODD pattern in a majority of those who are under the jurisdiction of a court. An unfortunate consquence of Oppositional Defiant Disorder is the lifestyle of blaming others instead of admitting the truth. By the time ODD youngsters have entered their teen years, they may have become chronic liars who rarely tell the truth or take responsibility for their own behavior.

Being Overly Touchy and Irritable

Oppositional Defiant Disorder causes a person to be so touchy and irritable that it is impossible for others to offer constructive criticism or advice. In Chapter 5 we read of Kim's instant irritability when the least hint of criticism triggered her self-defensive response. To keep from hearing anything that pressed her to improve, she lashed out verbally to stop such comments from her parents, teachers, or job supervisors. My childhood years living on a farm taught me the meaning of the question, "How do you pet a porcupine?" Answer: "Very carefully!" This sums up the problem of getting along with someone who is ADHD/ODD. Their prickly, overly touchy, irritable reactions cause others to draw back and keep a safe distance.

Being Overly Angry and Resentful

A persistent goal for parents and instructors of young children is to teach the social principle of forgiveness. We want youngsters not to carry grudges beyond a reasonable length of time. Social skills include the habit of turning loose of old anger. Oppositional Defiant Disorder does not learn this part of the Golden Rule. ODD persons go through life feeling angry and resentful. These dyslogical emotions are not based upon reality. Even when individuals who are ADHD/ODD are treated generously and fairly, they continue to make angry accusations and display active resentment. Parents, teachers, and job supervisors often find it impossible to change these negative feelings in individuals who hang onto old anger, brood about old hurts, and refuse to forgive or be forgiven. This characteristic of ODD quickly disrupts all relationships. Sooner or later, family members, classmates, teachers, and coworkers get enough. Rejection by others is the unfortunate outcome of a lifestyle in which a person harbors grudges without trying to build a more positive outlook.

Being Spiteful and Vindictive

Individuals who carry old anger soon long for revenge. A major earmark of Oppositional/Defiant Disorder is the active effort to get even. ODD individuals do not forgive, nor do they turn loose old grievances. They yearn to hurt real or imagined enemies. Gaining revenge is a motive that drives the imagination of ADHD/ODD persons day and night. As these overlapping syndromes live side by side, the ADHD/ODD individual begins to use language as a weapon against others. These persons load their conversations with sarcasm and putdown comments designed to hurt feelings and embarrass others. When adults try to correct such abusive verbal behavior, the ADHD/ODD youngster explodes in self-defense: "I don't care! She said it first!" Young adults like Kim go out of the way to say harsh things about others: "I don't care! I won't take that crap off anybody!" This lifestyle of speaking spitefully and seeking revenge isolates the ADHD/ODD person from normal social relationships. No one wants to spend time with someone who speaks hatefully of others and continually wants to get even.

Conduct Disorder

Conduct Disorder (CD) is much more aggressive than ODD. The CD syndrome involves "repetitive and persistent" intrusion into the privacy and basic rights of others. This means that from early childhood, the youngsters with CD develop habits of aggression that invade the lives of others. In Chapter 5 we met James, the hostile, aggressive, and destructive child who was unwelcome everywhere outside his home. Approximately 3 out of 10 persons diagnosed as ADHD also display several of the following symptoms of Conduct Disorder.

Aggression and Violence Toward Animals and People

Children with Conduct Disorder quickly become known as bullies. Everywhere they go, they intimidate others aggressively. They habitually make threats that frighten other children and cause concern in adults. These CD aggressors start fights, both verbally and physically. This lifestyle of bullying others includes threatening physical harm. To get their own way, individuals with Conduct Disorder brandish sticks, baseball bats, broken glass containers, stones or bricks, knives, and even guns.

These aggressors often are physically cruel to animals and people. They go out of their way to kick dogs and cats, cut tails off animals they catch, and slap or kick smaller children. It is not unusual for a person with CD to tie someone to a tree or lock them inside a small space, then abandon him or her for several hours or overnight. Individuals with CD rarely show remorse or guilt for their aggressive, intrusive behavior. James, whom we met in Chapter 5, never cried. No matter how severely he hurt or frustrated others, he felt no sorrow or saw any reason to apologize.

Destruction of Property

Setting Fires

A major compulsion of persons with Conduct Disorder is the urge to start fires. This should not be confused with normal childhood curiosity about how fires start and why things burn. Many children start one or two fires as they experiment with igniting something to see it burn. Children who develop normally learn from those events not to do so again. Conduct Disorder often includes a continuing compulsion to set fire to dry grass, trees, piles of lumber, abandoned tires, or abandoned buildings. Older adolescents and adults with CD frequently commit arson, burning large buildings or acres of forest.

Vandalizing Property

Persons with CD often have an impulse to destroy the property of others deliberately. Law enforcement officers continually are surprised by senseless acts of vandalism in which people smash windows in vehicles, destroy lawns and landscape structures, demolish playground equipment, desecrate burial sites in cemeteries, or spray grafitti in public places. This CD behavior toward private and public property reflects rage and hostility that is hard to contain.

Lying and Stealing

An unfortunate characteristic of Conduct Disorder is the habit of telling lies. This usually occurs in the context of conning someone to satisfy a self-focused desire. Individuals with CD rarely tell the truth about money, job performance, what they do privately, or their loyalty in relationships. Along with conning others and telling lies, these individuals also tend to steal. Stealing from others becomes a type of game that leads to shoplifting, forging checks for quick cash, charging purchases to another person's credit card, stealing the identity of others by secretly using their Social Security or bank account number, tricking a telephone operator into placing forbidden calls, or slipping books past the library security system. This compulsion to steal is a "catch me if you can" game. Adolescents and adults who are CD often break into a neighbor's house or into a local business, or invade private business data through computer hacking, just to see if they can do it without being caught. Stealing and lying are not based on need, except when a CD individual has become addicted to drugs or gambling and must steal to support the addiction. Rather, these behaviors are driven by impulses and compulsions.

Disobeying Rules

From early childhood, youngsters like James and Kim with tendencies for Conduct Disorder deliberately break the rules. This behavior is automatic. Whenever presented with a rule, the CD personality balks and rebels. Any restriction on this person's freedom triggers an automatic response: "You can't tell me not to. I'll do it anyway." Habitual disobedience starts early, with the child refusing to mind parental time limits. If the child must be home by 4 P.M., he or she stays out until 7 P.M. If a 12-year-old child is told to be home by 8 P.M., he or she stays out all night, which triggers a neighborhood search by police and worried parents. Running away from home is a major tendency for children with Conduct Disorder. Skipping school enters the picture as soon as the student has places to hide during the day. Escaping from adult confinement becomes a challenge that the person with Conduct Disorder cannot ignore.

Overlap of ADHD and CD

When ADHD overlaps with CD, it is not always easy to separate the two syndromes. One imitates the behavior of the other. The major difference is that ADHD is not a hateful pattern. The ADHD person is loose, poorly organized, forgetful, restless, and accidentally rude and intrusive. Yet he or she does not mean to hurt others. Those with ADHD are sorry when their mistakes come to their attention. On the surface, Conduct Disorder may resemble ADHD because the person is overly active, inattentive, focused on self, and unable to stay on a task from start to finish. However, CD patterns are hateful, aggressive, compulsive, and completely selfish. Whoever stands in the way of an individual with Conduct Disorder is at high risk of being hurt.

Multiplex Developmental Disorder

During the 1980s, neuroscientists who studied ADHD began to see a tag-along syndrome that appeared in approximately 5 out of 100 individuals with ADHD. In 1986 David Cohen introduced the term *Multiplex Developmental Disorder* (MDD) to describe a lifestyle of "odd and peculiar behavior" that creates lifelong difficulties in five areas: thinking, socializing, sensory perception, motor coordination, and connecting emotions and feelings to events (Cohen, Paul, & Volmar,1986). Following Cohen's lead, David Dinklage and David Guevremont at the University of Massachussetts Medical Center developed clinical guidelines for separating MDD from ADHD (Dinklage & Guevremont, 1990). For the first time, we had a way to distinguish between attention deficits with hyperactivity and a different syndrome that tags along with ADHD in 5% of the attention deficit population. On the surface, the way that individuals with MDD react to oral language often resembles schizophrenic behavior with startled looks, disbelieving facial expressions, fearful reactions, or aggressive self-defense as if the speaker has made a threatening comment. However, ADHD/MDD individuals do not meet diagnostic standards for being labeled as schizophrenic or psychotic because they do not hallucinate, hear voices, or have delusional thinking (Barkley, 1990). Later in this chapter we will learn about Diane Kennedy's research, which links ADHD, MDD, and other tag-along syndromes with autism. The following symptoms distinguish ADHD from MDD that actually may be a form of high-functioning autism, or a subtype of Asperger's syndrome.

Irregular Thinking

When we spend time with individuals who are MDD, it soon becomes apparent that their thought patterns are irregular. They do not think about life, other people, or events the same way most persons do. Those who study MDD often use the terms "odd," "weird," "eccentric," and "bizarre" to describe how MDD individuals think and talk. As in ADHD, thought patterns tend to be loose and disorganized, yet what the MDD person says begins to make sense if one listens carefully. In imitation of ADHD, MDD jumps track in midsentence, skips from an unfinished topic to something else, and leaves out words so that what is said is only "half said." When asked a question, the MDD listener often responds by saying something unrelated to the question. Sense of time is scrambled so that the MDD speaker does not tell events in chronological order. Something that happened 10 years ago may become mixed with what the speaker is saying about an event that occurred yesterday or today. The MDD person often speaks in symbolic language, using metaphors instead of telling facts.

Terry is typical of people with MDD. I first met Terry when he was 10 years old. Now at age 40, he is a successful entrepreneur who owns several thriving marinas on lakes in Texas and Oklahoma. At age 9, his pediatrician prescribed Ritalin to decrease Terry's hyperactivity, distractibility, and impulsive tendencies at school. At that time, Terry displayed the *DSM–III* diagnostic criteria for ADD+H (Attention Deficit Disorder with Hyperactivity). The day we met, his mother gave me a note from Terry's fifth-grade teacher, who was a graduate student in a seminar on reading disabilities I was teaching that fall. "In my 21 years as a classroom teacher," she wrote, "I have never met a student like Terry. I can't figure him out. He seems to have good reading skills, but when he tries to describe things or give oral answers, he doesn't make sense. Please help me to understand this boy, and give me some ideas of how I can help him in my classroom."

During the day that Terry and I spent together, I recorded part of what we did orally together. I asked him to tell me about his favorite thing to do when he was not at school. "Fish," he said. "I love to." Then he told me the following story:

> My grandma came to our house for supper last night. And a year before that, I went on a fishing trip with my granddad. We borrowed Uncle Bill's bass boat and I got a new Zebco rod and reel at Kmart. And I wanted to stay out all night, but my brother had to go to Sunday school. What was I talking about? Oh, yeah. We caught twelve big ones, and Grandma fried them last night and I ate two by myself. You know? Like eating half a watermelon by myself. Only it's a lot saltier. Did you know that fish fly sometimes? I heard that on the Discovery Channel. But watermelon is better because ten years ago I got real sick eating fried crawdads. When I was a little boy, Grandma used to fry chicken like that. You know. In a big old skillet with a lot of grease. Like putting too much butter on your bread. And five years before that, I caught a big catfish with my bare hands. And in my dream, it meowed like my uncle's old tomcat. You know.

Tag-Along Syndromes

Like a mockingbird does. Cats try to catch mockingbirds, but they shouldn't because mockingbirds eat lots of bugs. Some fish know how to fly. Or did I say that already? And squirrels can fly, but they don't have feathers. Did you know that Grandma has a feather bed I get to sleep on sometimes? When I was three. My Granddad knows how to fry squirrels, too, but I like watermelon better.

Through the rest of his school years, Terry and I stayed in touch. I was one of the few people he knew who enjoyed listening to his stories. Although I could not talk like that, I learned how to carry on fascinating conversations with this lonely bright boy who had very few friends at school or within his family. When he was 21 years old, Terry fell in love with Toni, a remarkable person who loved this man who "talked funny" but who was gentle, kind, and exceptionally generous. I guided them in working out strategies through which Toni became Terry's wise supervisor, the way Maria did for Robert in Chapter 5. With her help and guidance, Terry discovered his talent for developing a successful business related to water sports and fishing.

Seeming Odd or Weird

It is easy to understand why terms like "odd" or "weird" are soon applied to individuals who are MDD. Listeners usually lose patience with MDD speakers. Persons who are MDD rarely get to the point of what they are asked to tell. In the middle of telling, they jump track and start to talk about something that fascinates them, or something that occupies their imagination but has little or nothing to do with the subject at hand. They add so much irrelevant detail to their stories and scramble the sequence of events so often that others give up trying to listen.

As MDD individuals interact with others, they often misunderstand what others intend or mean. Persons with MDD tend to read too much meaning into what actually was said or done. This becomes a kind of perseveration that causes the brain to lock onto a minor issue and not turn it loose. The following chain of misunderstandings is typical of MDD:

MOTHER: "Jan, I want you to get ready to go to town with me. Come in the house and get cleaned up."

JAN: "Why are we going to town?"

MOTHER: "I have to buy some groceries, and we need to pick up our clothes at the cleaners."

JAN: "Why did you take groceries to the cleaners? Why didn't you take the groceries to the store?"

MOTHER: "Now don't start that with me, Jan. That isn't what I said."

JAN:	"Mom, why did you take the clothes to the grocery store? Did you take my blue dress? Why did you take my blue dress to the grocery store?"
MOTHER:	"I didn't take your blue dress anywhere, Jan. It's hanging in your closet."
JAN:	"I don't understand. Why did you take my blue dress to the grocery store? Why didn't you take it to the cleaners?"
MOTHER:	"Drop it, Jan. I'm not talking about your blue dress."
JAN:	"Mom, I don't understand. Why take my blue dress to the store? You know I need it to wear to Sunday school."
MOTHER:	"Oh, for heaven's sake, Jan! Drop it! Get ready to go to town with me."
JAN:	"But, Mom. I still don't understand. I need my blue dress for Sunday school. Why did you take it to the grocery store? Somebody might steal it, and I won't have it to wear Sunday."

Irregular Social Skills

This kind of sidetracking and perseverating when Jan misunderstands also occurs in social situations. For example, Jan came home from a birthday party to tell this story:

MOTHER:	"Did you have a good time at the party?"
JAN:	"No. I hated it. I don't know how to make a donkey."
MOTHER:	"What are you talking about, Jan? What do you mean, you don't know how to make a donkey?"
JAN:	"That's what I said. I can't make a donkey. And I hated that old party. It was boring. I don't know how to make a donkey. And the other kids started talking about me and laughing. I hate that old party!"

Jan's mother called the mom who had hosted the party. She learned that the children played the game Pin the Tail on the Donkey. Each child was given a paper tail and a pin. A blindfold was put over the child's eyes, and he or she had to guess where the tail should be pinned. Jan had made a big issue of putting on the blindfold. "She kept saying that she couldn't see how to make the donkey if her eyes were covered," the mother explained. "I didn't know what she meant. Finally Jan went off by herself to another room. Then it was time to cut the birthday cake." This misperception of a social event and the belief that others were talking about her are typical of MDD behavior.

Tag-Along Syndromes

Like most youngsters with MDD, Jan does not process social events in a normal way. Her great difficulty with the structure of language and the names of people, places, and things constantly trips her up as she tells about important events in her life. For example, for her 13th birthday, Jan's Uncle Carl took her to the wonderfully funny stage show *Joseph and the Amazing Technicolor Dreamcoat.* In her own way, Jan had a good time and could not wait to tell her grandmother: "We went to Joseph's many coat of colors," she reported. "And a week after that I'm going to camp." "That will be lots of fun," her grandmother said. "Do you have your things packed and ready to go?" "Well, I don't know about that," Jan replied. "I just have one duffle bag, and I don't think I can get two quarts of clothes in it."

MDD individuals do not read body language or social signals well enough to keep up with what goes on in social activities. The brain stem and midbrain do not filter and organize incoming data well enough to build accurate mental images. Persons like Jan fail to read facial expressions, body language, and gestures—physical clues that are essential for good communication. MDD individuals fail to pick up on subtle tones of voice that signal lighthearted teasing. They do not comprehend double entendres, the use of words that have double meanings. MDD persons live by literal, concrete meanings. They do not see or hear subtle variations in language and body posture. This causes them to miss the punch line in jokes and fail to see what is funny when laughter breaks out in the group. At social events, the MDD person is soon on the outside of the group and wanders off to do his or her own "weird" thing. MDD individuals often begin to daydream in the middle of a group activity. They become preoccupied with their own imagination and soon become unplugged from what the group is doing.

Struggle with Social Politeness

MDD individuals struggle with social politeness. They are unaware when they come too close, stand too close, or crowd others too much. Many MDD persons do not maintain eye contact, as most people do during conversation and active listening. Instead, they look away, glance around, and even turn to one side instead of looking into the speaker's face. An especially disruptive habit of most MDD individuals is their tendency to walk away during a conversation, or to get up and mill around the room during group discussions or classroom listening events. Persons like Jan do not learn how to keep secrets or be discreet about private information. They blurt out embarrassing comments or "news" with no sense that their comments are inappropriate.

A major problem for Jan's mother to handle is her daughter's unrealistic perception that she is popular among her classmates. Jan believes that everyone at school likes her and wants to be her best friend. In fact, her classmates think that she is "goofy" and "strange," and they avoid her whenever they can. This false belief that she is well liked leads Jan to spend much time on her cell phone calling classmates in the evening, thinking that they are glad to receive her call. The opposite is true. Several families have "caller ID" and don't answer the phone when they see Jan's name on the screen. Her long, rambling conversations seem to be pointless and "weird" to most of her classmates whom Jan thinks are her friends. A sad reality is that MDD individuals have few friends. A type of "social blindness" keeps Jan from understanding how to make or maintain friendships. She has no idea what social skills are required to share interests with others and treat others with respect.

Irregular Hygiene and Grooming

Partly to blame for not having friends is the MDD pattern of poor hygiene. Unless they are closely supervised and forced to practice personal hygiene, MDD individuals like Jan forget to brush their teeth, shower regularly, shampoo hair often enough, use deodorant, or change socks and underwear. Soon they offend others with bad breath and body odor, adding to their reputation for being "weird." MDD persons rarely have a good sense of choosing what to wear. Without supervision, they show up at school or social events wearing mismatched garments, or wearing things that are inappropriate. Many MDD individuals develop rituals in how they dress. They lock onto one or two favorite garments and refuse to wear anything else. It is not unusual to find individuals with MDD wearing the same shirt or blouse, the same jeans or sweatpants, or the same socks and underwear every day. They see nothing inappropriate in wearing worn-out sneakers to worship services or to a wedding. Ritual behavior includes odd or peculiar hairstyles. Many MDD individuals either pay no attention to the condition of their hair, or they stubbornly cling to outdated or bizarre hairstyles that attract teasing and criticism.

Disturbed Sensory Perception

MDD individuals often fail to perceive what goes on around them, or they may think that one thing occurred when the opposite actually happened. For example, Jan complains about loud noises when she is in large groups. She often covers her ears and begs for the loud noise to stop. Others nearby hear only low-level sounds and are bewildered by Jan's overreaction. Yet when she listens to music, she turns the volume up so high that everyone complains about the loudness of her music. After going shopping at the mall, Jan may complain for several hours about how loud all that noise was. Yet when her parents demand that she turn down the volume of her CD player, she insists that she can barely hear the music.

Since infancy, Jan has recoiled from being touched or hugged. "Oh!" she squeals. "You're hurting me!" Yet when she sees an adult cuddling her younger brother, she climbs onto the adult's lap, demanding to be hugged for several minutes.

Individuals like Jan often are phobic about having their heads under water during a shower or bath. This overreaction to water touching the hair triggers crying and shouting matches when adults insist the the child must bathe or shampoo. Yet Jan loves to go swimming and has a great time ducking her head under the water to blow bubbles. Likewise, MDD individuals often have panic attacks under bright lights, or when they see inflated balloons. It is not unusual for a hysterical emotional reaction to occur when Jan sees large areas painted in bold, bright colors or overly busy patterns in wallpaper or floor coverings. Yet she has decorated her room with vivid colors and always fills art projects with very busy patterns. The limbic system of the MDD individual cannot cope with certain types of stimulus from the environment without triggering excessive emotional reactions.

Irregular Motor Coordination

164

Many MDD individuals walk in a peculiar way that is more a shuffle than a stride. Body posture while sitting or standing often seems "odd." Arms hang or swing stiffly instead of in a normally relaxed way. Legs remain stiff while walking instead of flexing in normal rhythms. MDD persons tend to slouch instead of standing upright, both while walking and standing still. The body moves forward in a series of lurches instead of gliding forward with normal coordination. Most MDD individuals move along with a "weird" gait, more like loping than striding. Many persons with MDD develop eccentric rituals in the way they swing their arms, clasp and unclasp their hands, hunch their shoulders in circular motions, crane their necks again and again, or stamp their feet when they walk, as toddlers do instead of setting each foot down in a normal walking style.

It is not unusual to see MDD persons constantly looking to each side as they walk, as if expecting an attack from an enemy. This furtive, hunched posture causes them to lunge along in a pattern that attracts negative attention. At the same time, MDD individuals often make blowing noises with their lips or sucking sounds with teeth and tongue as they move about. They often develop habits of snorting through the nose while moving. These unusual habits brand these persons as "odd," "weird," "strange," or "peculiar."

Disturbed Emotional Expression

How the emotions are expressed is quite different in most individuals who are MDD. Emotional expression (called *affect*) follows different cycles than most people exhibit. For example, Jan rarely laughs, cries, or expresses affection when others do so. In family events or in the classroom, she remains outwardly passive and uninvolved in whatever emotions are flowing around her. At her grandmother's death, Jan did not cry or show any sign of grief. At class parties, she never joins in the robust laughter that often rocks the room. When a classmate is injured on the playground and several children begin to cry, Jan remains neutral and unemotional. However, at home she explodes emotionally over minor events that no one else thinks are important. "Mom, where is my pink sweater?" Jan calls out. "I don't know, Jan. Where did you put it yesterday?" Mom replies. Suddenly Jan bursts into tears and wails loudly: "You never help me find my stuff! You don't care if I lose my sweater!" Mom must stop what she is doing to take charge of this emotional situation so that Jan can finish getting ready for school. Her pink sweater was lying on her book bag, exactly where she laid it the night before. Not remembering where it was triggered a panic attack accompanied by sobs and excess emotion.

When Jan's grandmother died, she remained calm through the funeral proceedings. With dry eyes and no apparent emotion, she demanded answers to many misperceived issues about death and a funeral. However, two days after Grandmother's funeral, Jan became grief-stricken and inconsolable when she found a dead bird in the backyard. Her mother and father spent several hours guiding her through the grief that flared at the sight of a dead bird, but not at the experience of losing a beloved relative. Like many who are MDD, Jan tends to laugh at inappropriate moments. She rarely giggles or laughs when others are doing so, yet she disrupts movies and television shows by giggling and laughing in a "weird" way when someone is injured or abused. At school one day, a classmate suffered a broken arm in a playground accident. Jan burst into laughter that escalated out of control. Finally the teacher called her mother to come for her so the class could settle down from the accident.

Tag-Along Mood Disorders

> In diagnostic terms, interference with daily living is the critical line that separates personality from pathology.
>
> —Lucy Jo Palladino, in Hartmann, 2003, p. xiv

Central to the challenge of managing ADHD are cycles of mood swings that disrupt the individual's life. As Chapter 4 explained, ADD individuals tend to present the same passive mood most of the time. Most persons with ADHD are emotionally all over the place with no predictability from day to day of what moods to expect. Amen (2001), Andreason (2001), Barkley (1995), Jordan (1998, 2000a, 2000b, 2002), Restak (2002, 2003), Ratey and Johnson (1997), Weiss and Hechtmann (1993) and others have documented several mood disorder syndromes that are frequently found in the shadows of ADHD and ADD. Do attention deficit individuals with mood swings need medical or psychiatric intervention? Again we must consider the severity scale first seen in Chapter 2:

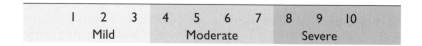

As a rule, individuals with mild or low moderate mood swing symptoms (Levels 4 or 5) would fit Lucy Jo Palladino's criteria of "not interfering with daily life." In most instances, these individuals can cope with mood changes if they are willing to accept advice from parents, teachers, friends, or job supervisors. Persons whose mood swings are above Level 5 require help through low-dosage medication, and diet modifications, which are described in Chapter 7.

Figure 6.2 presents the *Jordan Social-Emotional LD Mood Index,* which shows the range of emotions that often tag along with ADHD and ADD. An ideal balance of emotions (homeostasis) would be for a person's moods to stay steady over time between Levels 45 and 55 on this mood index. Normal fluctuations in body chemistry cause one's moods to rise or fall slightly, but always return to normal (Level 50). Individuals with ADHD tend to migrate from higher than normal happiness to lower than normal sadness. In determining when medical or psychiatric intervention is needed, we study the levels and duration of excess happiness (called *elation*) and sadness (called *depression*). If an underlying layer of long-lasting mood imbalance is not identified and treated, then other efforts to help ADHD or ADD individuals are not effective.

Balance of Optimism and Pessimism

In 1993, Vilayanur Ramachandran at the University of California in San Diego described how the right-brain and left-brain hemispheres work together to maintain emotional homeostasis, as described in Chapter 1. Ramachandran's research explained how the right brain "keeps the left brain honest" as the whole brain interprets emotions and feelings generated by events in our lives (Ramachandran, 1993). In a general way, the left brain regulates positive, optimistic emotions, feelings, and attitudes. As Chapter 2 explained, the left brain's executive function is cheerful, hopeful, and optimistic in looking ahead to what individuals should expect to happen next. In contrast, the right brain scans the environment to identify potentially harmful, unsafe events. Ramachandran sees the left brain as the optimistic brain whose talent is to urge "We can do it!" action. At the same time, the right brain is the pessimistic brain whose duty is to warn, "Not so fast. Let's be cautious." John Ratey and Catherine Johnson (1997) have described how the right brain uses its cautious/pessimistic point of view to balance the left brain's positive/optimistic feelings and emotions. A major characteristic of ADHD and ADD is lack of balance between higher and lower emotions and feelings. In Chapter 5 we met Kim and James, whose lives were chaotic because of lack of left-brain/right-brain homeostatis.

Manic/Depressive Disorder

Figure 6.2 shows the extreme range of a destructive mood swing disorder generally called *Manic/Depressive Illness* or *Bipolar Disorder*. This disruptive, sometimes life-threatening syndrome often hides beneath the hyperfocused surface of ADHD. Like Kim and James, many ADHD individuals live on an emotional roller coaster that swings them unwillingly from normally balanced emotions to soaring, frightening heights of elation, then downward to dark, sorrowful depths of depression. Figure 6.2 shows the subtypes of this form of mental illness, one that greatly complicates the lives of many individuals who are ADHD or ADD.

Bipolar I (Manic/Depressive) Disorder

As Figure 6.2 shows, there are several subtypes of manic/depressive syndrome. Bipolar I designates the roller-coaster form of this disorder that takes the individual up and down the mood swing ladder in cycles that change as time goes by. When Bipolar I symptoms swing up and down between Levels 30 and 70 on the mood index, the individual can manage to function in the classroom, at home, on the job, and in personal relationships. When Bipolar I symptoms swing below Level 30 and above Level 70, the individual must have medical intervention that stops excessive high and low mood swings so that the person's moods stay closer to normal (Level 50). Before Bipolar I is diagnosed and treated, most ADHD individuals with this tag-along syndrome often are beyond the reach of parents, teachers, job supervisors, or life partners.

The Range of Moods that Often Accompany ADHD, ADD, Dyslexia, and LD

Jordan Social–Emotional LD Mood Index

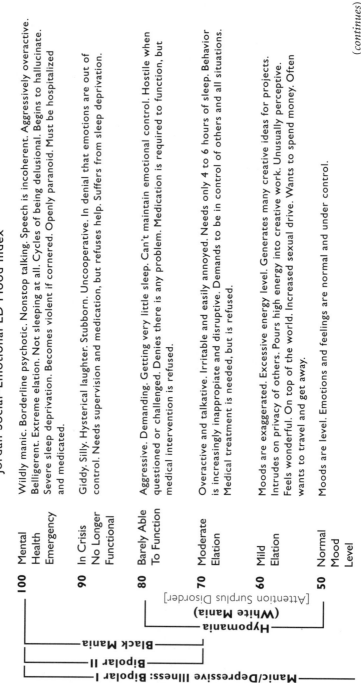

100	Mental Health Emergency	Wildly manic. Borderline psychotic. Nonstop talking. Speech is incoherent. Aggressively overactive. Belligerent. Extreme elation. Not sleeping at all. Cycles of being delusional. Begins to hallucinate. Severe sleep deprivation. Becomes violent if cornered. Openly paranoid. Must be hospitalized and medicated.
90	In Crisis No Longer Functional	Giddy. Silly. Hysterical laughter. Stubborn. Uncooperative. In denial that emotions are out of control. Needs supervision and medication, but refuses help. Suffers from sleep deprivation.
80	Barely Able To Function	Aggressive. Demanding. Getting very little sleep. Can't maintain emotional control. Hostile when questioned or challenged. Denies there is any problem. Medication is required to function, but medical intervention is refused.
70	Moderate Elation	Overactive and talkative. Irritable and easily annoyed. Needs only 4 to 6 hours of sleep. Behavior is increasingly inappropriate and disruptive. Demands to be in control of others and all situations. Medical treatment is needed, but is refused.
60	Mild Elation	Moods are exaggerated. Excessive energy level. Generates many creative ideas for projects. Intrudes on privacy of others. Pours high energy into creative work. Unusually perceptive. Feels wonderful. On top of the world. Increased sexual drive. Wants to spend money. Often wants to travel and get away.
50	Normal Mood Level	Moods are level. Emotions and feelings are normal and under control.

[Attention Surplus Disorder]
(White Mania)
Hypomania
Black Mania
Bipolar II
Manic/Depressive Illness: Bipolar I

(continues)

FIGURE 6.2. This wide range of mood disorders often coexists with ADHD, ADD, and dyslexia, or LD. Mood swings usually are part of the learning

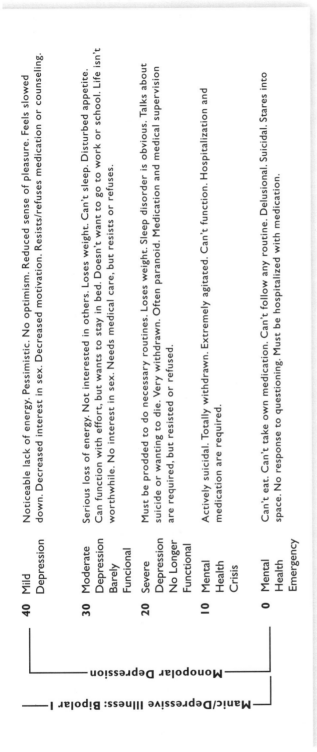

40	Mild Depression	Noticeable lack of energy. Pessimistic. No optimism. Reduced sense of pleasure. Feels slowed down. Decreased interest in sex. Decreased motivation. Resists/refuses medication or counseling.
30	Moderate Depression Barely Functional	Serious loss of energy. Not interested in others. Loses weight. Can't sleep. Disturbed appetite. Can function with effort, but wants to stay in bed. Doesn't want to go to work or school. Life isn't worthwhile. No interest in sex. Needs medical care, but resists or refuses.
20	Severe Depression No Longer Functional	Must be prodded to do necessary routines. Loses weight. Sleep disorder is obvious. Talks about suicide or wanting to die. Very withdrawn. Often paranoid. Medication and medical supervision are required, but resisted or refused.
10	Mental Health Crisis	Actively suicidal. Totally withdrawn. Extremely agitated. Can't function. Hospitalization and medication are required.
0	Mental Health Emergency	Can't eat. Can't take own medication. Can't follow any routine. Delusional. Suicidal. Stares into space. No response to questioning. Must be hospitalized with medication.

Monopolar Depression

Manic/Depressive Illness: Bipolar I

FIGURE 6.2. *Continued.*

Tag-Along Syndromes

The day I met 14-year-old Carlos was like standing in the wind blasts of a hurricane. His totally frustrated mother brought him to my office half an hour early for our appointment. She shoved her screaming son into my reception room and fled to her workplace. I came out of my office to confront an extremely angry, hostile adolescent who had no intention of cooperating with me that day. I stopped several feet away from Carlos and looked at him without speaking. He snarled like a trapped lion: "I hate being here! You can't make me do anything!" He was surprised when I absorbed his anger without responding. In a classic act of defiance, he folded his arms across his chest and glared at me. "I mean it!" he yelled. "You can't make me do anything!" I caught him off guard by saying nothing. Like most angry youngsters, his strategy was to engage me in a verbal fight that would let him control the situation. When I refused to fight back, he had no alternative plan of action.

For several minutes we stared at each other, then I smiled. Carlos was shocked. "You can't make me!" he declared again, but he dropped his arms and stuffed his fists into his pockets. I smiled again. By this time, Carlos was too bewildered to keep on being angry. "Let's find someplace to sit down," I said as I turned away. To show me that he had not been conquered, Carlos stomped his feet as he followed me into my office. He was surprised by what he saw. Nothing looked like school or like a doctor's office. Everywhere Carlos looked, he saw a quiet, comfortable place he recognized as being safe.

I sat at my large round table and smiled again. A dish of candy and chewing gum stood in the middle of the table. He watched me unwrap a piece of gum. Without a word, Carlos grabbed a piece of candy, then flopped down on the giant beanbag across the room from the table. "I don't want to be here," he grumbled quietly. His anger was gone. "I know you don't want to be here," I said, as I sat on the floor near the beanbag. "But I also know that you don't want to be at school. Why not?"

As if a dam had burst on a lake, I listened to a torrent of emotional pain and anger as Carlos spewed out his misery toward school, his parents, and all the "weird kids" who hated him. It was the first time in his life that an adult had listened to his feelings without interrupting or criticizing him. Finally he felt safe enough with me to let me inside his carefully guarded emotional fortress. When I asked Carlos why he had such strong negative feelings, he burst into tears and sobbed on his arm for several minutes. Through his sobs he spit out enough words to let me understand. "I can't read … Can't spell … I'm stupid … Hate school … Makes me feel so dumb … Kids are mean to me … Everyone hates me … Life sucks!" It was mid-morning before Carlos's emotions were calm. Finally when his anger was gone, he began to talk about himself. He described how sometimes he went crazy and climbed onto the roof of his home and tried to fly to a tall tree across the street. Several times he had climbed to the top of the city water tower and wondered what it would be like to jump 100 feet to the ground. Then he told me of times when he felt so sad he hid at the back of his closet with a blanket over his head. Several times he had run away from home to get even with his parents when they punished him. Many times he refused to get out of bed for two or three days on end. Finally he hid his face in his hands and whispered: "I'm crazy. I've never said this to anyone before, but I'm crazy. I'm no good, and I'm crazy."

Carlos had released the pent-up anger he had carried for many years. Finally he was ready to do some work with me. "Promise you won't make fun of my writing," he begged. "I'm a lousy writer. It drives my parents nuts when I make an F on spelling tests." I let Carlos lie on the beanbag to do some simple writing. I asked him to write the alphabet, days of the week, and months of the year. "That's a dumb thing to do!" he said. I agreed that for a person his age this might seem like a dumb thing to do. "But it will help me answer some important questions about why school is hard for you," I said. With a shrug, he wrote what is shown in Figure 6. 3. "I hated doing that," he said. "It makes me feel stupid."

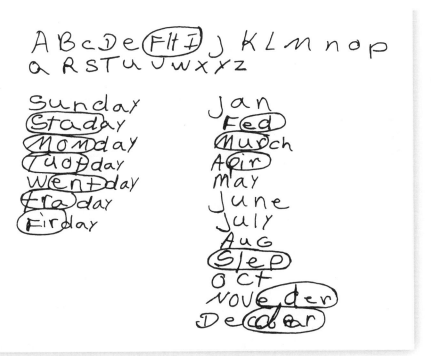

FIGURE 6.3. Carlos struggled hard to write the alphabet, days of the week, and months of the year. All his life adults had critized him for being "lazy," "a sloppy writer," "careless," and "not trying hard enough." In fact, this is an example of the best he could do because of undiagnosed dyslexia.

Tag-Along Syndromes

By then Carlos and I had been together for two hours. He paced my large office, looking at everything in the room. My office was filled with pictures, sculptures, and other pieces of handmade art. I explained that each art piece was a gift made by someone who had spent time with me. I told Carlos that all of this art was done by intelligent students who had found out about themselves by working with me. Finally I asked if he would let me find out how intelligent he was. "I told you I'm stupid!" he flared at me. "I told you I'm dumb!" "What if I find out you're actually very bright?" I asked. With a sneer, he said: "You can't do that!" "Yes," I replied. "I think I can." Reluctantly, Carlos decided that it would be OK. We spent another hour working through the *Wechsler Intelligence Scale for Children–Revised* (WISC–R; Wechsler, 1974). He was stunned when I showed him the results: Verbal IQ 124; Performance IQ 132; Full Scale IQ 130.

Carlos sat down on the beanbag and stared at me. Then his eyes filled with tears. "You're not joking me, are you?" he asked. Suddenly he rolled onto his stomach and beat the floor with his fists. "I've spent my whole life feeling stupid! You don't know how much I've hurt feeling so dumb! Now you tell me I'm very intelligent. This makes me so mad! Why didn't anyone ever tell me this before?"

Just then my receptionist rang to tell me that Mr. Santos was there to take Carlos home. "I don't want to leave," he said. "I want to stay here. Can't you tell my dad that you need me to stay this afternoon? I'll do a lot more work. Just tell him I need to stay."

In Chapter 5 we saw James Gilligan's model of "resurrection of self-esteem." For the first time in his school experience, Carlos had received unconditional acceptance, proof of his intelligence, and affectionate encouragement. As Gilligan demonstrated in his work with violent individuals, removing the toxic influence of shame brings new life to crushed self-esteem. That morning with me had been the first experience of joy that Carlos could remember. At last he had tasted unconditional success, and he was famished for much, much more.

My work with Carlos yielded multiple diagnoses of ADHD, dyslexia, and symptoms of bipolar mood disorder. He was fascinated to learn these facts about why he struggled with reading and writing skills in the classroom. An intuitive psychiatrist diagnosed Carlos as having severe Bipolar I Manic/Depressive Disorder. Soon they discovered the right balance of SSRI medication and a cortical stimulant (see Chapter 7). The wide mood swings disappeared at the same time the ADHD "noise" was eliminated, allowing Carlos to become a high-achieving student with modifications for dyslexia. Today at age 31, he is finishing his doctorate in clinical psychology. "You're getting to be an old man," he says each time he visits me. "I want to take your place helping kids like me."

Bipolar II: Hypomanic Personality

Figure 6.2 shows clusters of mood disorders that trap the feelings and emotions of many ADHD individuals toward the top of the mood scale. When an individual's emotions and feelings remain over time at Levels 60 and 70 on the mood index, a condition called *hypomania* takes charge of the person's life. This mood disorder also is called *white mania*. At this manic level of emotional intensity, hypomania is a disruptive disorder that cripples creative individuals with unfortunate emotional limitations. In her book *An Unquiet Mind*, Kay Jamison (1995) describes her lifelong challenge with hypomania:

> I simply did not want to believe that I needed to take medication. I had become addicted to my high moods; I had become dependent upon their intensity, euphoria, assuredness, and their infectious ability to induce high moods and enthusiasms in other people.... I found my milder manic states powerfully inebriating and very conducive to productivity. I couldn't give them up. (pp. 98–99)

Ratey and Johnson (1997) point out that white mania, or hypomania, allows individuals to feel "better than normal." During hypomanic cycles, persons think more rapidly than those who are in the normal range of emotional range (Level 50 on the mood index). In this state, individuals are more creative, and they score higher on IQ tests. During their white mania cycles, persons are friendlier, more fun to be with for brief periods of time, and more productive, enjoying cascades of fresh, new ideas. As Kay Jamison writes, it is very hard for anyone to give up these positive qualities in order to become "normal." In fact, those who experience hypomanic cycles rationalize why they do not need to change. They correctly argue that even though they are somewhat giddy and even silly, they do not become paranoid, as Bipolar II persons often do. They are never delusional, as Bipolar II individuals often are. They never need to be hospitalized for dangerous mood swings, and their white mania seldom destroys life or property through high-risk behavior.

This state of elation can be highly productive as creative ideas flow from the overly aroused noisy brain that never stops talking to itself. However, in spite of the continual flow of new ideas, individuals with hypomania often fail to succeed unless others can turn the flow of new ideas into reality. Hypomanic ideas are too loose and too poorly organized to follow through to completion. Adults with hypomania bombard their environments with hyperfocused behaviors that "drive others to distraction," as Hallowell and Ratey (1994a) have described it. Often it is impossible for hypomanic persons to manage a business, hold a marriage together, stay in school, or maintain good relationships with children and other relatives. Hypomania is so disruptive that others look for ways to avoid or get away from these aggressive individuals. Persons with hypomania actually are bullies, demanding to be in control of everyone and everything in their lives. They develop complex systems of control techniques that range from weeping in order to wear others down through guilt to furious tantrums that force others to agree just to have peace. As a child on my grandmother's farm, I learned the meaning of a bit of rural wisdom: "A dog can lick a skunk, but it ain't worth it." Those who must deal with hypomanic individuals give in rather than fight such controlling pressures. Winning such a battle of wits is not worth the emotional price one must pay to do so.

In separating the layer of hypomania from ADHD, diagnosticians look for seven major patterns that set white mania apart:

1. *Exaggerated self-esteem (grandiosity).* The hypomanic personality struts and prances with inflated ego and self-importance. This is self-advertisement on a grand scale. Outsiders see a person who is vain and arrogant, but who nonetheless is successful enough to be worthy of respect. The hypomanic personality is self-centered. This individual uses others without respecting the worth of others. In describing themselves in autobiographical sketches or during public presentations, persons in white mania cycles exalt themselves with grandiose phrases and exaggerated terms. They take credit for accomplishments that were achieved by others. Yet this self-centered individual displays a charismatic aura that attracts the loyalty of others. Hypomanic persons inspire followers to overlook the arrogant, self-focused lifestyle of the person who has placed self on an egotistical pedestal.

2. *Reduced need for sleep.* Individuals in white mania cycles have little need for sleep. It is not unusual for these high-energy persons to be wide awake again after three or four hours of rest. During these charged-up cycles, hypomanic individuals make phone calls at inappropriate times, waking others during normal hours of sleep or calling too early in the morning or too late in the evening. In the early part of the 20th century, Jimmy Durante, a famous comedian who rarely slept, rationalized to friends for his middle-of-the-night intrusions: "When Durante is awake, no bird sleeps." This hypomanic disregard for sleep often becomes a disruptive factor that strains relationships to the breaking point.

3. *Nonstop talking.* The impulse to keep on talking is called *hyperlexia.* Individuals with hypomanic personality are dreaded because of their habit of talking nonstop. Every thought the brain develops, no matter how trivial, is uttered in spoken words. Hyperlexic persons can-

not stop conversing, commenting, lecturing, or explaining. Even when they have nothing important to say, they say something to fill moments of silence. This hyperlexic tendency exerts verbal pressure in all situations. The manic speech flow interrupts sermons, classroom lectures, movies, and television viewing. Hypomanic persons constantly are on the telephone. They carry cell phones and pagers everywhere they go. They choose not to turn off their cell phones during concerts, worship services, or watching movies for fear of missing someone's call. They talk on their cell phones as they drive on busy streets and highways. They cannot refrain from making and receiving phone calls during restaurant meals or while standing in line at the airport or fast-food counter. Hypomanic individuals tend to become addicted to chat room communication on the Internet. They talk to the computer screen as they read messages. They replace speech with keyboarding as they spend hours interacting with others over the Internet. Nonstop talking from hyperlexic individuals drives everyone else "nuts." This characteristic of white mania is highly disruptive and soon triggers resentment and rejection from others.

4. *Racing thoughts and mental images.* Hypomanic individuals cannot keep their thoughts and mental images from racing. They often have the feeling that their brains are like a stock car race that never stops. This mental racing goes on and on, even during sleep. During white mania cycles, these persons find themselves pacing the floor rapidly, trying to keep up with racing mental images. Speech soon lags behind ideas that are speeding in the brain. Successful hypomanic persons develop a type of shorthand writing that lets them scribble chunks of ideas before the racing brain leaves important thoughts behind. It is not unusual to see these individuals whisper rapidly into a cassette recorder to preserve the good ideas their racing brains create.

5. *Distractibility.* It is impossible for hypomanic individuals to ignore what goes on around them. This intense awareness of one's surroundings is called *hyperfocus.* Eyes dart around to see what is happening or who is going by. Ears pick up every sound. The nose whiffs every odor. Internally, the racing brain hums to itself, talks to itself, and darts off on mental rabbit trails as memories are triggered by nearby events. The hypomanic brain cannot go from start to finish without becoming sidetracked. Too many side trails beckon with interesting things to be explored. Eye contact is lost, even when the person earnestly wants to listen. Sentences are left unfinished as the voice shifts to another topic. Tasks are left incomplete as cascades of new interests take the hypomanic attention elsewhere.

6. *Fixation on goal-directed activity.* In spite of being easily distracted, a major social problem of hypomania is the intensity of going after spe-

cific objectives. The hypomanic person is highly goal-directed, but these goals tend to be very narrow in focus. This goal-directed intensity quickly becomes obsessive. For example, at 4:30 P.M. the hypomanic boss decides that everyone in the office must go to dinner together tonight. With that single goal in mind, he or she starts an obsessive string of activities that must be handled now: Where should we go for dinner? Can we all get there by 6:30 P.M.? Everyone make arrangements to be part of the dinner group. Marge, get a babysitter. Joe, cancel your committee meeting on the church board. Dave and Flo, hurry the last office appointments so everyone is gone by 5:30. This flurry of unexpected activity places heavy stress on the office staff who had other plans for the evening, especially Marge, a single parent with two preschool children in daycare. The hypomanic boss is totally insensitive to the consequences of this intrusion into the private lives of his or her staff. The goal of everyone going to dinner tonight is the only issue of importance, regardless of incovenience to others.

7. *Compulsive high-pleasure activities regardless of consequences.* Hypomanic persons tend to forget responsibility as they indulge themselves in activities that yield high pleasure, regardless of consequences. The individual may go on an exciting shopping spree that adds thousands of dollars to credit card debt. It makes no difference that the person's financial position is close to bankruptcy. A hypomanic businessperson might go ahead with a high-risk investment in spite of urgent warnings from financial advisors. A married individual might get caught up in a spur-of-the-moment sexual affair with the spouse of a close friend because hormones are running high during this white mania episode. This is often called the "Scarlett O'Hara syndrome" after the famous moment in *Gone With the Wind* when the impulsive Scarlett says, "I'll think about that tomorrow. After all, tomorrow is another day."

Hypomanic personality imitates ADHD in several important ways: impulsivity, distractibility, racing thoughts, self-focus, short attention span, and hyperlexia. When ADHD overlaps white mania, it often is impossible to separate the syndromes completely. By itself, the ADHD personality is not arrogant or grandiose. ADHD individuals seldom devise schemes to use others. In fact, when persons with ADHD focus on the needs of others, they tend to be overly generous, truly wanting to help. Those with ADHD tend to be open to guidance on how to do better. When all the plugs stay in, the intelligence behind ADHD allows persons to achieve surprising goals. ADHD does not come and go in cycles. It is a constant factor, although attention deficits tend to diminish in severity as physical maturity takes place.

Bipolar II: Black Mania

The upper end of the mood index is called *Bipolar II: Black Mania* because of the severity of out-of-control emotions and feelings. In *An Unquiet Mind* Kay Jamison describes the terrifying mental state of black mania:

> Both my manias and depression had violent sides to them ... Being wildly out of control—physically assaultive, screaming insanely at the top of [my] lungs, running frequently with no purpose or limit, or impulsively trying to leap from [moving] cars.... I have, in my black, agitated manias destroyed things I cherish, pushed to the utter edge people I love, and survived to think I could never recover from the shame.... (p. 120)

The possibility of accidental suicide is a major concern for individuals who are in a state of black mania. As Jamison describes, she had irrational impulses to leap from moving vehicles. Numerous adolescents and adults I have counseled have described finding themselves at the top of water towers, on rooftops, on tall bridges, or at the edge of high cliffs about to jump. They were not trying to die. In their delusional Bipolar II state, they imagined that they could fly or "leap to the moon." Many high-speed, single-vehicle accidents occur when the driver is in a delusional black mania state. The driver imagines that the vehicle can fly over an approaching river, leap over a looming highway overpass, or pass under the bed of a truck.

The traffic problem of road rage often involves Bipolar II delusions. Recently a near-fatal road rage episode occurred near our home. An enormous truck-and-trailer rig was hauling several 2-ton coils of rolled steel. A much smaller pickup truck passed the large rig, then moved into the right lane ahead of the truck. This move triggered rage in the trucker's brain. Later he explained that he imagined the pickup truck driver had yelled insults as he "cut me off" in traffic. In his black mania state, the rig driver accelerated to 100 miles per hour and chased the pickup truck down the highway. Horrified drivers pulled onto the shoulder as the enraged trucker pursued his imagined persecutor. Finally, the large truck crashed into an overpass bridge rail. A 2-ton coil of steel dropped onto the highway below the overpass, destroying a section of the road while narrowly missing a passing vehicle. Later it was learned that the truck driver was under the influence of stimulants to keep him awake. He had no memory of driving 100 miles per hour or of chasing the smaller vehicle.

The violent mood swings of Bipolar II Black Mania pose a threat to the afflicted individual and to anyone nearby. At one end of this spectrum is the dark cavern of sorrow and grief that makes the person want to die. At the opposite end of this spectrum is the extreme state of giddy elation that makes the person want to jump over tall buildings, fly to the moon, or run over an imagined enemy on the highway. During deep depression, the individual is so withdrawn into a private emotional world that he or she cannot function as a member of the family, the workplace, or the classroom. At this level of emotion, death becomes a strongly attractive option that would stop the tortures of these terrifying mood swings. During manic elation, the individual reaches a state of mind often called madness. The manically out-of-control individual cannot function on the job, at home, in learning situations, or in personal relationships. Accidental suicide or violent death frequently mark the early end of life for individuals during black mania cycles. In this emotional state, they lose all sense of danger and engage in high-risk activities. When ADHD is part of the Bipolar II equation, life often becomes so out of control that the person must be hospitalized for his or her own protection.

Chronic Depression and ADD

A different kind of excessive emotion frequently tags along with ADD. Long-lasting, ongoing depression below Level 30 on the mood index is called *monopolar depression*. When ADD is mild, depression also tends to be mild. Individuals with ADD below Level 5 on the severity scale tend to live with sadness that does not diminish through mood-lifting cycles. This constant sadness is like fog over a landscape. It is expressed quietly through sighing and sad, wishful thinking that often appears in drawings or sorrow-tinged poetry and stories. This mild depression that lingers in the shadow of ADD is not dangerous. There is little thought of dying. This form of depression centers more on the disappointment of unfulfilled desires. Fantasy images surrounding mild depression are of sad events or sad imaginary characters whose wishes never come true. Nighttime dreams center around themes of loneliness or being abandoned, but not of frightful events. This level of depression seldom expresses itself in crying. Instead of having a normal balance between optimism and pessimism, these individuals live with an excess of sadness, which causes them to interpret life pessimistically.

As ADD symptoms move above Level 5 on the severity scale, the level of depression tends to increase. An ADD person at Level 6 to 7 on the severity scale tends to live with high moderate depression, shown at Level 30 on the mood index in Figure 6.2. In the same way that high moderate ADD interferes with academic learning or job performance, this level of sadness interferes with emotional well-being. High moderate depression involves active daydreams of a sad, pessimistic nature. This individual seeps tears that often surprise outsiders. Why is Aaron crying? In this state of high moderate depression, Aaron does not sob, yet tears often stream down his face during class time, family events, and especially when he is alone. As he stays alone for long periods of time, Aaron wonders about the blessings of death he has heard adults describe when older persons have "gone to heaven." Wouldn't it be better if he could go to heaven, too? In heaven he would not be lonely or sad. He could be with his grandparents who used to love him so much. As Aaron's thoughts shift to school, his sadness is heavy inside his chest because he feels left out. He never is chosen for playground teams. Teachers rarely select him to do popular things like carry a note to the office or lead the class to lunch. When Aaron thinks of his family, he focuses on the many moments when adults reprimand him for being forgetful, or losing his things, or not making better grades. As these sorrowful daydream images capture his attention, Aaron begins to weep silently. "Life is so sad," he thinks with a deep sigh as tears drip down his cheeks.

Children who grow up with these invisible feelings rarely attract enough adult attention to receive help. It is not unusual for youngsters like Aaron to pass through childhood, adolescence, and into adulthood without the underlying chronic depression being recognized or healed. Adults tend to focus on the ADD patterns presented in the ADD checklist in Chapter 4 without seeing the tag-along layer of depression. ADD individuals with lifelong depression often keep their chronic sadness a secret.

Severe ADD tends to come with the tag-along layer of severe depression. When ADD is above Level 7 on the severity scale, depression tends to hover around Level 20 on the mood index. This excess of negative, pessimistic feeling robs the individual of hope. There is no hope of making good grades, or of being happy like everyone else. There is no hope of having friends, being elected team captain, or being a popular leader of the class. There is no hope that parents will stop nagging and scolding about forgetfulness, laziness, and other shortcomings. At this point of hopelessness, the ADD person with severe depression wants to die. Thoughts of death permeate daydreams, imagination, fantasy thinking, and nighttime dreams. Severely depressed ADD individuals speculate on how they might die. Daydreams are filled with detailed plans for how death might be accomplished. Fantasy thinking builds imaginary scenarios in which the person who has died watches relatives at the funeral and overhears what they say. When this level of sorrowful emotion is reached, suicide becomes increasingly likely. Feelings of sadness and grief become intense. Individuals at this level of depression live with a frightening tightness of the chest, as if hands were squeezing the heart and lungs. They become short of breath with heart racing and blood pressure soaring. Yet these depressed individuals rarely reach out to anyone for help. They suffer in silence, victimized by daydreams of dying and nightmares of death. Alone, they sob into the pillow, or muffle sounds of weeping under a blanket. This extremely private suffering is commonly described by ADD individuals who survive suicide attempts and at last find a compassionate counselor who understands.

The Devastation of Shame and Depression

At the heart of chronic depression is the corrosive presence of shame. Persistent depression distorts emotional reality so that it becomes impossible for the person to be realistic about his or her self-worth. Like a constant voice in the background, depression whispers the litany of shame: "You're dumb. You're ugly. No one likes you or wants to be around you. There's no use trying because you will fail anyway. No one loves you because you're so worthless." This destructive emotional litany saturates the individual's self-image with shame. As shame takes deeper root in the person's thoughts and feelings, hope dies. This severe depression steeped in shame snuffs out any hope that life ever will improve.

I met Mark soon after he entered 10th grade. At age 16, he was the most shame-filled, deeply depressed person I had ever seen. He never had done well in school, in spite of continual encouragement and support from his parents. His school years had been so miserable that he grew up thinking about how to kill himself. Only his intense fear of going to Hell kept him from attempting suicide. By third grade he had become withdrawn, sullen, and angry. No matter how hard his parents and teachers tried to cheer him up and encourage him, Mark's attitude snarled back: "Leave me alone!" He entered high school with few academic skills, no friends, no hope, and a constant wish to die. A few weeks after he entered 10th grade, one of Mark's teachers took special interest in this lonely, withdrawn student. With exceptional intuition and kindness, she looked beneath his sullen surface and saw signs of language disability and deep sadness. She convinced Mark's parents to have their son evaluated for possible learning disability and emotional problems.

Mark entered my office sandwiched between his parents, who walked beside him as human shields, protecting him from the world that he perceived to be threatening and unfriendly. Mark sat between his mom and dad around my circular conference table. At age 16 he was 6 feet, 5 inches tall, with an athletic build and such a handsome face he reminded me of several movie stars. In that first meeting, he scarcely spoke, and he avoided eye contact with me. His mother did most of the talking on his behalf. I learned that as Mark reached age 15, he had begun to talk openly about wanting to die. He had stopped trying to do school assignments unless his mother was by his side. He no longer attended religious services with his family. When visitors came, he shut himself in his room. He avoided all school events, and he refused to read. He spent many hours sitting before his television with the sound turned off.

As Mark's parents and I talked quietly, he began to glance at me, then quickly look away. Whenever I spoke his name, he looked my way but refused to make eye contact. He sat with head bowed, hands folded tightly in his lap, and body stiff in a rigid posture. As our conference continued, I saw Mark's body begin to relax. Finally his posture was normal, and he separated his hands in a comfortable way. He listened intently to what his parents and I discussed, but he did not take part in our conversation except to nod "yes" or shake his head "no."

I was surprised when Mark agreed to come again so that he and I could work alone. During our first private visit, he chose to sit beside me close enough to let our arms touch now and then. I placed a tablet and pencil on the table and asked him to write the alphabet, days of the week, and months of the year. Figure 6.4 shows his work. As he wrote, I noticed that his face became flushed and he was breathing harder. I asked if he would mind writing some words I would dictate. He said it would be OK.

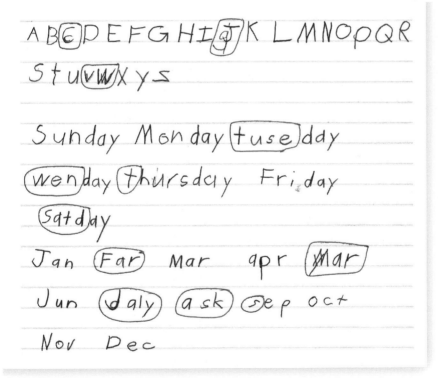

FIGURE 6.4. This was the best that 16-year-old Mark could do writing the alphabet, days of the week, and months of the year. He entered high school struggling at this level of encoding dysfunction. The layers of undiagnosed dyslexia and chronic depression had crushed his self-esteem and self-confidence.

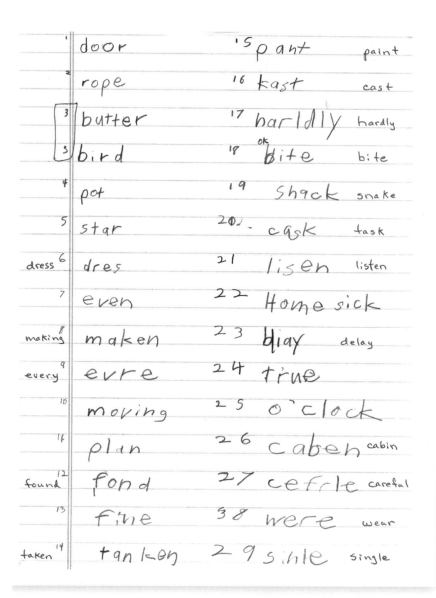

1. door
2. rope
3. butter
3. bird
4. pot
5. star
dress 6. dres
7. even
making 8. maken
every 9. evre
10. moving
11. plin
found 12. pond
13. fine
taken 14. tanken

15. pant — paint
16. kast — cast
17. hardly — hardly
18. bite (ok) — bite
19. shack — snake
20. cask — task
21. lisen — listen
22. Home sick
23. dlay — delay
24. true
25. o'clock
26. cabeh — cabin
27. cefrle — careful
38. were — wear
29. sihle — single

FIGURE 6.5. This dictated spelling activity triggered a panic attack that dropped Mark to his knees with chest pain. He was deeply humiliated when his third-grade literacy skills were revealed by this activity.

Figure 6.5 shows the dyslexic patterns that emerged during those encoding (writing) activities.

As Mark finished writing the last word, he was trembling. His eyes were filled with tears, and he was breathing rapidly with shallow gulps for air.

Suddenly he cried out and clutched at his chest. To my surprise, he fell to his knees and bowed his head low. I knelt beside him and encircled his shoulders with my arms. "I'm having a heart attack!" Mark choked. "No, Mark," I said. "You aren't having a heart attack. You're having a panic attack that makes your chest feel tight." Slowly he relaxed in my embrace, then he began to cry. "I'm so ashamed!" he sobbed over and over. "I'm so ashamed! I can't do anything right!" I held him for several minutes while his sobs released the tension that had triggered those physical signals of too much emotional stress.

When Mark was relaxed again, we talked about times when such panic attacks occurred. "They started when I was in third grade," he remembered. "I was so ashamed. I knew I was stupid because I couldn't do anything the other kids could do. I didn't tell anyone about my attacks because I was afraid they would make me go to a doctor. But all my life, sometimes it drops me to my knees and makes me feel like I'm about to die. It hurts so much. And I'm all alone and nobody knows what's happening to me. I'm too ashamed to let them know how dumb and stupid I am."

Finally Mark was ready to sit at the table again. "What's wrong with me, doc?" he asked. "I know I'm dumb, but why can't I learn to read and spell like everybody else?" I showed Mark several maps of the brain, and we talked about where emotions and feelings come from and how the brain learns and thinks. He was fascinated with that straightforward information about himself. Then we talked about dyslexia and how it made reading, writing, and spelling so hard and fearful for him. We also talked about his lifelong difficulties keeping his attention focused without drifting off into daydreams. "Will I ever get over all this?" he asked. I explained that a certain kind of medication called antidepressant, and another kind of medication called cortical stimulant, might help his brain chemistry become balanced. He agreed to see a psychiatrist who specialized in treating mood disorders and attention deficits in adolescents.

That doctor was himself moderately ADD and dyslexic. Mark could not believe that a doctor could be so understanding. After taking his new medications for two weeks, he came to see me again. Mark entered my office with a broad smile. Then he laughed. Suddenly he lifted me off the floor in a huge embrace while he laughed and chuckled. Finally he put me down so we could talk. "I'm like a new guy," he said with a twinkle of joy in his eyes. "My brain works better than it ever did before. I've decided that life isn't so bad, after all. I had no idea that this is the way most people feel all the time."

Mark had experienced Gilligan's "resurrection of self-esteem" described in Chapter 5. With his feelings of depression transformed into new hope and self-confidence, Mark could not wait to finish finding out about himself. He was eager for me to evaluate his intelligence. I have seldom seen such intellectual excitement as we worked through the *Wechsler Adult Intelligence Scale* (WAIS; Wechsler, 1974). Figure 6.6 shows Mark's very wide subscore

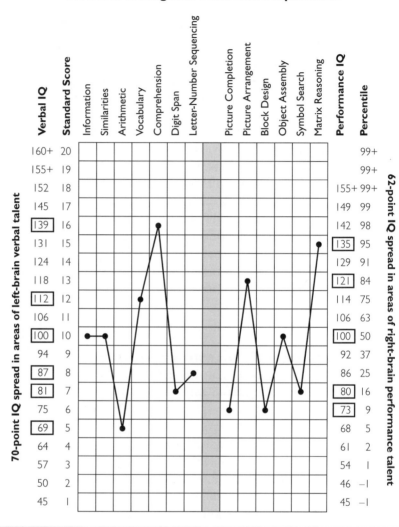

Wechsler Intelligence Scale Score Equivalents

FIGURE 6.6. After Mark's self-confidence had been increased, he was ready to work through the *Wechsler Intelligence Scale for Adults, Revised* (WAIS–R). He was astonished to discover that his highest areas of intelligence ranked him within the very superior range of mental ability. He always had believed that he was "dumb" because of his dyslexic struggle with literacy tasks. This kind of very wide spread between top and bottom scores indicates underlying learning difficulty (LD) that interferes with classroom performance.

Overcoming Attention Deficit Disorders in Children, Adolescents, and Adults

scatter that usually signals ADD, dyslexia, or both. He was intrigued as I explained the concept of different neurological talents. He touched his IQ profile, feeling the high IQ areas as well as the lower IQ subtests. "So this is why I've never felt good at school," he said quietly. "I just thought I was too dumb to learn. I've always been so ashamed of being dumb. Now I guess I'll have to change my mind about myself." For the first time in his life, through correct medication and frank information about himself, Mark experienced the joy of emotional peace. He rapidly caught up in academic learning and later earned a university degree in computer science.

High Functioning Autism

> When I was a child, the ringing school bell hurt my ears like a dentist's drill hitting a nerve.... If there is too much background noise, I cannot hear what's happening in the foreground. Constant noise is very tiring for people with sensory oversensitivity. A sound that would be small to a normal person may sound like a blast to a person with autism.... I know one college student who is driven to distraction because she can see the sixty-cycle flicker of the fluorescent lights and can hear the electric wiring humming in the walls.... Tactile oversensitivity is another problem that is shared by people with autism and ADHD. Scratchy petticoats rubbed my nerve endings raw. It was like having coarse sandpaper in my underwear. As a child I could not understand why [others] ... tolerated the scratchy wool that I could not stand.
>
> —Temple Grandin, in Kennedy, 2002, pp. xi–xii

> I now recognize that those of us treating [ADHD] too often miss Asperger's syndrome, especially when it is simultaneously present with [ADHD].
>
> —Paul T. Elliott, in Kennedy, 2002, p. 168.

Diane M. Kennedy's comprehensive book *The ADHD/Autism Connection* (2002) focuses our attention on the following diagnostic categories in *DSM–IV–TR* with the question "Are these all within the autistic spectrum?"

Pervasive Developmental Disorders

299.0	Autistic Disorder
299.80	Rett's Disorder
299.10	Childhood Disintegrative Disorder
299.80	Asperger's Disorder
299.80	Pervasive Developmental Disorder NOS

Attention-Deficit and Disruptive Behavior Disorders

314.xx   Attention-Deficit/Hyperactivity Disorder
.01   Combined Type
.00   Predominantly Inattentive Type
.01   Predominantly Hyperactive-Impulsive Type
314.9   Attention-Deficit/Hyperactivity Disorder NOS
312.xx   Conduct Disorder
.81   Childhood-Onset Type
.82   Adolescent-Onset Type
.89   Unspecified Onset
313.81   Oppositional Defiant Disorder
312.9   Disruptive Behavior Disorder NOS

Bipolar Disorders

296.xx   Bipolar I Disorder
296.89   Bipolar II Disorder
301.13   Cyclothymic Disorder
296.80   Bipolar Disorder NOS

Since the mid-1990s, genome research has produced a stream of new information about genetic involvement in all of these disorders (Attwood, 1998; Blakemore-Brown, 2002; Kennedy, 2002; Klin et al., 2000; LaHoste et al., 1996; Rowe et al., 1998; Smalley et al, 1998; Wing, 1997, 2001). Gene markers for hundreds of physical and emotional conditions often overlap, indicating that many sources of human malaise are cross-linked by genetics and biochemistry.

Chapter 1 described how brain information is carried across synapse junctions by neurotransmitters, especially *serotonin, dopamine, norepinephrine (noradrenaline),* and *acetylcholine.* Each of these neurotransmitters plays a critical role in how the brain functions. These and other brain chemicals team together to govern how we learn, remember, think, decide, wait, take action, and so forth. Chapter 1 explained how the gene DRD4 and its variations (alleles) fail to regulate dopamine well enough to maintain full attention, eliminate distraction, and control impulses. Below are examples of how certain genes and chromosomes are cross-linked in several types of brain-based disorders:

Neurotransmitter	Gene Mutation	Resulting Disorder
Serotonin	5-HTT(iii)	ADHD
		Autism(iv)
		Bipolar(v)

	TPH	Autism(vi)
		Bipolar(vii)
	5HTR2A	ADHD
		Autism(viii)
		Bipolar
Dopamine	DRD2	ADHD(ix)
		Autism(x)
	DRD4(xi)	ADHD(xii)
		Bipolar(xiii)
	DRD5	ADHD
		Autism(xiv)
	DAT1	ADHD
		Autism(xiv)
	TH	ADHD(xvii)
		Autism
		Bipolar(xviii)

This evidence of how certain genes are involved with several types of disorders raises the question: Are the tag-along syndromes described in this chapter actually part of the same autistic spectrum? Growing knowledge of autistic brain syndromes suggests that all of the disruptive behaviors described in this chapter may actually be layers of high functioning and very high functioning autism.

187

What Is Autism?

For 25 years, the Judevine Center for Autism in St. Louis, Missouri, has led the way in meeting the needs of children, adolescents, and adults who are autistic. The following definition of autism is derived from research by the Judevine Center staff:

> Autism is the absence of some normal behavior and a collection of odd behaviors taken to the extreme. Most children with autism look normal and are often unusually attractive. Impaired communication is a primary symptom. People with autism do not understand social exchanges, the clues that are given through body language or voice tone. They do not indicate shared social understanding. Often, they avoid looking at others. Autism is a multifaceted communication and sensory impairment that impedes the processing of information. Autism is seen in three primary symptoms: 1) a pervasive lack of response to others, 2) abnormal speech patterns, and 3) insistence on

sameness and overreaction [ritualized behavior]. In its mildest forms, autism resembles a learning disability. In its most severe forms, the person can be self-injurious, repetitive, and exhibit highly unusual and aggressive behavior. Many persons who are autistic demonstrate significantly advanced skills in music, math, or jigsaw puzzles while being significantly delayed in other areas.

—Judevine Center for Autism, February 16, 2004

If new research confirms that the tag-along syndromes described in this chapter indeed are subtypes of autism, this scale indicates where they would rank in severity of autistic symptoms:

1	2	3	4	5	6	7	8	9	10
Asperger's		ADHD		ODD CD			Bipolar II: Black Mania		
				Bipolar II: White Mania					
		ADD Bipolar I				MDD	Rain Man		

Asperger's Syndrome

In Chapter 5 we met Nate and his surrogate, Roy. Hiding beneath Nate's severe ADD was a form of very high functioning autism known as Asperger's syndrome. In childhood, Nate was indeed eccentric, with bizarre behaviors that baffled his mother and other relatives. In adulthood he has become a successful computer scientist specializing in designing ingenious computer programs. Yet he continues to have surprisingly inadequate social skills. As an adult, Nate is "weird" in virtually every social sense. In a university classroom, he sets the curve for high grades in computer science and math courses. On the job, he amazes his supervisors and colleagues with his ingenious skills in devising new computer programs. Yet he lives alone, a contented recluse who still talks to Roy at night. His apartment is littered with piles of soiled clothes and scattered books and papers. His kitchen and bathroom areas are offensive. Yet the work space around his three computers is immaculate. With his computers, Nate lives a highly ordered, ritualized life that gives him great satisfaction. Even though he forgets to change his socks and underwear for days at a time, this eccentric man copes with ADD at a level of success that brings respectful praise from satisfied clients and employers.

Asperger's syndrome is distinctive from ADD. The following behaviors, which are typical of Asperger's syndrome, trigger comments that label persons like Nate as "weird," "eccentric," "strange," and sometimes "obnoxious."

1. *Awkward gross motor coordination.* From early childhood, individuals with Asperger's syndrome tend to be awkward as they stand, walk, run, hop, skip, or play ball. This poor motor coordination produces a stiff, awkward body posture that keeps the individual from relaxing in normal ways. For example, at social events Nate stands around with stiff body posture. His arms hang at odd angles instead of relaxing down the sides of his body. His legs do not bend and flex in normal ways. When he sits, Nate's body continues to appear stiff and awkward. At table for a meal, his arms and legs cannot find a relaxed position. Even when Nate goes to bed, his body does not settle into a typically relaxed posture.

2. *Flat tone of voice.* Individuals with Asperger's syndrome do not speak in normally fluent ways. The voice tends to be flat and monotone without the usual rising and falling tonal inflections. Sometimes the voice slips into a sing-song pattern (called *prosody*). When persons like Nate enter a stream of conversation, they take on a pedantic tone of voice that sounds like a stilted lecture. Speech is slow and deliberate rather than flowing and spontaneous. Very quickly this monotonous, flat, or sing-song vocal pattern becomes boring to listeners. Others soon find excuses to move away from this lecturing voice that drones on and on.

3. *Failure to read social signals.* A major problem of Asperger's syndrome is the person's failure to notice or read social signals from others. All of his life, Nate has stood too close to others. From early childhood his mother tried to teach him not to stand so close when he talks or listens. "Don't get up in peoples' faces," his mother said a thousand times. But Nate never has learned this simple social skill. Those with Asperger's syndrome do not have a built-in sense of distance in social situations. As he interacts with others, Nate is blind to social signals that mean "Back away" or "Give me a break" or "Not now." Persons like Nate barge into private space without recognizing the rudeness of such behavior. This blindness to personal space becomes offensive when Nate develops body odor because he failed to shower, when his socks begin to smell after the fourth day of being worn, or his breath is bad because he does not brush his teeth.

4. *Awkward at small talk.* In spite of having a high IQ and an excellent academic record, Nate has never learned how to make small talk in social interactions. When he and I meet for one of our cherished visits, he cannot think of little things to say. At work, at parties, or at church events, he hangs around awkwardly, not knowing how to enter the flow of conversation. By the time he thinks of an appropriate comment, the conversation has moved on to another topic. After he entered college, Nate tried a few times to date girls, but he could not think of anything to say on a date. Soon word spread on campus that girls should avoid this weird man. "He gives me the creeps, staring at me that way without

saying anything," his dates reported to friends. This quickly closed the door to dating during his college years.

5. *Slow thinking and responding.* A major characteristic of Asperger's syndrome is slow mental processing. It is impossible for Nate to hurry as he thinks. When he has all the time he needs, his brain produces brilliant thoughts, but if he must hurry, he is lost. As Nate talks with me, he has all the time he needs. In this context, he amazes me with his intelligent thinking and problem solving. Slow thinking is a handicap for Nate when he is under pressure to respond rapidly.

6. *Excellent recall of trivial detail.* Individuals with Asperger's syndrome have extraordinary recall of detail. Nate astounds his friends and colleagues by his knowlege of trivial details related to computer science. He knows bits and pieces of information about computers that others have never heard before. His idea of a good time is to tell all he knows about computer science. Soon he has lost his audience, even those who are also gifted with computer technology. As Nate takes center stage reciting his immense store of trivial detail, his monotonous voice drones on and on as if he is delivering a lecture. Listeners slip away, leaving one or two captive persons who have not managed to escape this boring experience. Unfortunately, Nate does not recognize the strong signal this departure represents. His habit is to follow the last person, trying to corner him or her into hearing the rest of his pedantic recital. Yet Nate is respected for having such an astonishing fund of knowledge. He is the one to ask when anyone needs obscure information about computer science. However, his colleagues know that it will take all day for Nate to tell them what they need to know.

7. *Limited sense of humor.* Individuals with Asperger's syndrome think in literal, concrete terms. Their brains handle facts but their thought patterns do not respond to humor. It is very difficult for Nate to catch the meaning of a joke. He is baffled by friendly teasing. When others laugh, he wonders why. Sometimes he tries to memorize a joke so he can join in storytelling in the snack bar. Yet his effort to tell a joke or funny story is embarrassing. It takes too long for him to find his words, he adds too many trivial details, and he forgets the punch line. Before he finishes telling the joke, others have stopped listening or moved away. Nate tries to analyze humor the way he analyzes a computer problem. He does not understand how humor works.

8. *Narrow range of interests.* Because the Asperger's brain deals with trivial details in a literal fashion, individuals like Nate lock onto only a few topics of interest. As he passed through adolescence, his talks with me guided him toward the specialized logical thinking that is required for understanding computer science. Once he discovered his talent for this narrow field, he became a computer specialist. As he entered early adulthood, he also developed an obsessive interest in creating crossword

puzzles. Now his only interests are computer programming and how words interface in visual patterns. His only reading relates to these two interests. His only conversation is about these two areas of expertise.

9. *Obsessive splitting.* A major characteristic of Asperger's syndrome is the obsessive impulse to split hairs. The Asperger's brain requires that details must be perfectly aligned. Any detail that is incorrect or out of place drives Nate up the wall. Oddly, this obsession with detail does not connect to his living space or personal hygiene. The obsession to split, then split the splits, is an unfortunate social problem. Nate cannot refrain from correcting others as they make mistakes. During a lecture, he interrupts to correct the speaker, regardless of how this disrupts the class process. After a worship service, he shows the minister a list of errors the speaker made in quoting scripture or in grammatical usage. I witnessed this Asperger's pattern when Nate invited me to attend a conference at which he presented a new computer program. When we attended someone else's lecture, the speaker showed a cartoon to illustrate the issue of stress in overcrowded situations. In the cartoon, a little man was squeezed into an elevator that was packed with passengers. The point of the presentation was to stimulate group discussion on the issue of social crowding. As the group began to respond, Nate stood up. "There are too many people on that elevator," he said in a loud voice that interrupted the group activity." "I beg your pardon," said the startled presenter. "The law says that only twelve people may get on an elevator," Nate declared in his monotone pedantic voice. "There are thirteen people in that picture." A growl of irritation swept the room. "Oh, shut up!" someone said. "Sit down, you jerk!" another voice muttered. Nate had no idea why his interruption was inappropriate, or why so many people were upset at what he had done.

10. *Triggers dread in others.* Soon after Nate is hired for a new job, enrolls in a university class, or joins a singles adult group, he triggers dread in others. His habits of poor hygiene, obsessive splitting, boring style of talking, and awkwardness in social skills quickly mark him as someone to avoid. Nate has no idea why this happens. When he and I discuss this issue, I develop visual outlines that pinpoint socially inappropriate issues that isolate him from others. For example, I might write a list of specific Asperger's tendencies that others find objectionable.

- Your socks smell bad.
- You have bad breath.
- Your clothes are dirty.
- You hair needs shampooing and combing.
- You stand too close.

Most of us would be shocked and insulted by such candor. For Nate's literal brain, these are unemotional facts he can understand. With this kind of visual aid, he can see himself in these behaviors that cause others to stay away. I remember an especially challenging time with Nate when he cried as he told me of his loneliness. "Will you help me learn how to get along with other people?" he sobbed. Together we constructed a list like the one shown below. Beside that offensive list, I wrote a new list of personal hygiene rituals for Nate to analyze:

You forget to bathe.	Take a shower every day.
You forget to use deodorant.	Use deodorant after every shower.
You forget to change socks and underwear.	Put on clean socks and under-wear after every shower.
You forget to shampoo your hair.	Shampoo every time you shower.

Nate took this advice literally. He taped this list to his bathroom mirror and created a new set of rituals to replace the offensive ones. Later one of Nate's colleagues asked me what I had done to Nate. "He's different," the man said. "Now he smells clean and his hair looks nice. The trouble is, he insists on taking two showers every day and changing his clothes twice a day. Now we can't get him to relax from doing these new rituals." For the first time in his life, Nate understood why others always had pulled away from him socially. His colleagues began to include him in their activities, now that his personal hygiene was acceptable. "We can put up with Nate's weirdness now that he smells OK," his friends agreed.

11. *Inappropriate social habits.* Persons with Asperger's syndrome do not develop appropriate social habits. Awkward body coordination, poor conversational skills, narrow range of interests, absent sense of humor, and blindness toward social signals keep Nate from learning how to "dance the tribal dance." He has no idea how to dress appropriately, or how to handle food and beverages in social situations. His eating habits are sloppy as he smacks and slurps loudly while eating. He talks with his mouth filled with food. He thinks nothing of blowing his nose on a napkin or picking food from his teeth with a fingernail. When gas builds up, he belches loudly or offends those nearby by discharging intestinal gas. He shows up at social events wearing soiled sweatpants, old athletic shoes, and a grungy T-shirt with an inappropriate message emblazoned on front and back. No matter how often we discuss these issues, his Asperger's brain does not learn new social habits.

12. *Ritualized behavior.* The Asperger's brain must be highly structured to make sense of the world and to survive in society. This requires rituals that do not change. As a child, Nate invented Roy, the doll who became his ritual companion. As he grew older, Nate drove his mother

to distraction by obsessive rituals in how he dressed, ate meals, and kept his room. As an adult, he is highly ritualized in the clothing he wears. Nate's dress ritual is to wear T-shirts with messages for others to read. In his closet, 31 T-shirts hang in alphabetical order according to the first word of the shirt's message. He wears these shirts in alphabetical order, starting with A on the first day of the month, then progressing through the alphabet until the end of the month. Nate wears a certain brand of running shoes. He has seven pairs of shoes that he wears in numerical sequence each day of the week. His trousers are a certain brand of jeans, all green in color. He eats meals one food at a time. As he finishes one food, he turns his plate to the next item, then turns again to eat the next serving, until his meal is finished. If anyone intrudes into Nate's rituals and moves his things, he becomes confused and angry. Immediately he puts everything back in its ritual order. It is impossible for him to share space with a roommate or a coworker because of this obsessive need to keep his life strictly ordered his own way.

13. *Stubbornness.* All his life, Nate has been a quietly stubborn person. His behavior is called *passive/aggressive,* described in Chapter 4. On the surface, it appears that he does nothing when others press him to act, hurry, or respond. Inwardly, his emotions and feelings become quite active as his Asperger's brain chooses not to cooperate. Individuals with passive/aggressive tendencies absorb a great deal of pressure and insult. At first glance, it appears that they pay no attention to ouside pressure. However, persons like Nate begin a slow-burning resentment toward whomever is applying pressure. As the Asperger's brain decides to ignore the intrusion, invisible emotions begin to churn. Low-level anger begins to surge toward an outburst. At a certain point, this surge of anger explodes and the person becomes engaged in a shouting match, sometimes flinging things around the room or shoving the intruder away. These outbursts usually startle outsiders who do not see these aggressive episodes coming.

14. *Controlling others.* Outsiders often are surprised to hear Asperger's individuals described as controllers. Their passive behavior hides a personality trait that compels them to control every situation, if possible. When I first met Nate and his mother, I quickly recognized his success in controlling the household. Every time Nate's ADD/Asperger's behavior brought his mother to tears, he was in control. Each time his stubbornness triggered a shouting match, he was in control. Every family reunion he disrupted placed him in control as his mother left the event early to take him home to his safe, private space. As an adult, Nate strives to control others through his expert knowledge of trivial detail. On the job, he guards information that others need, sharing it only when it becomes clear that they need his help. Then he forces them to pay the price by

Tag-Along Syndromes

tolerating his obsessive, ritualized behavior. The habit of standing too close to others is a control technique. Even when this triggers negative reactions, Nate has gained control of where others stand or when they move away. Having control is a major source of emotional satisfaction for Nate.

15. *Boring personality.* At a national conference on learning disabilities, Martha Denckla presented new information from her research on autism and Asperger's syndrome. Someone in the audience asked: "Dr. Denckla, how would you best describe Asperger's?" Without hesitation, Denckla replied: "Boring! Boring! Boring!" At first this seemed a rude response, insensitive to the struggles of persons like Nate. Yet Denckla was candidly accurate. A major characteristic of Asperger's syndrome is the quality of being boring. The slow-paced, monotone speech patterns are boring. Listening to an endless recital of trivial detail about an obscure topic is boring. Tolerating hair-splitting interruptions of group discussions is boring. Spending an evening with an Asperger's individual is boring. Without question, Denckla's description was accurate. Following one of Nate's boring presentations, a weary colleague commented: "A little Asperger's goes a long way."

16. *Rationalizing.* One of the most annoying characteristics of Asperger's syndrome is the person's automatic habit of rationalizing. I have never seen Nate admit being wrong unless he first goes through an elaborate explanation of why it was not his fault, why someone else was to blame, and why his own behavior was not the problem. If I wait long enough, he eventually confesses that his behavior might not have been perfect. Yet he never fully acknowledges his responsibility without listing reasons why someone else should take the blame. This tendency to rationalize is part of the narrow range of logic that drives the Asperger's brain. Rationalizing is a form of splitting hairs. Persons like Nate cannot face life without this support system of rationalization. To say simply "It was my fault" denies Nate the satisfaction of analyzing every possible detail the way he creates a new computer program or develops a new crossword puzzle.

17. *Creativity within a narrow range of talent.* Nate is one of the most creative persons I know within the narrow landscapes of computer science and crossword puzzles. Within these boundaries, he has few equals. For example, his intensely focused talent has produced ingenious computer programs that greatly improve literacy skills for dyslexic individuals. Nate's creativity with computers will leave a beneficial mark on the world. Unfortunately, there is no flexibility to permit him to expand his horizons socially or intellectually.

18. *Works best alone.* Asperger's individuals rarely are effective team members. Asperger's syndrome results in too many social limitations to

permit persons like Nate to fit into work groups, committees, or leadership teams. Fortunately, Nate's unique talent with computer science makes him a valued employee on projects that he can do alone. Working by himself in his ritualized private space is the only way he can be productive.

19. *Poor leadership ability.* A sad reality of Asperger's syndrome is the fact that individuals like Nate cannot be effective leaders. No matter how hard they try, their eccentric ways alienate others too quickly to permit leadership qualities to emerge. When an Asperger's individual is named to a leadership position, he or she becomes an autocratic, dictatorial ruler rather than a leader. The first thing such a person does is to develop a rule book. Then the Asperger's supervisor enforces the rules in a literal fashion. Soon the workforce or staff are upset by arbitrary decisions that are based on picky adherence to rules rather than personal merit. When persons like Nate are assigned to supervisory roles, group morale deteriorates rapidly. Asperger's leaders cannot generate group loyalty. Their type of leadership is arbitrary and inflexible to the point of being offensive. The habits of rationalizing, splitting hairs, and living by rituals are demeaning to the personal dignity of others. These Asperger's patterns soon become threatening to the personal freedoms of others.

Visual Perception Disorder

Toward the end of the 1880s, physicians and educators in Europe were perplexed by the fact that certain individuals with normal vision (20/20 acuity) became "word blind" when they looked at black print on white paper under bright light. In spite of having 20/20 visual acuity, those persons declared that when they tried to read, they saw the kinds of distortions shown in Figures 6.7 through 6.12. In these distortions, the print begins to swirl, shift back and forth, move up and down, fade in and out, or fall off the edge of the page. This visual perception phenomenon was called *word blindness.* Separate classrooms were established in European countries where word-blind students were taught to compensate for this visual perception disability (Broadbent, 1872; Hinshelwood, 1896, 1900). The phenomenon of word-blindness was first studied in the United States by Samuel T. Orton (1925, 1928, 1937). However, it was not until the 1970s that the first solution for word-blindness was discovered by Helen Irlen, a psychologist working with dyslexic adult readers at Long Beach Community College in California. Irlen discovered that if struggling readers placed sheets of colored spotlight filters on their book pages, the print often stopped moving and the print distortions frequently disappeared. During the 1980s Irlen perfected a standard method for identifying word blindness that she called *scotopic sensitivity syndrome.* In her book *Reading by the Colors* (1991), she named

(*text continues on p. 198*)

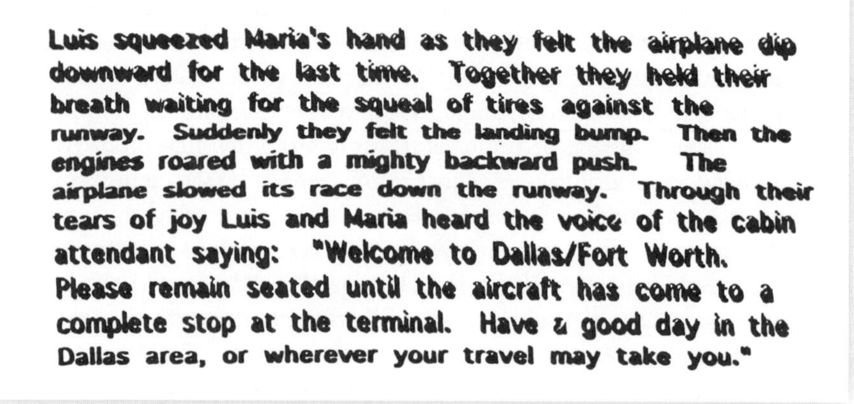

Luis squeezed Maria's hand as they felt the airplane dip downward for the last time. Together they held their breath waiting for the squeal of tires against the runway. Suddenly they felt the landing bump. Then the engines roared with a mighty backward push. The airplane slowed its race down the runway. Through their tears of joy Luis and Maria heard the voice of the cabin attendant saying: "Welcome to Dallas/Fort Worth. Please remain seated until the aircraft has come to a complete stop at the terminal. Have a good day in the Dallas area, or wherever your travel may take you."

FIGURE 6.7. Without warning the page blurs out of focus, then comes back into focus. This pulsing effect places great strain on the eyes. The reader can make the print clear for a moment by widening the eyes, or by squinting the eyes almost closed.

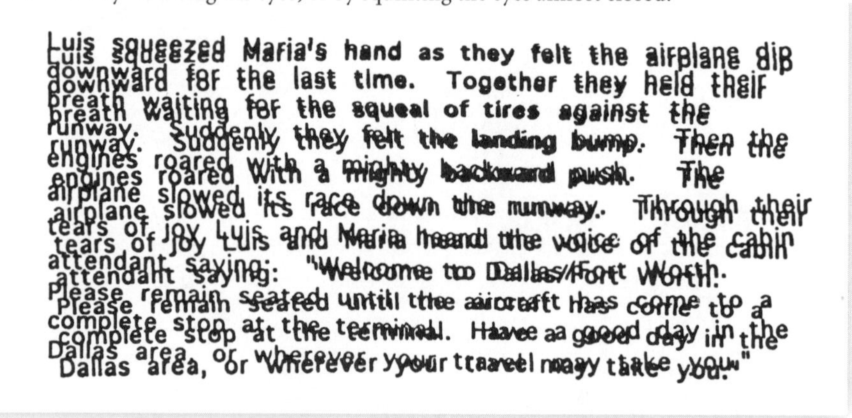

Luis squeezed Maria's hand as they felt the airplane dip downward for the last time. Together they held their breath waiting for the squeal of tires against the runway. Suddenly they felt the landing bump. Then the engines roared with a mighty backward push. The airplane slowed its race down the runway. Through their tears of joy Luis and Maria heard the voice of the cabin attendant saying: "Welcome too Dallas/Fort Worth. Please remain seated until the aircraft has come to a complete stop at the terminal. Have a good day in the Dallas area, or wherever your travel may take you."

FIGURE 6.8. Lines begin to swirl like a wheel rotating as the eyes focus on a particular word.

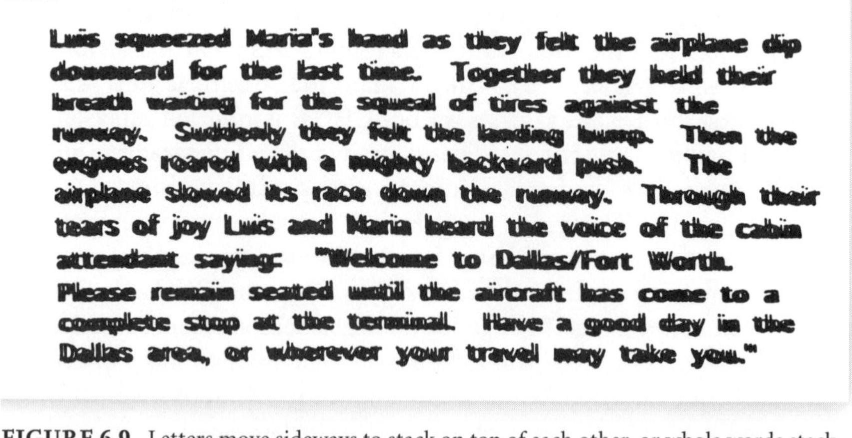

Luis squeezed Maria's hand as they felt the airplane dip downward for the last time. Together they held their breath waiting for the squeal of tires against the runway. Suddenly they felt the landing bump. Then the engines roared with a mighty backward push. The airplane slowed its race down the runway. Through their tears of joy Luis and Maria heard the voice of the cabin attendant saying: "Welcome to Dallas/Fort Worth. Please remain seated until the aircraft has come to a complete stop at the terminal. Have a good day in the Dallas area, or wherever your travel may take you."

FIGURE 6.9. Letters move sideways to stack on top of each other, or whole words stack, then move apart. This produces a smudged effect that makes reading impossible.

Overcoming Attention Deficit Disorders in Children, Adolescents, and Adults

Luis squeezed   Maria'shandasthey   felttheairplanedip
downwardfor   thelasttime.Together   theyheldtheir
breathwait   ingforthesqueal of tir esagainstthe   runw
Suddenlythey   feltthelandingbump.   Thentheengi   nes
roaredwithamig   htybackward push.   Theairplaneslow
itsracedowntherun   way.Throughthe   irtearsofjoy   Luis
andMariaheard   thevoiceofthecabin   attendantsaying
"WelcometoDal   las/Fort Worth.Plea   seremainseated
untiltheaircr   afthascometoacom   pletestopatthe   ga
Haveagood   dayintheDallasarea,or   whereveryour   trav
maytake   you."

FIGURE 6.10. Words move sideways, creating a "river" effect, as if small rivers are cascading down the page. These rivers change rapidly as words continue to move back and forth.

Luis squeezed Maria's hand as they felt the airplane dip
downward for the last time. Together they held their
breath waiting for the squeal of tires against the
runway. Suddenly they felt the landing bump. Then the
engines roared with a mighty backward push. The
airplane slowed its race down the runway. Through their
tears of joy Luis and Maria heard the voice of the cabin
attendant saying: "Welcome to Dallas/Fort Worth.
Please remain seated until the aircraft has come to a
complete stop at the terminal. Have a good day in the
Dallas area, or wherever your travel may take you."

FIGURE 6.11. Inside portions of words slowly fade away, then come back. This "washout" effect greatly increases reading difficulty for word-blind individuals.

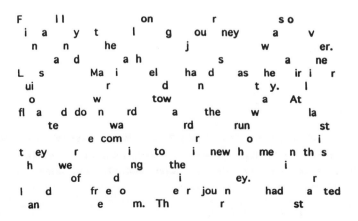

FIGURE 6.12. Some Irlen syndrome readers see lines ripple up and down, like a flag in the wind. Laying a marker below each line often stops this ripple effect.

Tag-Along Syndromes

this visual perception phenomonen *Irlen syndrome*. The Irlen method of eliminating scotopic sensitivity (word blindness) has opened the door to reading for countless children, adolescents, and adults around the world.

Still, no one knew why adding color to reading reduced or eliminated the print distortions of word blindness. During the 1990s, brain imaging research began to explain what causes scotopic sensitivity and why adding color corrects the problem for certain individuals (Eden, 1996; Lehmkuhle et al., 1993; Livingstone et al., 1991). This research discovered a missing link in the *magnicellular pathway*, which carries visual information from the retina of each eye to the *lateral geniculate nucleus* in the brain stem, shown in Figure 6.13. When neurons within the magnicellular pathway develop normally, two types of vision transmission cells work together as a team. The larger *magno cells* rapidly transfer light impulse data for luminance contrast, space, depth perception, movement, motion, and position in space. These "vision particles" reach the brain stem first and wait while

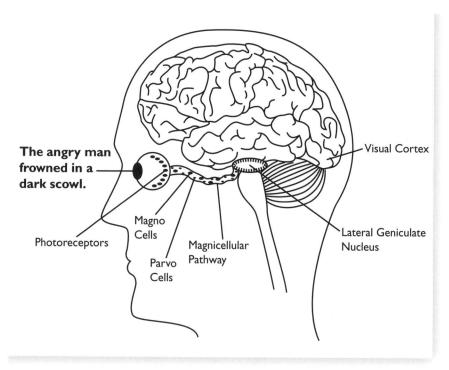

FIGURE 6.13. Between the retina of each eye and the visual cortex where the brain interprets what the eyes see is the magnicellular pathway. This visual pathway contains pairs of cells that work together to pass visual data from the eyes to the brain. Incomplete neural development within the magnicellular pathways causes the brain to see distorted images, especially black print on white paper. These twisting, moving, blurring visual images are called scotopic sensitivity syndrome, or Irlen syndrome.

the smaller *parvo cells* more slowly transfer data related to color, shape, curvature, form, and still images. The lateral geniculate nucleus is designed to blend these vision particles into mental images that the higher brain can recognize.

In word-blind individuals, the magno cells are incomplete. This deficit in neuron formation transmits moving, twisting, sliding distortions to the higher brain like those shown in Figures 6.7 through 6.12. These unstable visual impressions force individuals with scotopic sensitivity to glance away from printed information, instead of looking at it steadily. If they keep on looking at black print on white paper, their eyes are overwhelmed by glare coming from the white background as well as the constantly changing visual impressions. Brain imaging research by Margaret Livingstone has demonstrated that adding the right color (or colors) to the printed page while reducing the level of light shining on the page "fills in" the missing segments of magno cells. This stops the print distortions. Using fMRI brain imaging, researchers watch scotopic magnicellular pathways change from abnormal to normal when appropriate light levels and colors are added to a word-blind person's visual processing (Livingstone, 1993).

Word blindness triggers a cascade of behaviors that often imitate ADHD or ADD. Soon after the affected individual starts to read under bright light, both eyes begin to sting or burn. They squint to shut out bright light. After a few minutes, both eyes begin to hurt or feel uncomfortable. Many readers with scotopic sensitivity lean over their work to shade pages from overhead light, or they hold a hand up to the forehead to shade the eyes. Word-blind individuals often want to wear a baseball cap in the classroom to shade their eyes. Print begins to blur in and out of focus in a pulsing pattern (see Figure 6.7). Many word-blind readers see a swirling pattern like a turning wheel (see Figure 6.8). Words and lines of print often stack on top of each other, then separate (see Figure 6.9). Rivers of space start to run down the page as words slide sideways, then come back together (see Figure 6.10). Letters begin to flicker or blink on and off, causing inside portions of words to fade away, then return (see Figure 6.11). Scotopic sensitive readers often see colored halos surrounding words, along with colored "speckles" flashing on the page. Sometimes they see words sliding off the edge of the page. At a certain point of visual stress, whole lines ripple up and down like a flag waving (see Figure 6.12).

Many word-blind readers lean down close with the nose almost touching the page, then lean back away from the page. They might lift a book up close to the face, then put it back on the desktop. They start to shift and turn their bodies in different directions in an attempt to view the page from different angles. After a few minutes, a distinctive headache develops across the forehead (frontal headache), then moves over the temple regions (temporal headache). When Irlen syndrome individuals keep on trying to read, they often develop a headache at the back of the head and down the neck (occipital headache). As these word-blind patterns set in, the reader begins to fidget, squirm, glance away, and appear to be ADHD. When Irlen syndrome is corrected by color and lower level light, symptoms of ADHD often disappear. The tag-along syndrome of poor visual perception often is mistaken for ADHD.

Learning Disabilities

In the book *Overcoming Dyslexia in Children, Adolescents, and Adults* (2002), I have documented close links between ADHD, ADD, and learning disabilities (LD), especially various subtypes of dyslexia. My research through 47 years of diagnosing and remediating dyslexia indicates that 65% of those who are dyslexic also have ADHD or ADD. In looking at LD patterns in attention deficit individuals, Russell Barkley (1995) estimated that 20% to 30% of those with ADHD also have LD in math, reading, or spelling. During 25 years of research with LD adults, Laura Weisel (1992, 2001) has found ADHD or ADD symptoms in 45% of her clients who have reading disabilities. In researching learning disabilities in adjudicated delinquents in the state of Arkansas, Caroline Pollan and Dorothy Williams (1992) found that 46% of that population had significant symptoms of ADHD or ADD and dyslexia. Learning disabilities often tag along in the shadow of attention deficits. Of the LD patterns that imitate ADHD and ADD, the most commonly seen are types of dyslexia.

What Is Dyslexia?

Dyslexia now is the most thoroughly researched type of learning disability.

—Drake Duane, March 1985

Twenty years ago, Drake Duane, a neuroscientist with the Mayo Cinic, reviewed 100 years of research of dyslexia and concluded that enough was known about this type of learning difficulty to establish support programs in America's school systems to treat dyslexic learners. Since that time, further brain research has added to the enormous body of scientific literature devoted to dyslexia, which is described in Chapter 6. Yet the issue of dyslexia remains highly controversial among educators, who rarely use that label with students who struggle with reading, writing, and spelling. For example, in 1986 the Texas state legislature amended the Texas Education Code with Section 38.003, which established a new category of special education called dyslexia. That legislation mandated that every child within the Texas public schools be evaluated for dyslexia. In 1998, further legislation required every Texas school district to employ a "dyslexia teacher" who is specially trained and certified in working with dyslexic learners (Moses, 1998). However, in the states that border Texas, dyslexia is not included in the official definitions of learning disabilities, leaving dyslexic learners without support in spite of constant struggle with literacy skills.

In her book *Overcoming Dyslexia: A New and Complete Science-Based Program for Reading Problems at Any Level* (2003), Sally Shaywitz presents in simple language the brain-based causes for dyslexia, along with strategies for helping individuals overcome this reading disability. Shaywitz writes from the point of view of a wise, compassionate neuroscientist who yearns to see educational systems provide appropriate help for these struggling learners. In my books *Jordan Dyslexia Assessment/Reading Program* (2000b) and *Overcoming Dyslexia in Children, Adolescents, and Adults* (2002), I write from the point of view of one who is dyslexic, a challenge I have faced all my life. Each of these books provides a wealth of information about what causes dyslexia, how it interferes with classroom learning, its impact on the lives of dyslexic individuals, and how we can help dyslexic learners become successful. In presenting our information about dyslexia, Shaywitz and I avoid technical, clinical terminology such as *eidetic* and *diseidetic,* which is often used by researchers to identify subtypes of dyslexia. Instead, our goal is to explain dyslexia in simple language that does not require advanced clinical knowledge of this learning challenge.

Dyslexia Does Not Fit
the Left-Brain Linear Style of Learning

Those of us who are dyslexic are misfits inside traditional classrooms, where the curriculum is built upon a rigid, inflexible model of teaching and learning called *left-brain linear style.* Figure 1.15 shows the perceptual orientation of most classroom teaching, in which thoughts are expected to flow in a left-to-right/top-to-bottom direction. Long-term memory and classroom problem solving also must flow in this perceptual direction. Students who do not follow this left-brain linear requirement are "wrong." To succeed in today's educational environment, young learners must quickly become fluent in processing classroom information from left to right and top to bottom. This curriculum standard assumes that the left brain development of all students entering formal learning is ready to acquire the left-brain skills shown in Figure 6.14. To succeed inside the left-brain linear box, youngsters in kindergarten must begin to master these basic literacy skills:

Decoding printed symbols	Recognizing letters and numerals. Connecting sounds to letters. Reading printed and handwritten language. Interpreting printed and handwritten math information.
Encoding language and math symbols	Controlling finger movements for penmanship. Spelling correctly from memory. Using correct grammar and punctuation. Using vocabulary correctly. Connecting meaning to printed or handwritten information.
Building long-term memory for word meanings	Learning new vocabulary. Using vocabulary correctly in speaking and writing.
Mastering math and arithmetic concepts	Building long-term memory for rapid math computation: adding, subtracting, multiplying, dividing, using fractions and decimals.

Sally Shaywitz's brain imaging research has mapped how the left brain reads. Figure 1.13 shows the eight-step loop that produces reading in most individuals. The left-brain linear model of education assumes that all persons can learn to read like this. However, at the turn of the 21st century, the controversial point of view emerged that *reading, spelling, and writing are unnatural inventions* that not everyone can learn to do beyond a limited skill level.

> Programmatic research over the past 35 years has *not* supported the view that reading development reflects a *natural* process that children learn to read as they learn to speak, through natural exposure to a literate environment.... If learning to read were natural, there would not exist the substantial number of cultures that have yet to develop a written language, despite having a rich oral language. If learning to read unfolds naturally, why does our society have so many youngsters and adults who are illiterate?
>
> —G. Reid Lyon, January/February 2000

> We have just reviewed 5,500 years of evidence to show that writing systems are inventions, and that humans do not spontaneously and

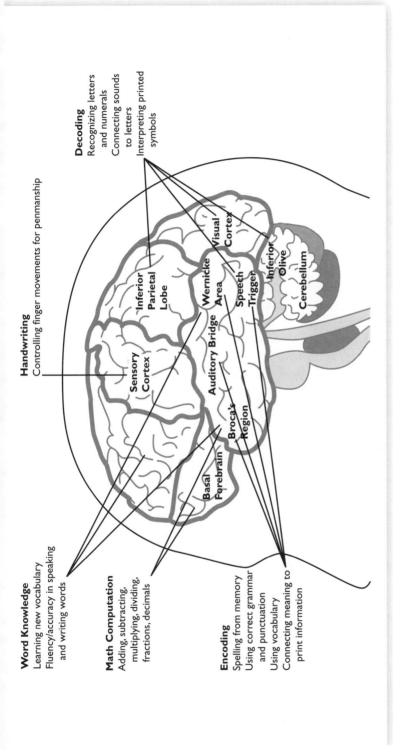

FIGURE 6.14. The left-brain model illustrated in Figure 1.15 assumes that when children enter first grade, their left brains will be ready to master these language skills on the schedule set by the school curriculum. Approximately 4 out of 5 youngsters are ready for this language learning. However, 1 out of 5 is not. Most of these individuals are dyslexic. When dyslexia exists, many "bridges are out" along these information highways that must function well for the student to master literacy skills.

Word Knowledge
Learning new vocabulary
Fluency/accuracy in speaking and writing words

Math Computation
Adding, subtracting, multiplying, dividing, fractions, decimals

Encoding
Spelling from memory
Using correct grammar and punctuation
Using vocabulary
Connecting meaning to print information

Handwriting
Controlling finger movements for penmanship

Decoding
Recognizing letters and numerals
Connecting sounds to letters
Interpreting printed symbols

Sensory Cortex

Inferior Parietal Lobe

Wernicke Area

Visual Cortex

Auditory Bridge

Speech Trigger

Inferior Olive

Cerebellum

Broca's Region

Basal Forebrain

Tag-Along Syndromes

effortlessly develop writing systems or find it easy to learn them. We
have seen that the alphabet is a particulary 'nonnatural' writing system.
Reading is definitely not a biological property of the human brain.
—Diane McGuinness, 1997, p. 117

Overall, the human population follows a pattern in which a certain per-
centage become fluent readers, some achieve average reading ability, and
some never become fluent with decoding/encoding language. To become
fully literate, an individual must be born with enough potential plasticity
of the brain to build neural pathways for fluent reading, spelling, and written language skills. To learn to read, write, and spell, the left brain must
grow neurons in response to years of classroom stimulus in what we call
reading readiness training.

During my career with struggling learners, I have seen a ratio of success and failure in achieving literacy skills. Two out of five (40%) people are
born with natural neurological talent to become fluent at reading, spelling, and writing. These individuals have natural neural plasticity to shape
left-brain regions into the "literate brains" shown in Figures 1.13 and 6.14.
These persons become gifted/talented readers and writers who set the curve
for the rest of us. The next two out of five (40%) people are born with
enough neurological talent to become "average" at reading, spelling, and
writing. After years of classroom stimulus, they are able to do necessary
(functional) literacy work, but they do not read or write for pleasure. The
remaining 1 out of 5 usually is dyslexic. For us, learning to read, write, and
spell is an overwhelming challenge. If we labor long enough with literacy
skills, some of us who are dyslexic figure out how to become literate, especially through keyboard writing and computer-based learning. Unfortunately, many dyslexic individuals do not. The generally held assumption
that "everyone can learn to read" is not true. Through heroic effort with
specially designed multisensory, interactive methods, most dyslexic individuals can achieve basic skills between third- and fifth-grade literacy level.
This is called *functional literacy.* It is unfortunate that today's left-brain linear style of teaching causes many of these individuals to fall through the
cracks of the educational system.

Figure 6.15 shows the left brain regions where dyslexia occurs. After
half a century of dyslexia research and a lifelong struggle to overcome this
learning disability, I have identified the five subtypes of dyslexia shown in
Figure 6.15. Genome research of genetic markers for dyslexia has shown
that the tendency (predisposition) for this language processing challenge
is passed down generational lines by chromosomes 2, 3, 6, 15, and 18
(Fisher & DeFries, 2002; McGuinness, 1997; Pennington & Gilger, 1996;
Scarborough, 1998; Shapiro, Accordo, & Capute, 1998; Shaywitz, 2003;
Sternberg & Spear-Swerling, 1999).

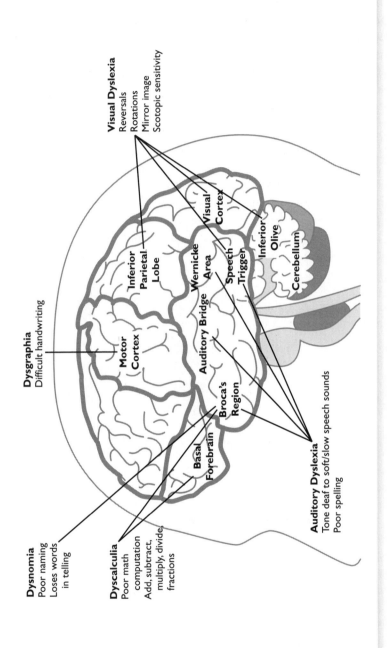

Dysnomia
Poor naming
Loses words
in telling

Dyscalculia
Poor math
computation
Add, subtract,
multiply, divide,
fractions

Dysgraphia
Difficult handwriting

Visual Dyslexia
Reversals
Rotations
Mirror image
Scotopic sensitivity

Motor
Cortex

Inferior
Parietal
Lobe

Wernicke
Area

Visual
Cortex

Auditory
Bridge

Speech
Trigger

Inferior
Olive

Broca's
Region

Cerebellum

Basal
Forebrain

Auditory Dyslexia
Tone deaf to soft/slow speech sounds
Poor spelling

FIGURE 6.15. These five subtypes of dyslexia occur when neuron formations are incomplete throughout these regions of the left brain. When genetics passes dyslexia down the family line, it is not unusual to find individuals who have all five of these subtypes of dyslexia. It is rare to find only one subtype alone.

Tag-Along Syndromes

Visual Dyslexia

My label *visual dyslexia* is a simple way of describing the subtype of dyslexia in which the brain reverses letters and numerals, flips them upside down, and scrambles their sequence in reading and writing. Visual dyslexia refers to the "glitches" that occur in the left-brain visual cortex and parietal lobe when individuals are required to interpret (decode) written language and math symbols. Visual dyslexia is not a problem with eyesight. Most persons with visual dyslexia have normal vision (20/20 acuity). The problem arises from confused orientation with left to right, and top to bottom. The dyslexic brain wants to interpret details backward and upside down. For example, individuals with visual dyslexia never are fully sure which direction several letters in the Roman alphabet should face. All their lives, they mistake *d* and *b*, *p* and *q*, *M* and *W*, and *u* and *n*. They often stumble over which way numerals should face *(3, 5, 6-9, 7)*. Double digits often are reversed: for example, 12 is written as 21. To read, write, and spell, persons with visual dyslexia must pause, back up, search their memories, then try again. Mirror image also causes many words or syllables to be read backward: *stop* for *post, won* for *now, tub* for *but, Apirl-April, bran-barn.* Persons with visual dyslexia continually misread words they see in print: *Altus* for *Tulsa, exist* for *exit,* or *hummingbird* for *hamburger.* Dyslexic individuals tend to reverse left/right, up/down or top/bottom. For dyslexic individuals, remembering the directions north, east, south, west frequently is impossible unless they use a rhyme, such as "Never Eat Sour Watermelon." While ADHD persons face similar challenges, their symptoms often disappear during adolescence and early adulthood. In dyslexia, these tendencies to reverse and scramble mental images often remain for life.

Figure 6.14 shows where reading begins at the back of the left brain in the parietal lobe and visual cortex of the occipital lobe. Visual dyslexia is caused by incomplete dendrite pruning throughout these regions of the left brain, where symbols reverse, flip upside down, or scramble out of sequence. Figures 6.16 and 6.17 show a portion of the *Jordan Dyslexia Assessment Inventory,* which asks the individual to write the alphabet, days of the week, and months of the year with no visual cues on the walls or in nearby books. These activities reveal how visual dyslexia interferes when individuals attempt to write this basic information. Figures 6.18 and 6.19 show how visual dyslexia interferes with reading activities as letters change position or direction. Approximately 65% of those who have these encoding and decoding struggles also are handicapped by the scotopic sensitivity (word-blind) symptoms shown in Figures 6.7 through 6.12. More than half of all individuals with visual dyslexia also have the tag-along layer of ADHD.

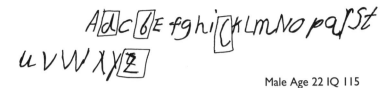

Male Age 22 IQ 115

Male Age 41 IQ 119

Female Age 36 IQ 133

Female Age 27 IQ 127

FIGURE 6.16. Each of these intelligent adults struggled for several minutes to write the alphabet. They whispered to themselves, backed up and started again, touched the paper as they wrote, and relied on multisensory techniques (see/say/hear/touch) to recall the letters in sequence. None of these individuals was sure that he or she had written the alphabet correctly. *Note.* From *Jordan Dyslexia Assessment/Reading Program* (2nd ed., p. 26), by D. R. Jordan, 2000, Austin, TX: PRO-ED, Inc. Copyright 2000 by PRO-ED, Inc. Reprinted with permission.

Auditory Dyslexia

Since the term *dyslexia* was coined in the 1880s, teachers have wondered why certain students never learn phonics. Regardless of how much drilling and tutoring is done, some learners never connect sounds to letters in spelling or reading. These "tone deaf" individuals have normal hearing, yet they do not learn to "hear" vowels and soft consonants that are the

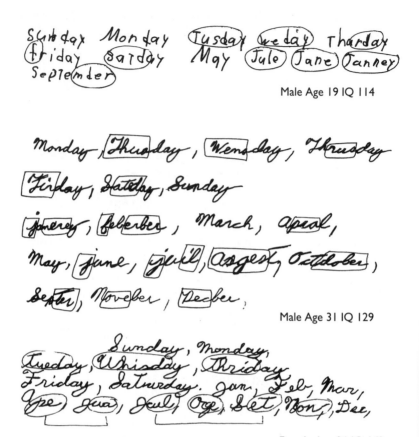

Male Age 19 IQ 114

Male Age 31 IQ 129

Female Age 26 IQ 142

FIGURE 6.17. In spite of high intelligence, each of these adults struggled for several minutes to write the days and months from memory. They whispered to themselves, continually erased and changed, and grew increasingly frustrated as time went by. Each person exhibited strong negative emotions and talked about how hard school always was. *Note.* From *Jordan Dyslexia Assessment/Reading Program* (2nd ed., p. 27), by D. R. Jordan, 2000, Austin, TX: PRO-ED, Inc. Copyright 2000 by PRO-ED, Inc. Reprinted with permission.

building blocks of words. During the 1980s, Paula Tallal, a neurobiologist at Rutgers University, and her colleagues discovered a missing link in the auditory pathway between the limbic system and higher brain regions that process oral language (Tallal, Miller, & Fitch, 1993). Figure 6.20 is a diagram of the auditory pathway from the middle ear, where speech sounds are converted into electrical codes. These codes are fired to the medial geniculate nucleus, where coded speech is filtered and organized. Finally this

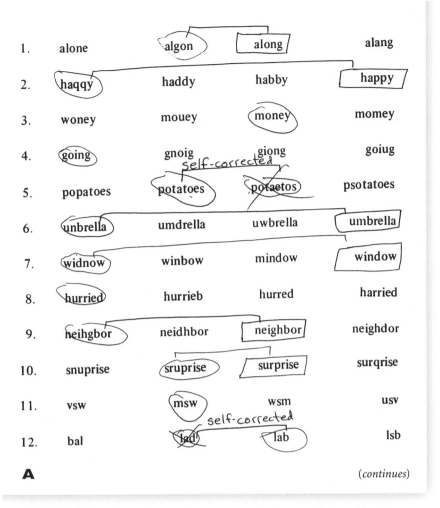

1.	alone	algon	along	alang
2.	haqqy	haddy	habby	happy
3.	woney	mouey	money	momey
4.	going	gnoig	giong	goiug
			self-corrected	
5.	popatoes	potatoes	potaetos	psotatoes
6.	unbrella	umdrella	uwbrella	umbrella
7.	widnow	winbow	mindow	window
8.	hurried	hurrieb	hurred	harried
9.	neihgbor	neidhbor	neighbor	neighdor
10.	snuprise	sruprise	surprise	surqrise
11.	vsw	msw	wsm	usv
		self-corrected		
12.	bal	lad	lab	lsb

A

209

(*continues*)

FIGURE 6.18. These exercises show how an 11-year-old girl struggles with symbol sequence and (A) left-to-right and (B) top-to-bottom directionality as she matches words in daily school activities. *Note.* From *Slingerland Screening Test for Identifying Children with Specific Language Disability,* Form C, by B. H. Slingerland, 1984, Cambridge, MA: Educators Publishing Service. Copyright 1984 by Educators Publishing Service. Reprinted with permission.

oral language data is sent to the left brain, where speech codes are turned into "brain language." Between the medial geniculate nucleus and the parietal and temporal lobes is a pathway of auditory cells that work in pairs. Some of these cells process soft/slow language sounds (vowels and soft consonants). Other cells process hard/fast language sounds (hard consonants). Auditory dyslexia (tone deafness) occurs when the soft/slow auditory cells do not "hear" the softer, slower sounds of our language.

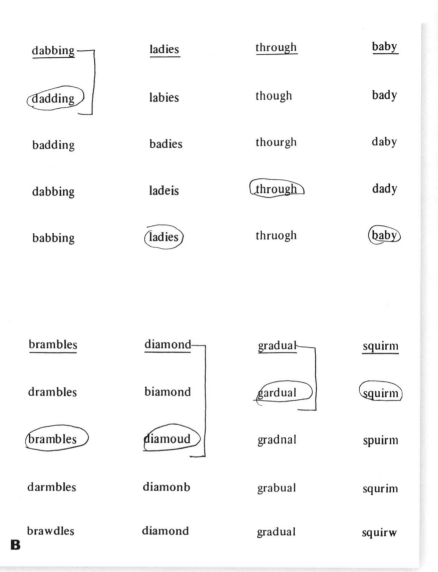

dabbing	ladies	through	baby
dadding	labies	though	bady
badding	badies	thourgh	daby
dabbing	ladeis	through	dady
babbing	ladies	thruogh	baby

brambles	diamond	gradual	squirm
drambles	biamond	gardual	squirm
brambles	diamoud	gradnal	spuirm
darmbles	diamonb	grabual	squrim
brawdles	diamond	gradual	squirw

B

FIGURE 6.18. *Continued.*

For example, all spoken words are made of sound chunks called *pho-nemes*. When we talk, we utter hard/fast, soft/slow phonemes in specific sequences. For example, the word *cut* is created by the sequence hard/fast /k/, soft/slow /u/, hard/fast /t/. Persons with auditory dyslexia are tone deaf to the soft, slow middle sound /u/. Tone deaf individuals cannot develop good spelling from memory because they do not hear all of the speech sounds in correct sequence. Figure 6.21 shows how auditory dyslexia appears in

Mark the word just like the word you saw on the card.

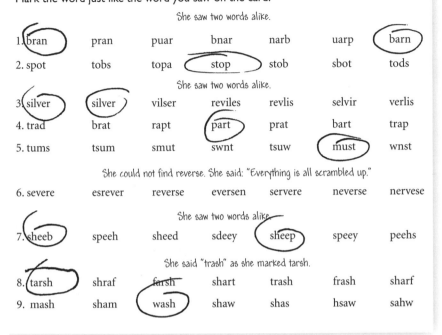

She saw two words alike.

1. (bran)   pran   puar   bnar   narb   uarp   (barn)

2. spot   tobs   topa   (stop)   stob   sbot   tods

She saw two words alike.

3. (silver)   (silver)   vilser   reviles   revlis   selvir   verlis

4. trad   brat   rapt   (part)   prat   bart   trap

5. tums   tsum   smut   swnt   tsuw   (must)   wnst

She could not find reverse. She said: "Everything is all scrambled up."

6. severe   esrever   reverse   eversen   servere   neverse   nervese

She saw two words alike.

7. (sheeb)   speeh   sheed   sdeey   (sheep)   speey   peehs

She said "trash" as she marked tarsh.

8. (tarsh)   shraf   farsh   shart   trash   frash   sharf

9. mash   sham   (wash)   shaw   shas   hsaw   sahw

FIGURE 6.19. This 21-year-old dyslexic woman worked hard to match words. She whispered and touched each word, spelling it to herself. Finally she circled her choice of what matched the word she had seen on a card. She continually said: "Oops! That's not right. Uh-uh. I got it backwards. Let's see. It had *d*. Wait, was it *b*?" Even with this practice, her memory could not maintain left-right, top-bottom orientation. *Note.* From *Jordan Dyslexia Assessment/Reading Program* (2nd ed., p.27), by D. R. Jordan, 2000, Austin, TX: PRO-ED, Inc. Copyright 2000 by PRO-ED, Inc. Reprinted with permission.

writing as a 9-year-old boy with auditory dyslexia wrote what he thought he heard his teacher say.

Dysgraphia

The first discussion of chronic poor handwriting appeared in 1869, when the English neurologist Henry Charlton Bastian published his studies of written language deficits in adults who had suffered left-brain trauma from accidents, strokes, or seizures. Such brain trauma produces language loss called *aphasia* (Bastian, 1869). Bastian described illegible penmanship as *dysgraphia*. Others used the term *agraphia*. Illegible handwriting can result from brain injury to the motor cortex. However, dysgraphia that is linked to dyslexia is not the result of brain damage. Dysgraphia usually is

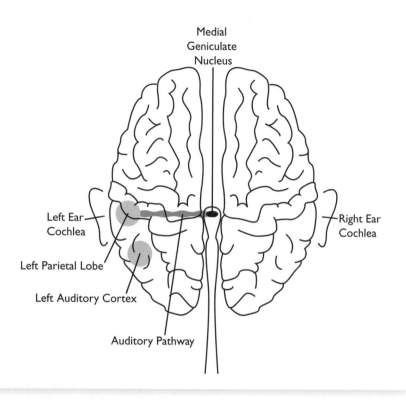

Medial
Geniculate
Nucleus

Left Ear—
Cochlea

Right Ear
Cochlea

Left Parietal Lobe

Left Auditory Cortex

Auditory Pathway

FIGURE 6.20. The cochlea in each middle ear gathers speech sounds that are changed into electrical codes. These sound codes are sent to the medial geniculate nucleus in the brain stem. The medial geniculate nucleus organizes the soft/slow and hard/fast sound chunks into word patterns, then fires that data to the parietal lobe, which sends it on to the auditory cortex. The auditory pathway between the brain stem and parietal lobe has two types of cells that work as a team. Larger cells process the soft/slow speech sounds of vowels and soft consonants. Smaller cells process the hard/fast sounds of hard consonants. Auditory dyslexia occurs when underdeveloped larger cells do not transfer the soft/slow speech sounds in the right sequence. The auditory cortex receives only part of the original oral speech. This makes it impossible for the dyslexic person to connect sounds to letters in listening, reading, and spelling.

part of the genetic predisposition for dyslexia. It is passed down genetic lines along with visual dyslexia and auditory dyslexia.

Figure 6.22 shows the regions of the left-brain primary motor cortex that control voluntary muscle activity over the whole body. As infants and toddlers reach developmental milestones on schedule, neural pathways become hardwired to perform lifelong motor tasks. Figure 6.22 shows the developmental sequence that starts in infancy with tongue control as sucking reflex and ends during early childhood with leg control for elaborate gross

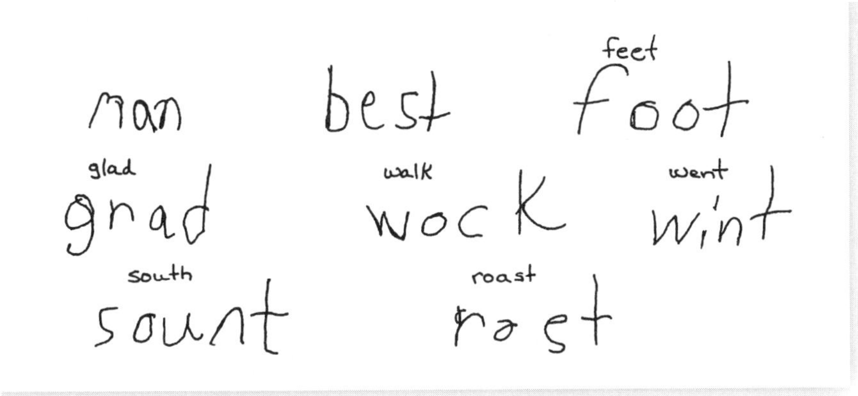

FIGURE 6.21. This very intelligent 9-year-old boy struggles hard to succeed on weekly spelling tests. After practicing all week at home with these words, this was the best he could do on the Friday written spelling test. Later the teacher learned that home spelling practice was done orally. When he tried to write what he could say correctly, these dyslexic patterns interfered.

motor activity, such as hopping, skipping, running, climbing, leaping, and racing. In most youngsters, neural maturity within the motor cortex prepares the fingers and hands for the fine motor coordination required for handwriting. When dysgraphia exists, this developmental milestone within the primary motor cortex fails to emerge.

In classrooms and workplace situations where literacy is judged by the neatness of one's penmanship, individuals with dysgraphia are at a serious disadvantage. Not everyone who writes poorly is dysgraphic. There are many reasons why an individual might not develop attractive penmanship. In today's educational environment, a main reason for poor handwriting skills is lack of consistent, structured practice in penmanship skills in most elementary school classrooms. Lack of handwriting stimulus leads to unpruned dendrites within the motor cortex where finger dexterity is controlled. Having "sloppy" handwriting does not always mean that a person has dysgraphia. The following checklist of handwriting deficits shows the unique signature of dysgraphia that is part of the dyslexic syndrome.

_____ Cursive and manuscript styles are mixed together
_____ Lowercase and capital letters are mixed together
_____ Writing is too large for the space provided
_____ Words and lines of writing are jammed together
_____ Letters or numerals are written backwards or upside down
_____ Letters or numerals are rolled halfway over

Tag-Along Syndromes

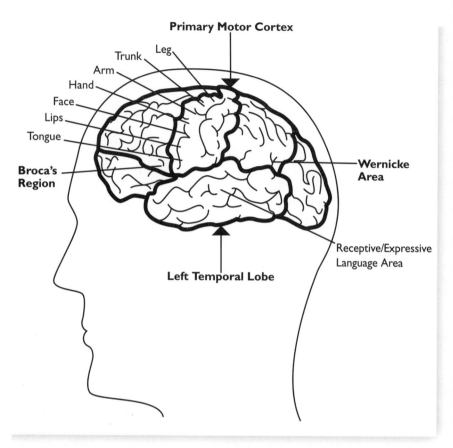

Primary Motor Cortex

Trunk
Leg
Arm
Hand
Face
Lips
Tongue

Broca's Region

Wernicke Area

Receptive/Expressive Language Area

Left Temporal Lobe

FIGURE 6.22. When brain regions develop normally, neurological talents emerge in an orderly developmental sequence. Within the primary motor cortex, muscle control emerges in the sequence shown above, beginning with tongue movement during early infancy and ending with coordination of leg movements during early childhood. At the same time, specialized regions of the left frontal lobe (Broca's Region) and left temporal lobe (Wernicke Area) learn to process receptive and expressive oral language. When neural wiring fails to develop within the hand/arm control regions of the motor cortex, a handwriting disability called dysgraphia makes it impossible for the individual to become competent with penmanship.

_____ Letters or numerals are made from several small fragments of pencil strokes

_____ Writing floats above the line, then cuts down through the line

_____ Writing wanders away from the left margin

_____ Writing skips lines and does not follow numbered lines

_____ Size of writing changes from small to very large in the same writing space

A major challenge for individuals who are dysgraphic is copying or drawing geometric shapes. Figure 6.23 shows the struggle of an intelligent 11-year-old boy to copy simple shapes. Figure 6.24 shows the dysgraphic inability of a boy in third grade to reduce the size of his handwriting to fit the space provided on worksheets. Figure 6.25 illustrates why dyslexia

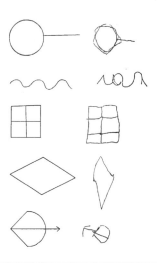

FIGURE 6.23. This was the best that an 11-year-old boy could do to copy these simple shapes. Dysgraphia forces him to use too-large pencil strokes that cannot maintain coherence of the models he sees. As his pencil turns corners and changes direction, he loses his mental image of where the pencil goes next. *Note.* From *Jordan Dyslexia Assessment/ Reading Program* (2nd ed., p. 37), by D. R. Jordan, 2000, Austin, TX: PRO-ED, Inc. Copyright 2000 by PRO-ED, Inc. Reprinted with permission.

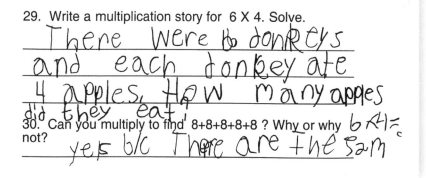

FIGURE 6.24. This 9-year-old boy excels in math and in oral language activities. However, when he tries to do worksheet assignments, he cannot fit his writing into the space provided. He becomes deeply frustrated when he runs out of writing space before he encodes all of his knowlege or ideas. He receives a lot of criticism from adults who think he does not try hard enough to write neatly.

Tag-Along Syndromes

and dysgraphia trigger emotional outbursts when this extremely intelligent 11-year-old girl must do handwritten assignments. When she can tell orally or write through her keyboard, her language skills are advanced and fluent. When she must do handwriting, this ragged penmanship humiliates her and triggers angry outbursts. Figure 6.26 shows the backward strokes in the writing of a 9-year-old girl who is dysgraphic. The arrows trace her struggle to follow the left-to-right and top-to-bottom orientation required inside the left-brain linear box. Figure 6.27 shows the dysgraphic effort of an 11-year-old boy to write a story. His penmanship actually is a series of broken pieces strung together to form letters. He also rolls letters

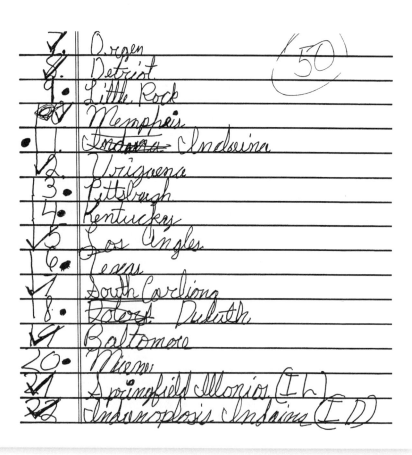

FIGURE 6.25. This 11-year-old girl earned Full Scale IQ 142 on the *Wechsler Intelligence Scale for Children*. When she is free to write through her computer keyboard, her written language skills are at a ninth-grade level. However, when she must write by hand, her penmanship is barely legible and exposes her underlying dyslexic patterns. She experiences cycles of depression because she cannot produce the high quality of writing by hand that she can do fluently through her keyboard.

partway over toward the left, causing the letter *a* to look like the letter *g*. Figure 6.28 shows the struggle of a 13-year-old dysgraphic boy to write a story about his favorite experience. Figure 6.29 shows how an intuitive teacher translated his story by separating the words and lines. In my experience with several thousand dysgraphic individuals, I have found ADHD or ADD in more than half of this segment of the dyslexic population.

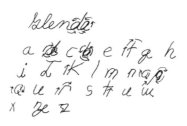

FIGURE 6.26. Tracing over this 9-year-old girl's handwriting reveals the fluctuations that occur within her brain as she copies or writes. Tracing re-creates the physical stress that triggers frustration and dread in every writing task this child is asked to do.

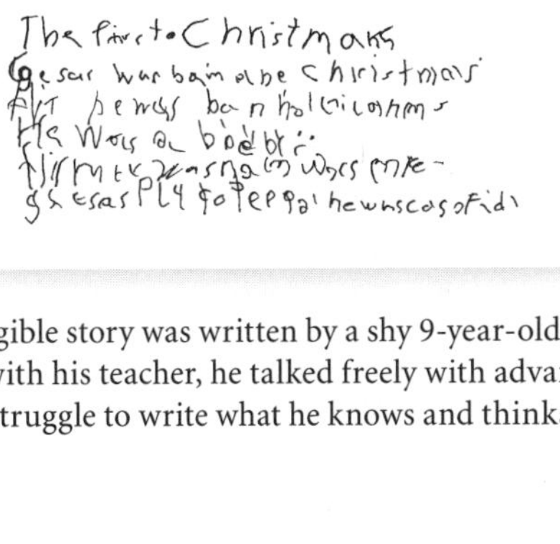

FIGURE 6.27. This illegible story was written by a shy 9-year-old boy who rarely spoke in the classroom. Alone with his teacher, he talked freely with advanced vocabulary and oral language skills. His struggle to write what he knows and thinks illustrates severe dysgraphia.

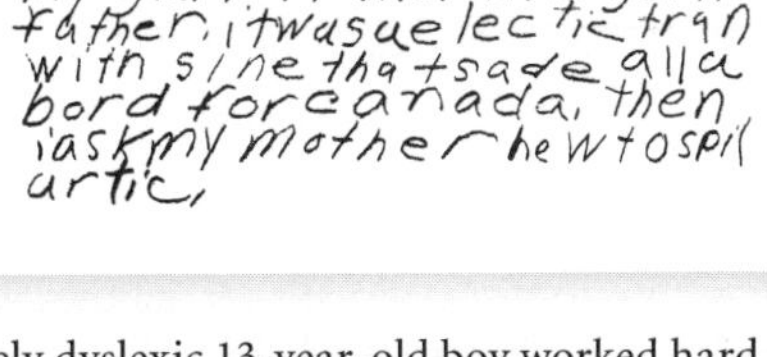

FIGURE 6.28. A severely dyslexic 13-year-old boy worked hard to write this story, only to have it rejected by adults because it made no sense. An intuitive teacher copied it onto the spacing grid shown in Figure 6. 29. She was surprised to see an intelligent story emerge as the words and lines were separated.

Tag-Along Syndromes

When handwriting remains at this level of struggle, most of these persons give up trying. They no longer focus attention on writing tasks, and they disrupt the class by becoming restless, bored, and irritable.

Dyscalculia
The fourth subtype of dyslexia that often exists beneath the layers of poor reading, spelling, and handwriting is an inability to remember the

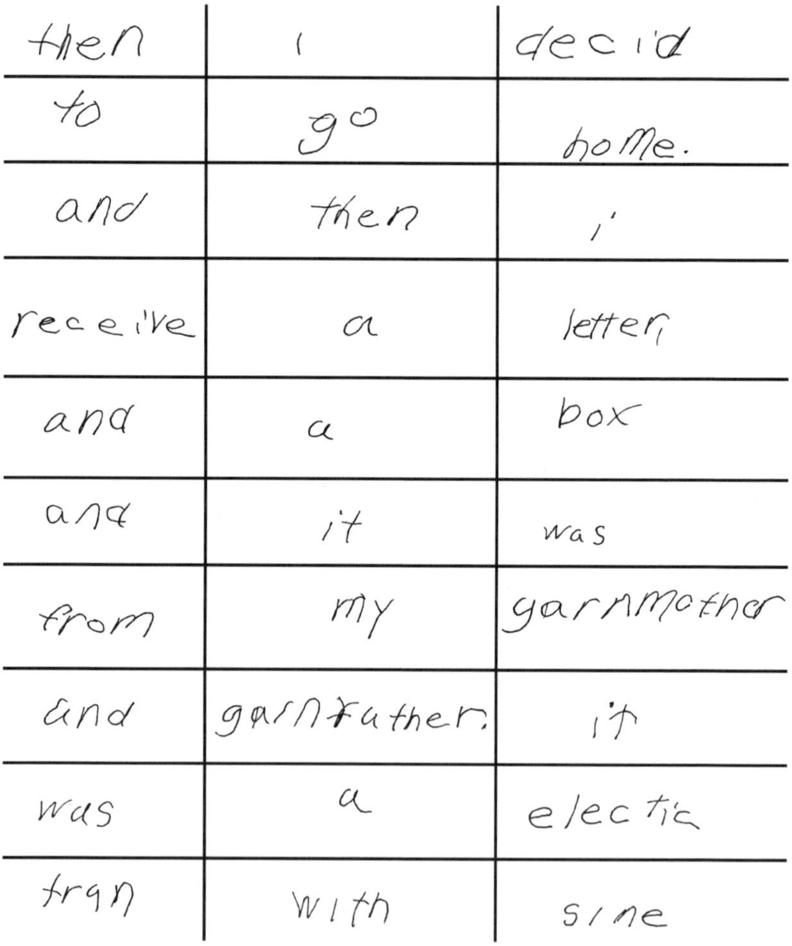

then	(	decid
to	go	home.
and	then	;
receive	a	letter,
and	a	box
and	it	was
from	my	garnmother
and	garnfather.	it
was	a	electic
trqn	with	sine

FIGURE 6.29. Separating words and sentences reveals the message that the dysgraphic writer of Figure 6.28 wanted to convey. Extra space around each word lets the writer correct errors before writing the story again.

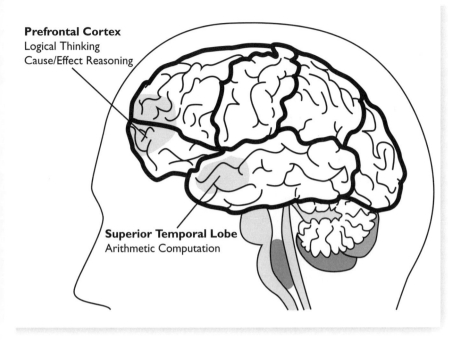

FIGURE 6.30. These regions of the left brain team together to learn the computation skills of basic arithmetic and math. Incomplete neuron development in these regions makes it impossible for the higher brain to build permanent memory of math and arithmetic facts and procedures. This is called *dyscalculia*.

facts, concepts, and procedures of basic math and arithmetic. This is called *dyscalculia*. Figure 6.30 shows the regions of the left brain where arithmetic computation skills (addition, subtraction, multiplication, division, fractions) originate. Incomplete neuron development in these left-brain regions creates "number dyslexia" the way that other regions of the left brain create dyslexia for reading and spelling. Ironically, many individuals with dyscalculia later become talented with types of higher mathematics that are processed mostly in right-brain regions that are not dyslexic. Among such individuals was Albert Einstein, who could not master basic skills of arithmetic computation. By age 13 he was dismissed from school and labeled "dunce." As Einstein entered adolescence, he began to excel in higher mathematics that did not require arithmetic computation. In his early 20s, his extraordinary right-brain talent for abstract math reasoning led him to conceptualize the formula $e = mc^2$, which opened profoundly important new areas of science and mathematics.

Tag-Along Syndromes

The following checklist shows the signature of dyscalculia, which often tags along with ADHD or ADD.

_____ Cannot remember simple facts about addition, subtraction, multiplication, division, fractions, or decimals.

_____ Cannot build long-term memory for arithmetic functions.

_____ Must use a multisensory method to work math problems. Must see/say/touch at the same time (count fingers, whisper over and over, use a calculator).

_____ Must use scratch paper to practice, rehearse, or doodle in order to figure out number relationships.

_____ Cannot shrink size of handwriting to fit into spaces on worksheets.

_____ Writes clusters of marks on scratch paper, then counts them to find sums or totals.

_____ Continually loses the direction in carrying and borrowing.

_____ Misreads math signs. Thinks "times" for + or "add" for ×.

_____ Writes numerals backward.

_____ Continually erases or writes over first answers.

_____ Sometimes manages to do correct problem solving if given enough time to work at own pace.

_____ Becomes overly frustrated when pressed to work problems in a hurry.

Figures 6.31 through 6.33 show how dyscalculia emerges in math activities. As these individuals struggle with math dyslexia, their behavior becomes restless, frustrated, and often disruptive. They exhibit very short attention span in math activities. They cannot keep up with classmates who learn new math information quickly. They misunderstand math terminology used by teachers and other students. They fail to complete assignments or do homework satisfactorily. On the surface, the behavior of students with dyscalculia imitates ADHD and ADD.

Dysnomia

The fifth subtype of dyslexia is lifelong difficulty understanding, remembering, and correctly using words in speaking and writing. This struggle with vocabulary and sentence structure is called *dysnomia*.

A prominent civic leader in the American Southwest was noted for the dyslexic signature of his speech. One day he met a relative of someone who recently had died. "Was that you or your brother who

From a classroom math assignment
Reversed Numerals

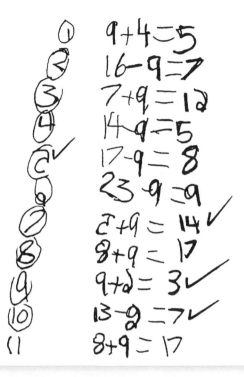

FIGURE 6.31. Multiple layers of visual dyslexia, dysgraphia, and dyscalculia trigger major struggle as this 9-year-old boy tries to do math assignments. Using a hand calculator eliminates more than half of the dyslexic interference in doing classroom math work. His accuracy and fluency in math work double when he no longer has to struggle with handwriting.

was killed in that wreck?" he asked. Another time this dyslexic man said, "I can see the writing on the handwall." One day he posted a notice in his workplace: "There will be no before drinking till after the job." At a company party he commented to a friend, "That guy over there keeps watching me like I was a hawk." At a dinner party he noticed a woman who was somewhat overdressed for the occasion. "She ain't exactly no fried chicken," he said to a friend. One day he amazed his office staff when he said, "If the phone answers for me, tell them for a few minutes that I've gone for down the street coffee."
—Dale Jordan, 2000, p. 45.

Tag-Along Syndromes

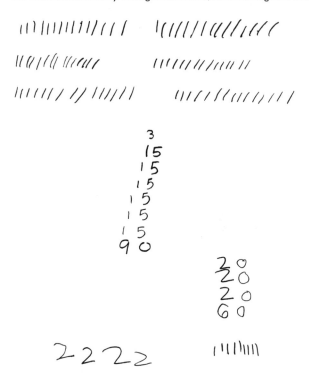

She found the answers by writing marks in sets, then counting each mark.

FIGURE 6.32. Students with dyscalculia try various ways to compensate for not remembering math facts on command. To do this simple math assignment, this 14-year-old girl had to do trial-and-error practice on scratch paper. After nine years of formal school experience, she still cannot do math from memory.

This subtype of dyslexia presents a challenge in building long-term memory of the names of things (nomenclature). The tone deafness of auditory dyslexia, plus the directional scrambling of visual dyslexia, prevent these individuals from hearing, pronouncing, and using words accurately. In Mrs. Jolly's classroom, we met Jacob and saw his dyslexic struggle with writing and spelling (see Figures I.4 and I.5). At home, his dysnomia creates frustrating moments for the family. For example, during a New England winter storm, his dad said: "Jacob, go check the furnace and see if it's OK." A few minutes later, his dad was frustrated to find the boy in the kitchen

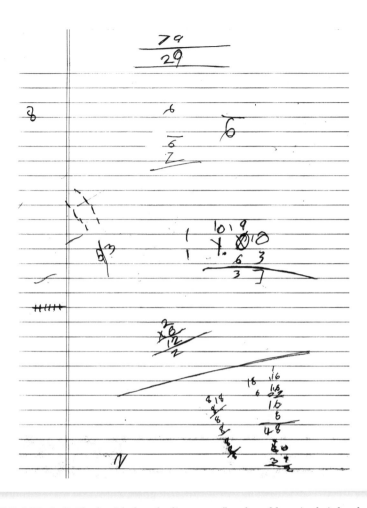

FIGURE 6.33. Individuals with dyscalculia cannot "work problems in their heads." To develop mental images of number relationships, they must use a multisensory technique in which they see it/say it/write it over and over. These students must use scratch paper to practice various possibilities as they do math assignments. They must have all the time they need without feeling pressure to hurry. Using a hand calculator more than doubles the accuracy and productivity of persons with dyscalculia.

searching through the shelves. "What are you doing?" his dad asked. "I said go check the furnace." Jacob had heard "thermos" and thought he was supposed to find it in the kitchen. He does not know that these are different words. Most individuals who are dyslexic do not distinguish between "ideal" and "idea," causing them to say: "I've got a really good ideal how to do that." They do not know that these different words exist. Along with mishearing similar sounding words, Jacob does not immediately connect meaning to what he hears. He continually interrupts when others are speaking: "Huh?" or "What do you mean?" It is very difficult for him to perform on vocabulary tests. He rarely succeeds on tests that ask him to select the correct meaning from three or four choices. As he learned to take his own shower, Jacob asked which "tallow" he should use. Whenever he heard a siren coming down the street, he shouted: "Here comes a truckfire!" When he and his grandmother went shopping, he tugged at her sleeve and said: "Grandma, my tie is unshoeing." In telling his friends about his family's vacation, Jacob said: "We're going to Mervont." On Sunday morning, he talked about "going to Skunday Sool." One of Jacob's dysnomia moments became a favorite slogan for his family. As he yawned heavily one evening, he said: "I'm very tryer. I want to go to bed."

One day Mrs. Jolly made a list of Jacob's dysnomia moments in interpreting what she said:

What Mrs. Jolly Said	What Jacob Heard
leopard	leprosy
pity	picky
curiosity	cures
grief	grease
compare	repair
rose	roll
gulf stream	gull stream (later, golf stream)

These kinds of tongue-twisters are earmarks of dysnomia, which is closely linked to auditory dyslexia. In formal language situations when Jacob is expected to use words correctly and pronounce them accurately, he becomes embarrassed, frustrated, and emotionally upset if anyone teases or corrects him. Under classroom pressure to use oral language fluently, Jacob unplugs his attention and drifts away into daydreaming. If he encounters too much stress, he bursts into tears and flares in tantrums. Beneath the surface of his behavior are overlapping layers of dyslexia and ADHD.

ADHD and ADD Are Many Things

This chapter reveals the complex potential layers that must be recognized if ADHD and ADD are to be treated successfully. These comorbid issues seldom are identified through standard test scores alone. Parents and teachers face the challenge of discovering the multiple reasons why Luis, Anna, and Jacob cannot fit inside the left-brain linear box without consistent help that embraces all of the layers of their learning differences.

The Role of Diet and Medication in Overcoming ADHD and ADD

Chapter

7

⤙ ⤙

Does Diet Matter for ADHD and ADD?

Some mental health professionals believe that changing one's diet can have a positive impact on individuals with ADD—for example, eliminating or cutting back on all chemical additives in food and all processed or naturally occurring sugars. Although most professionals do not believe that ingested foods can *cause* ADD, many believe that certain foods exacerbate the problem in a person who already has the condition.

225

—James L. Thomas, 1996, p. 140

The evidence to date suggests that there is a small group of children who have multiple physical and behavioral difficulties in addition to symptoms of ADHD who may benefit from dietary intervention. The children most likely to respond are those who are quite young and who suffer from myriad problems besides ADHD, including allergies, sleep disorders, and a variety of neurological problems.

—Barbara Ingersoll and Sam Goldstein, 1993, p. 163

Diet has a smaller part to play in the treatment of ADD than popular mythology might suggest. Diet never causes ADD, though in a minority of ADD and non-ADD children, certain foodstuffs may make their behavior more active and possibly more irritable. There seems to be little evidence that diet directly affects attention, impulsivity or insatiability. Sugar has not been shown to cause bad behavior. If parents wish to try a diet, they have our full support. All we ask is that they do it properly, under the supervision of a specialist doctor or dietitian.

—Christopher Green and Kit Chee, 1994, p.93

The 20th century ended with these kinds of cautious, somewhat skeptical attitudes among most physicians and psychologists about the role of diet in the treatment of ADHD or ADD. However, as we entered the 21st century, new understanding of the impact of diet on brain functions was emerging.

Recent studies by [Keith] Conners ... point to a link between carbohydrate intake and hyperactivity and suggest that protein may lessen the effect that carbohydrates may have in increasing hyperactive behavior.

—Harvey C. Parker, 1996, p. 17

Diet matters. Pay attention to it.... Give people a lot of sugar (or substances like bread that are easily broken down to sugar) in the morning and they will act as if they have ADD.... In order for children and adults to focus, they need to have nutritious food that enhances energy and concentration. Especially for people with ADD, the solution is a higher-protein, lower-carbohydrate diet ... the exact opposite of the way that most people eat.

—Daniel G. Amen, 2001, p. 212

Diet Often Matters for ADHD and ADD

For two reasons, 1973 was a memorable year in my life. That year I left university-based clinical work with struggling learners to join my wife in private practice with dyslexic, ADHD, and ADD individuals of all ages. Immediately we plunged into the world of frustrated parents, struggling youngsters, disruptive adolescents, and discouraged adults who could not get their lives in order. Also in 1973, pediatrician Benjamin Feingold in San Francisco became a national media sensation with his proposal that hyperactivity and attention deficits are related to food allergies, as well as to chemical additives and sugar. Through national talk shows and other media, the public heard Feingold claim that 50% of ADHD behavior could be reduced or eliminated by removing trigger foods, sugar, and chemicals from the child's diet. Like a thunderstorm breaking over the city, our diagnostic center was deluged by excited parents who wanted Dr. Feingold's kind of help with disruptive youngsters like James and Kim, whom we met in Chapter 3. Soon hundreds of Feingold diet chapters had formed across the country with parents exchanging recipes they insisted had reduced hyperactivity in themselves and their offspring. Our staff became sharply focused on behaviors that might be related to food and beverage intake. As we saw in Chapter 3, James became a new person when trigger foods were eliminated from his diet.

Feingold Kaiser-Permanente Diet

In 1975 Feingold published his widely read book *Why Your Child Is Hyperactive*. For the first time, we could separate media hype from what Feingold actually proposed. The book revealed that Feingold's concepts of diet control for ADHD and ADD had been misrepresented. Unfortunately, initial publicity that reduced the Feingold diet to inaccurate sound bites had left an indelibly bad impression in the minds of many physicians and mental health providers. For example, pediatrician Paul Warren had this to say about the long-term effect of the Feingold diet:

> As we've watched Feingold graduates—the kids who were treated through the diet—mature down through the years, we've not often been able to see many significant differences. In other words, it appears that special diets do not work for the vast majority of children upon whom they are tried, particularly in the long term.
> —Paul Warren, 1995, p. 72

To this day, Ben Feingold's contribution to managing ADHD behaviors through diet is seriously underestimated. The Feingold K-P diet divided foods into two groups of foods to be advoided. Group 1 consisted of foods that contain natural salicylic acid (salicylate foods). In nature, this family of natural plant chemicals appears in many foods. Among fruits containing salicylic acid are apples, apricots, blackberries, strawberries, oranges, cherries, raspberries, gooseberries, peaches, plums, and grapes. Any food or beverage product that contains grape extract, such as grape juice, wine, sweeteners, flavors, or coloring agents processed from grapes brings salicylic salts into the body. Certain vegetables also are a source of salicylic salts, such as tomatoes, cucumbers, and bell peppers. Today's popular fast foods include many items containing tomato sauce and catsup, along with all kinds of cucumber pickle products. Feingold contended that hyperactive, disruptive behavior often is triggered by eating or drinking salicylate foods or beverages.

Group 2 in the Feingold K-P diet consisted of chemical additives that saturate prepared foods in grocery stores and on restaurant menus. Partly in response to the surge of public interest in Feingold's theories, in 1975 the Food and Drug Administration began to remove several chemical dyes, preservatives, and flavoring agents from the nation's food chain. However, one must read labels very carefully to find food products that do not contain chemical additives. Prepared foods continue to contain such chemical additives as sorbates, sulphites, benzoates, nitrates, nitrites, antioxidants, and propionates. In addition, artificial coloring agents are added to virtually every kind of prepared food product, including freshly packaged meats.

As the Feingold diet gained popularity, several other diet plans emerged to treat ADHD, ADD, and other types of disruptive behavior. In his books *Improving Your Child's Behavior Chemistry* (1976) and *Feed Your Kids Right* (1979), pediatrician Lendon Smith presented a simple, commonsense diet he thought would increase attention span and reduce hyperactive/disruptive behavior. Smith also presented behavior management guidelines that answered many questions for parents of ADHD and ADD children. During the 1980s, pediatric allergist William G. Crook gained national attention through his books *The Yeast Connection: A Medical Breakthrough* (1986) and *Help for the Hyperactive Child* (1991). Crook contended that many individuals suffer from a toxic condition caused when the yeast *Candida albicans* invades the body immune system and irritates the central nervous system. Crook instructed parents to follow a diet that eliminated sugar, chemical additives, and all foods and beverages that tend to trigger allergic reactions in children. This dietary program included taking antifungal medication, especially *nystatin.* Crook also specified supplemental doses of vitamins, minerals, and fatty acids. Through her book *Is This Your Child? Discovering and Treating Unrecognized Allergies* (1991), pediatrician Doris Rapp emerged as a popular authority on hidden food and environmental allergies that trigger ADHD, ADD, and other disruptive disorders. Rapp presented strict diet programs along with careful attention to environmental sources of allergies that interfere with learning and social behavior. A major voice in the national discussion of whether diet matters with ADHD and ADD has been C. Keith Conners. His thoughtful books *Hyperkinetic Children: A Neuropsychosocial Approach* (with K. C. Wells, 1986) and *Feeding the Brain: How Foods Affect Children* (1989) set the tone for unemotional, rational consideration of the effects of foods and beverages on brain functions in learning and behaving.

Intolerance to Foods

Lost in the public debate over these diet plans was the important distinction between allergic response to food substances and the critical issue of cytotoxic intolerance for specific foods and beverages. Careful reading of

Feingold's work discloses that he did not claim that allergies to Group 1 or Group 2 foods cause hyperactivity and disruptive behavior. Nor did Feingold contend that sugar by itself is a major culprit, as many parents believe. The Feingold model was based upon disruptive body chemistry reaction to certain food substances called *food intolerance*. The clinical term for this often catastrophic reaction is *cytotoxic*. Many children, adolescents, and adults have dramatic intolerance for certain foods or beverages. This is similar to being poisoned when a toxic substance enters the bloodstream. Being food intolerant (cytotoxic) is not the same as being allergic. An allergy triggers a chain of defensive body chemistry responses that rid the bloodstream of the irritating substance (mold, dust, food substance). A rash may appear, nasal passages become congested, eyes water, and the person sneezes or coughs. Yet an allergic condition seldom makes the central nervous system ill. In contrast, intolerance for food substances poisons nerve pathways and causes swelling of brain tissues. This triggers or exaggerates disruptive physical and emotional reactions.

An example of the often severe effect of food intolerance is described by Thom Hartmann, who is ADHD:

> Many people of northern European ancestry carry the gene [for celiac disease] in which the body's immune system reacts to the gluten protein in wheat, rye, and barley as if it were cholera or some other pathogen. I had never had a problem with these foods until, at the age of fifty, I was in Australia and contracted dysentery from contaminated water. Although antibiotics eventually knocked out the dysentery, for the next year I continued to have symptoms of a milder, cholera-like illness that went away only when I eliminated all wheat, rye, and barley from my diet ... for the rest of my life, I must totally avoid bread, pizza, and so many of the other foods that are common in a typical Western diet.
>
> — Thom Hartmann 2003, p. 66

The Impact of Diet on Unwellness

Following World War I, neurologist Samuel T. Orton spent many years studying families of dyslexic individuals (Orton, 1925, 1928, 1937). Long before we learned that dyslexia is a genetic disorder, Orton's research documented how the whole body is involved when dyslexia exists in families. He described a range of physical patterns that are seen in relatives of dyslexic persons. For example, Orton found that a majority of the blood relatives of dyslexic individuals begin to show gray or white streaks in their hair during their late teens or early 20s. Many of these relatives are gray- or white-haired by age 30. Approximately 13% of dyslexic family members are left-handed, compared with 3% of the general population. Dyslexic families display many more allergies than nondyslexic groups, including allergic sensitivity to the environment, food substances, and beverage ingredients. In particular, individuals with dyslexia tend to be intolerant of whole milk. The cytotoxic condition of lactose intolerance creates intense gastric distress along with swelling of the brain. Orton found that many persons with dyslexia have toxic reaction to wheat gluten, resulting in unwell symptoms that include swelling of joints and inflammation of large muscle neurons.

Orton discovered that dyslexic families include increased numbers of relatives with autoimmune disorders, such as lupus in women and arthritis and fibromyalgia in men. On the typical American diet that is high in carbohydrates, dyslexic individuals tend to live with large muscle distress, inflammation of joints, and gastritis that keeps the lower intestinal tract in a state of irritation that often becomes irritable bowel syndrome or colitis. Dyslexic individuals and their blood relatives are prone to develop Crohn's disease (polyps protruding into the digestive tract). Dyslexic families have lifelong problems with flatulence (gas buildup within the small intestine). Orton speculated that this syndrome is caused by lack of digestive enzymes in the lower bowel. Toward the end of his professional career, Orton concluded that dyslexia is a whole body issue that requires changes in one's diet to avoid lifelong discomfort and borderline poor health from food intolerance, especially for gluten and whole milk.

230

The Role of Salicylate Foods in Autoimmune Disorders

Since 1964 R. Paul St. Amand, an endocrinologist at the University of California in Los Angeles, has investigated the relationship between diet and autoimmune disorders, especially fibromyalgia. His research has focused on the cytotoxic impact of salicylate foods on the central nervous system. St. Amand has documented how salicylates trigger the debilitating symptoms of fibromyalgia, including pain in large muscles, chronic fatigue, inflammation of joints and muscle fibers, insomnia, disorientation, chronic bladder problems, and vaginal infections (St. Amand, 1999). St. Amand's research has linked adverse reaction to salicylate substances with these types of chronic malaise:

Fatigue	Impaired memory	Impaired concentration
Nervousness	Chronic pains	Occipital headaches
Anxiety	Restless legs	Bladder infections
Insomnia	Frontal headaches	Skin rashes

Panic attack	Depression	Pungent urine
Weight changes	Gas/bloating	Constipation
Diarrhea	Leg cramps	Ringing ears
Abnormal tastes	Eye irritation	Nasal congestion
Brittle nails	Hunger tremors	Heart palpitations
Faintness	Sugar craving	Salt craving

Samuel Orton's earlier research revealed that many individuals with dyslexia suffer from autoimmune disorders. Chapter 6 describes the frequent overlap of ADHD and dyslexia. This comorbid relationship between attention deficits and dyslexia gives the research of Feingold and St. Amand added importance. St. Amand's remedy for fibromyalgia is twofold. First, all sources of salycilate salts are eliminated. This includes avoiding several classes of fruits, vegetables, and most spices. Virtually all cosmetics and soap products, such as aloe and balsam, contain salicylates, (see Appendix 1 in St. Amand's book *What Your Doctor May Not Tell You About Fibromyalgia*). Along with this elimination diet, patients also take daily doses of *guaifenesin*, an inexpensive medication often available without prescription. St. Amand's current work affirms Ben Feingold's teaching 30 years ago that many ADHD individuals have adverse reaction to salicylate foods.

America's Dietary Revolution

231

The 21st century began with a virtual revolution in America's eating habits. Numerous new diet plans emerged to turn the traditional food pyramid upside down. For most of the 20th century, Americans were advised to eat mostly carbohydrate foods with limited amounts of protein. On this diet, which emphasized starches and grain products, obesity, Type II diabetes, and ADHD increased dramatically, especially in children. In 2003 pediatrician Julian Stuart Haber wrote the following:

> Recently, several authors have argued that Attention Deficit Hyperactivity Disorder (ADHD) is a myth. Nothing could be further from the truth. It is a very real entity [that] has been called by many different names over the past fifty-five years.... As many as 15% of our children and adolescents are receiving medical treatment for ADHD ... is no question that the number of children diagnosed with this disorder is increasing ... the use of stimulant medications in preschool children between two and four years of age has tripled.
> —Julian Stuart Haber, 2003, p. xiii

A major new voice in the impact of diet on ADHD is psychiatrist Daniel G. Amen, who is redefining diagnosis and treatment of ADHD (he calls it ADD) through the Amen Clinic ADD Brain Enhancement Program (Amen, 2001). Diagnosis is based upon brain imaging through SPECT (single photon emission tomography), along with body chemistry analysis and elimination of trigger food substances. Amen's point of view is summarized in this statement:

> Dietary interventions are important in treating all types of ADD. Food can be used like medicine. It can have a powerfully positive effect on cognition, feelings, and behavior, but it can have a negative effect as well. In fact, the right diet can decrease the amount of medication needed. However, the wrong diet will do the opposite.
>
> —Amen, 2001, p. 224

The Amen Clinic ADD Brain Enhancement Program emphasizes a diet based upon four groups. This diet plan eliminates all forms of sugar (fructose, lactose, sucrose, corn syrup, glucose), caffeine, alcohol, and white wheat products.

1. *Plenty of water* — At least eight 8-ounce glasses of water each day.
2. *Healthy proteins* — Only complete protein such as fish (especially farm-raised salmon and tuna); chicken or turkey; very lean cuts of beef; milk, low-fat cottage cheese, or low-fat string cheese; soy-based foods; protein powder.
3. Complex carbohydrates — Fruits, especially apricots, oranges, kiwi, tangerines, pears, grapefruit, apples. All vegetables except carrots (due to high sugar content). Beans, especially black beans and kidney beans. Whole grains, but no white bread or bread with added sugar.
4. Unsaturated fats — Olive oil, canola oil, grapeseed oil, avocados, nuts (Brazil nuts, macadamia nuts, almonds, cashews, pistachios). No peanuts, pecans, or walnuts.

High-Protein/Low-Carbohydrate Diets

By 2004 high-protein/low-carbohydrate diets had been adopted by enough Americans to create economic problems for grain producers and manufacturers of bread and pasta products. Meanwhile, sales of animal protein sources soared. As yet, no scientific studies have been done to determine how this national dietary shift affects ADHD or ADD. However, a stream of anecdotal reports and testimonials from satisfied individuals fill the news and talk shows, telling how life has improved through turning the food pyramid upside down.

Family Diet

During my 20 years in private practice with ADHD, ADD, and dyslexic individuals and their families, my staff and I witnessed countless episodes of food or beverage intolerance that triggered outbursts of tantrums, aggression, rebellion, hyperactivity, mood swings, or depression. With our dyslexic clients and their families, we verified Orton's observations of the link between gluten, whole milk, and unwellness, including fibromyalgia and chronic gastritis. Whole milk proved to be a major trigger for many ADHD and dyslexic individuals. Removing or strictly limiting milk intake frequently reduced hyperactivity, irritability, gastritis, distractibility, and oppositional behavior. This change in diet often increased attention span, improved sleep, and fostered better social relationships without medication. We met many individuals who could not tolerate products made from grapes or tomatoes, or foods containing gluten. When they gave up pizza, spaghetti dinners, white bread burgers and sandwiches, catsup, or beverages containing grape extracts, their lives improved enough to make such sacrifices worthwhile. We watched as many families changed their habits in grocery buying and food consumption to avoid foods that triggered inappropriate behaviors and unwell aftermath. As Feingold pointed out, the entire family must agree to follow the new eating plan. Most families who made those dietary changes found that everyone felt better, once they got past the grouchy withdrawal period of eliminating trigger foods and beverages. In spite of the controversies surrounding the Feingold diet, the Atkins diet, and similar dietary programs, the fact remains that many ADHD and ADD individuals struggle with intolerance for certain food substances. The quality of their lives improves significantly when cytotoxic substances are eliminated from the diet.

The Emotions and Feelings of Diet Control

Despite the lack of scientific evidence that any dietary component is a major cause of ADHD, many people continue to believe that manipulation of children's diet can influence their behavior. It may

be that adherence to a very controlled diet … yields a benefit because the extra attention the child receives helps him to control his
inborn tendency toward inattentiveness and overactivity. In addition,
a dietary explanation allows parents to view the child as 'ill' rather
than 'bad,' thus reducing some of the social and emotional stress on
the child.

—Lisa J. Bain, 1991, pp. 58–59

Physicians and mental health providers who are devoted to the scientific
method tend to require measurable objective facts before they trust new
ideas. This point of view usually discounts subjective, anecdotal testimonials from those who benefit from new or unusual treatment methods (Bain, 1991; Ingersoll & Goldstein, 1993; Warren & Capehart, 1995;
Wender, 2000). For most of my career in diagnosing and remediating dyslexia, ADHD, and ADD, the issue of diet control was mostly pragmatic. My
point of view has been that if manipulating diet helps struggling families
and individuals, then "go for it" and be thankful for whatever benefits they
enjoyed. As I entered middle age, I began to suffer from mysterious cycles
of large muscle distress, frequent "fuzziness" in thinking and remembering, inability to sleep longer than four or five hours at night, chronic fatigue that felt like I was carrying a heavy load on my shoulders all the time,
and moderate depression. By age 55 I was struggling hard to maintain private practice and conduct staff training seminars throughout the Western
Hemisphere. I spent a fortune at a world-famous medical center where
none of the specialists diagnosed the problem. By my 59th birthday, my
intuitive family physician suggested that I might be suffering from fibryo-
malgia. I was so unwell I had to retire from private practice. After a few
months of rest, I joined a university staff to lead teams in developing workplace programs for adults who were ADHD, ADD, and dyslexic. As that
work progressed, the symptoms of muscle distress, chronic fatigue, severe
malaise, and depression returned. At age 65, I was forced to retire again,
thinking that my years of productive work were over. When I turned 66,
a friend convinced me to try the controversial Atkins diet, which called
for eliminating all starches and eating mostly protein foods with small
amounts of red, green, or yellow vegetables and fruits, but nothing white
or brown. Within 6 weeks after starting this new diet regime, my symptoms of fibromyalgia decreased by 60%. This radical change in well-being
revealed that by middle age, I had become acutely intolerant of gluten,
similar to Thom Hartmann's experience described above. Eliminating all
grains and starches from my diet dramatically improved my life. We discovered that our children also have intolerance for gluten. Scientists might
discount my personal experience as being too subjective and anecdotal.
However, the joyful emotions I gained from turning the food pyramid

upside down are beyond my ability to express. The issue of diet influence on ADHD, ADD, and dyslexic individuals remains deeply personal and worth considering.

The Role of Medication in Reducing ADHD and ADD

The issue of whether to prescribe medications for ADHD or ADD has always been controversial. In Chapter 3 we met James, whose behavior was out of control. His parents were torn between personal conviction that it was somehow "wrong" to control children through medication and their desperation to have a normal family life. James suffered from overlapping behavior disorders. In the shadow of ADHD lurked Oppositional Defiant Disorder (ODD) and intermittent episodes of Conduct Disorder (CD). In Chapter 3 we also met Kim, whom I knew as a difficult child, a rebellious adolescent, and a dysfunctional young adult. During her school years, Ritalin reduced disruptive behavior enough to let her finish high school and be reasonably happy and stable. On her 18th birthday, Kim rebelled against medication, and her parents helplessly watched her life fall apart. Those who object to stimulant medication for youngsters do so out of fear of possible side effects. Yet the side effects of unrelieved ADHD and ADD can be far worse than the mild side effects some individuals experience from medication.

During the 1990s Russell Barkley and his research associates at the University of Massachussetts Medical Center documented why we must follow the standard of *differential diagnosis* in separating the layers of ADHD from tag-along syndromes (Barkley, 1990). This approach to seeing each layer of an individual's challenges usually leads to *multiple diagnosis* with dual medication along with appropriate diet change. Often it is necessary to include talk therapy. In 1995 Barkley and his research team reported that 65% of those diagnosed as ADHD also had ODD, while 30% also had CD (Barkley, 1995). In 1992 the research team of Gilger, Pennington, and DeFries documented the comorbid relationship between attention deficits and dyslexia (Gilger, Pennington, & DeFries, 1992). My clinical experience with struggling learners found that 65% of those with dyslexia also have ADHD or ADD. Laura Weisel (1992, 2001) found 42% overlap of ADHD or ADD and some type of LD. Carolyn Pollan and Dorothy Williams (1992) documented 45% overlap of LD, ADHD/ADD, and disruptive behavior disorders in school dropouts, adjudicated adolescents, and adult males serving prison sentences. If we do not carefully see these tag-along syndromes that also need treatment, then medicating only one layer of challenge may unleash unacceptable mood disorders that are not treated.

Cortical Stimulants for ADHD and ADD

When the cortical stimulant medications Dexedrine and Ritalin first appeared halfway through the 20th century, little was known about long-term effects of such treatments. Because high dosage strengths of both medications reduce appetite, Dexedrine and Ritalin became overprescribed in weight loss programs. At high dosage levels, all medications overload the brain and disrupt normal body functions. Because of early abuse of these stimulants, a wave of fearful rumors erupted, causing many professionals and individuals to see these medications as harmful and to be avoided.

But as worldwide research began to show, when cortical stimulants are used at low dosage strength, addiction does not occur, children's growth is not slowed down, and health is not affected. The key to using cortical stimulants wisely is to use the lowest possible dosage strength that reduces the disruptive symptoms of ADHD or ADD. As with every medication, not everyone responds to the same treatment. Some individuals are allergic to all of the treatments described below. For example, 3 out of 100 persons cannot tolerate the effects of Ritalin. However, 97 out of 100 individuals do respond well. When used correctly, these medications do not touch the pleasure centers in the brain where drug addictions originate. Correct administration of cortical stimulants does not lead to addiction of these substances. If parents follow the medical guidelines in monitoring daily doses, these cortical stimulants are among the safest medications ever produced.

Enhanced Executive Function

Chapter 2 describes the role of the neurotransmitter dopamine in maintaining executive function. A major cause of ADHD is too little or too much dopamine in the prefrontal cortex. Cortical stimulant medication is designed to increase the supply of dopamine enough to arouse drowsy executive function. The presence of cortical stimulant stabilizes the presence of dopamine, allowing the prefrontal cortex to function normally while the medication is active in the brain. Barkley and his colleagues have reported a wide range of effectiveness in treating ADHD with cortical stimulant medication (Barkley, 1990, 1995). Their success rate ranged from 50% to 95%, depending upon how well tag-along syndromes were medicated through differential diagnosis. If underlying layers of behavior disorders were not taken into account, 50% of their ADHD patients improved with cortical stimulant medication alone. However, when behavior or mood disorders were simultaneously treated by mood control medication, 95% of their ADHD patients improved. Treatment for ADD follows a similar range of success. If an ADD individual is treated with cortical stimulant without recognizing underlying depression, the success rate is about 30%. When tag-along depression is treated with antidepressant medication along with a cortical stimulant for ADD, the success rate rises to 55%.

Low Dosage Strength

All cortical stimulants are measured in milligrams. One milligram (mg) equals 1/30,000th of an ounce. The key to success in using cortical stimulant medication is to keep dosage strength as low as possible. In 1989 Harvey Parker developed the Standard Ritalin Dosage Chart that continues to guide physicians in prescribing cortical stimulants: *low dosage*—0.3 mg per kilogram (2.2 pounds) of body weight; *medium dosage*—0.6 mg per kilogram of body weight; *high dosage*—1.0 mg per killogram of body weight. For example, a child who weighs 88 pounds (40 kilograms) would be given 12 mg for low dosage, 24 mg for medium dosage, or 40 mg for high dosage. Occasionally we see an unusual brain chemistry pattern that requires twice as much, or half as much, medication than others need to reduce ADHD or ADD symptoms. A rule of thumb is that cortical stimulant should not make the person feel different. As increased flow of dopamine arouses the drowsy prefrontal cortex, executive function quietly takes charge of the limbic system, allowing outsiders to see decreased ADHD or ADD symptoms with increased ability to stay focused without distraction, restlessness, or irritability. The person taking the medication should not feel nervous, strange, or weird. In most individuals, hyperactivity declines so that body action approaches normal level for the person's age. If hyperactive individuals become passive and placid, the brain has been overmedicated and cannot learn effectively. The goal of cortical stimulant medication is not to eliminate hyperactivity. The goal should be to reduce or eliminate the distracting "noise" throughout the brain. As this occurs, the level of hyperactivity declines but may not be eliminated altogether.

Rebound from Medication

While taking cortical stimulant medication, most ADHD individuals spend a reasonably quiet, productive day at school or at work. As the school day or workday ends, some of these individuals explode with release of pent-up energy. This is called *rebound* as the day's medication disappears from the brain. Parents often suffer through frantic evenings as rebound energy turns the child into an erupting volcano. Rebound tends to run its course by bedtime, although some rebounders do not calm down until midnight. Some families choose to live with uncontrolled hyperactivity, impulsivity, and insatiability rather than endure the rebound after stimulant medication "wears off." Unfortunately, unmedicated ADHD youngsters tend to rebound all day at school as well as at home. This places teachers in intolerable situations trying to maintain classroom order in the presence of disruptive behavior. Many youngsters who rebound also have tag-along intolerance for certain food substances. When trigger foods are eliminated from their diet, rebound from medication usually diminishes or disappears.

Increase in Usable Intelligence

The most important benefit from cortical stimulant medication is that the person's intelligence is more fully usable in organized, focused, productive ways. Figure 7.1 shows the benefit of Ritalin for a 19-year-old man with ADD. He had been an underachiever all his life. With a cortical stimulant, his intelligence became much more usable and productive. With low-dosage strength Ritalin, he became a high achiever as he finished his college education. As a cortical stimulant reduces distraction, others see positive results in all aspects of the individual's life. Two prominent pediatricians have described the benefits when cortical stimulant medication is effective:

> When ... stimulant drugs are effective, they improve many symptoms of the syndrome. ADHD children generally (1) become calmer and less active; (2) develop a longer span of attention; (3) become less stubborn and easier to manage (they "mind" better); (4) are often more sensitive to the needs of others and much more responsive to discipline and the wishes of others; (5) have longer fuses and fewer or no temper tantrums; (6) experience fewer emotional ups and downs; (7) show a decrease in impulsivity, waiting before they act, and may begin to plan ahead; (8) demonstrate an improvement in school performance; (9) improve their handwriting; and (10) become less disorganized.
> —Paul H. Wender, 2000, p. 74

> [T]reatment with these medications, used at appropriate dose levels, results in increased alertness, decreased activity levels, and decreased impulsivity in 70 to 80% of the children properly diagnosed with attentional and related problems.
> —Julian S. Haber, 2003, p. 100

Possible Side Effects of Medication

All medications have the potential for causing side effects in some individuals. As with intolerance for certain food substances, some persons cannot tolerate certain chemical compounds that create medicines. Side effects tend to be greater with amphetamines than with methylphenidates, which are described below. When side effects occur, they often disappear within two to three weeks as body chemistry adjusts. The most common side effect of cortical stimulants is reduced appetite. However, there is no danger of malnutrition because the body continues to process food normally.

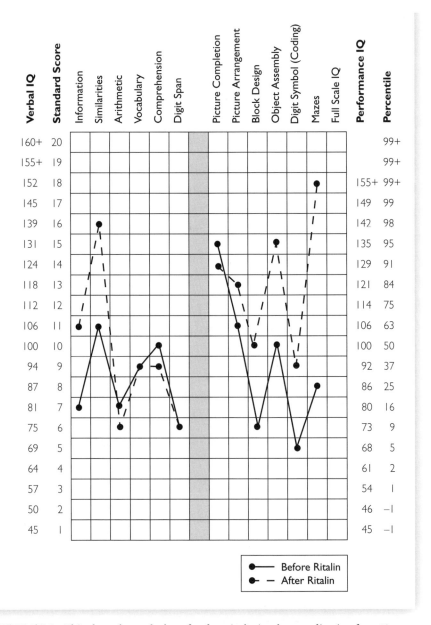

FIGURE 7.1. This chart shows the benefit of cortical stimulant medication for a 19-year-old man who never had done well in school. As he planned to enter adult education, he asked me to advise him on what to do. I had known him since he was 9 years old, but I never could convince his parents to try medication to reduce his ADHD patterns. As a young adult, he agreed to try Ritalin for one semester. The solid line on this *Wechsler Adult Intelligence Scale* shows the level of his usable intelligence before ADHD patterns were reduced. The dotted line shows the difference when medication stablilized his ability to stay focused without distraction. With this benefit from cortical stimulant, he finished college with the best grades he had ever earned.

Some individuals have trouble falling to sleep or staying asleep all night. Occasionally the medication triggers headaches or stomachaches. These transient side effects usually disappear by the second week. If the medication includes the levoamphetamine molecule, the individual might develop mild tics. If so, the person can switch to a different cortical stimulant without that chemical ingredient. It is not unusual for underlying depression or mood swings to become pronounced as cortical medication takes effect. If so, dual medication with an antidepressant is required.

Should the Person Have Drug Holidays?

One of the most frequently asked questions by parents is "Should I stop giving this medication on weekends and holidays? What about during the summer?" This depends upon the child. Some individuals need cortical stimulant during the school day or workday but not at other times. However, most persons who respond well to medication at school or on the job should continue to take it on weekends and holidays. This is because without it, the benefit of medication—elevating dopamine to achieve good executive function—disappears overnight. Each new day begins with disruptive symptoms active again. If medication is taken only during the week, the old ADHD or ADD symptoms are in charge on weekends and holidays. This causes disruptive up-and-down swings in the person's lifestyle that undermine the helpful benefits of medication. It does no good for an individual to swing back and forth from being productive and sociable at school or at work to being disruptive and in conflict on weekends and holidays.

Amphetamine Derivatives

Dexedrine

The use of medication to control symptoms of inattention, hyperactivity, and learning difficulties began in Portland, Oregon, in 1937, when Charles Bradley prescribed Benzadrine (Bradley, 1937). Benzadrine contained both the left and right sides of the amphetamine molecule *levoamphetamine* and *dextroamphetamine*, which are mirror images of each other. Until the mid 1950s, Bradley demonstrated that Benzadrine was effective with a majority of individuals whose symptoms later were called ADHD. However, there were so many side effects from Benzadrine that it did not become a popular treatment for attention deficit disorders. In the 1960s scientists discovered that if they eliminated the levo side of the amphetamine molecule, the remaining dextroamphetamine helped reduce inattention and hyperactivity without the side effects of Benzadrine. That molecular adjustment led to the development of the medication Dexedrine, which became popular during the 1960s and 1970s.

Today's chemical formulation of Dexedrine causes few side effects. Dexedrine takes effect in about one hour and lasts about five hours in the brain. Dexedrine is twice as powerful as Ritalin, making the dosage strength much less than Ritalin. Two forms of Dexedrine are available. Five mg tablets often are prescribed three times a day for maximum dosage of 15 mgs every 24 hours. Also available are Dexedrine spansules, which are administered once a day. These spansules are composed of time-release beads that dissolve slowly in the digestive tract, gradually releasing the medication over a period of eight hours. This eliminates the noon dosage that often creates problems at school or in a family's busy lifestyle.

Adderall
During the 1990s a new form of amphetamine Adderall became available to treat ADHD and ADD. This new cortical stimulant is twice as powerful as Ritalin. Adderall contains four amphetamine salts, including levoamphetamine. Only a few individuals have negative side effects from Adderall. When the tablet form is used, two doses a day are required. Each dose lasts about five hours. In 2001 the time-release Adderall XR became available. The medication is contained in tiny beads that dissolve at different rates over nine hours. This medication seems to trigger more side effects than the time-release spansules of Ritalin, Metadate, and Concerta, which are described below. If an individual tolerates Adderall XR well, the advantage of the spansule form is that only one dose is given each day with breakfast. Parents are cautioned that Adderall XR does not work well with a high-fat breakfast, such as bacon and eggs. Fat in the meal prevents the medication from being absorbed from the small intestine.

Methylphenidate Derivatives

Ritalin
Ritalin was first synthesized in 1955 as a short-acting form of dextrolevomethylphenidate. It begins its work in the brain within 30 minutes and is gone from the brain after four hours. It requires a second dose at noon, and often a third dose in late afternoon to avoid rebound during the evening. As a rule, Ritalin has fewer side effects than Dexedrine. Two time-release forms are available. Ritalin SR takes longer to have effect, and it puts only half as much medication into the brain as regular Ritalin. Therefore, this form is less effective than regular Ritalin, as well as causing more frequent rebound, agitation, and mood swings. Ritalin LA is a capsule containing time-release beads called "sprinkles." As the capsule melts, half of the beads release a normal dose of Ritalin that takes effect in 30 minutes. The rest of the beads dissolve four hours later. One morning dose of Ritalin

LA lasts about nine hours. This medication provides a good day at school or work, but it is gone from the brain during the evening, when homework usually is done. If a person cannot swallow a capsule, the beads can be sprinkled on a teaspoon of applesauce, followed by a glass of water.

Focalin

Focalin is a new short-acting form of methylphenidate that is designed to eliminate most side effects of cortical stimulants. Focalin begins its work in 30 minutes and is effective for five hours. Focalin is twice as powerful as Ritalin and is used when an individual cannot tolerate other medications. Focalin also is safe to use as a late afternoon booster because it does not keep the person awake at night. A time-release spansule form of Focalin is expected to be available in 2005.

Metadate CD

This generic methylphenidate comes in a time-release capsule containing two sets of sprinkles. One third of the beads dissolve immediately, like Ritalin and Concerta. Over the next eight hours, the remaining beads gradually release their dosage through a membrane in the capsule. Metadate CD is effective for about nine hours. For those who cannot swallow a capsule, these beads can be sprinkled over a teaspoon of applesauce at breakfast.

Concerta

Concerta became available in 2000. This is the first true long-acting medication to treat ADHD. Concerta delivers methylphenidate through a time-release system called OROS. Concerta comes in a nondissolvable capsule that is coated with Ritalin that dissolves immediately after swallowing. This begins to take effect within 30 minutes. Inside the capsule is a pastelike form of methylphenidate. A tiny hole in the top of the capsule permits molecules of the medication to escape into the digestive tract. The bottom of the capsule contains sponge-like material called an expander. As the capsule passes through the lower intestine, the walls of the capsule permit fluid to enter the expander. As the expander enlarges, molecules of methylphenidate are pushed out of the capsule and absorbed into the bloodstream. This OROS system meters the discharge of medication for 12 hours. Concerta is engineered to control ADHD or ADD symptoms for a full day at school or work. The medication still is effective during the evening for homework. About an hour before normal bedtime, the brain is free from the medication. Concerta cannot be taken by individuals who suffer from gastrointestinal reflux (GER), pyloric stenosis (restricted esophagus), Crohn's disease (polyps in the intestinal tract), surgically altered intestinal tract, or any disease that interferes with gastrointestinal absorption.

Pemoline

Cylert has the same effect as Ritalin, but it seldom is prescribed because of the potential to cause damage to the liver. A physician must monitor Cylert closely through frequent blood tests to make sure that the liver remains healthy. Cylert rarely is prescribed for children. It is reserved for use by adolescents and adults when no other type of medication is effective.

Atomoxetine
Strattera

This drug became available in 2000 as an alternative to the cortical stimulants described above. Strattera is a nonstimulant that blocks reuptake of the neurotransmitter norepinephrine. This increases alertness while decreasing random muscle activity. In addition to decreasing ADHD and ADD symptoms, Strattera also decreases anxiety and depression when they coexist with ADHD or ADD. The main side effects are trouble sleeping and decreased appetite. Normal appetite returns within three months for most individuals who keep on taking Strattera.

Antidepressant Medication for Mood Disorders

The cortical stimulant medications for ADHD or ADD are designed mainly to regulate dopamine, which is essential for executive function. Some of these cortical stimulants also boost the supply of norepinephrine, a neurotransmitter that works to maintain balance of higher brain functions. A different neurotransmitter, serotonin, is dominant in maintaining balanced emotions and feelings that originate in the midbrain (limbic system). Figure 6.2 shows the very wide range of moods that are governed mostly by serotonin. As we have seen in earlier chapters, many individuals with ADHD or ADD live with imbalance of emotions and feelings. These underlying mood disorders must be treated along with cortical stimulant medication to establish the best possible balance between higher brain and midbrain functions. Only a few of these mood regulators have been designed for children. Without mood control medications specifically designed for children, physicians face the challenge of helping youngsters who suffer from the mood disorders described in Chapter 6. Through careful trial and error at low dosage levels, it is not hard to find an antidepressant that is effective with school-age youngsters.

Serotonin-Specific Antidepressants

A wide range of medications to relieve depression and other mood disorders are designed to maintain a full supply of serotonin in the midbrain.

These are called SSRI (selective serotonin reuptake inhibitor) medications. Currently in use are Celexa (citalopram), Prozac and Sarafem (fluoxetine), LuVox (fluvoxamine), Paxil (paroxetine), and Zoloft (sertraline). These medications are designed to lift moods out of depression or bring moods down from hypomania (see Chapter 6). Often it is necessary to do trial-and-error experimentation with two or more of these medications to find the one that best fits each person's body chemistry without side effects. As the SSRI medication begins its work, a positive mood emerges with more open happiness, less anxiety, and less worry or fretting. Social relationships improve, as does life at home, at school, and at work. Antidepressants are slow to enter the brain and reach their peak effectiveness. Once the brain is fully medicated, the effect lasts around the clock until the next dose is taken. SSRI medications are used to reduce symptoms of chronic major depression, dysthymia (cycles of depression that come and go), bipolar disorder, obsessive-compulsive disorder (OCD), and eating disorders.

These medications must be taken consistently. Missed doses trigger headaches, nausea, muscle aches, stomachaches, poor sleep, and emotional overflow with bouts of crying, nervousness, and sadness. Withdrawal from SSRI medications must be gradual under a doctor's supervision. Side effects often appear, such as slower heart rate, dry mouth, constipation, cycles of blurred vision, and trouble urinating. Because the brain builds up tolerance for these medications, most individuals must change to a different SSRI every year or two.

244

Secondary Amine Tricyclic Antidepressants

When SSRI medications are not effective, a second class of antidepressants is available to regulate mood disorders. These medications work with two neurotransmitters (serotonin and norepinephrine) to reduce symptoms of major depression and anxiety disorders: Norpramin (desipramine), Pamelor and Aventyl (nortriptyline), and Vivactil (protriptyline).

Tertiary Amine Tricyclic Antidepressants

When none of these medications is effective, a third class of antidepressants is available to regulate mood disorders. These medications work with three neurotransmitters at the same time: serotonin, dopamine, and norepinephrine. These tricyclic antidepressants are helpful in reducing symptoms of anxiety disorders, obsessive-compulsive disorder, major depression, chronic pain, and insomnia. The most widely used tricyclics are Elavil and Endep (amitriptyline), Anafranil (clomipramine), Adapin and Sinequan (doxepin), Tofranil (imipramine), Surmontil (trimipramine), and Wellbutrin (bupropion).

Alpha-Adrenergic Receptor Agonists (AARAs)

Chapter 6 described several overly disruptive syndromes that often put individuals in danger, such as rage disorders, conduct disorder, and severe Oppositional Defiant Disorder. When ADHD comes with aggression, rebellion, or harmful resistance to authority, these medications often reduce or eliminate the aggressive behavior. AARA medications were developed to modify or eliminate the tic symptoms of Tourette's syndrome and the runaway behaviors of obsessive-compulsive disorder. As time went by, AARA medications were also found to reduce ADHD or ADD symptoms when comorbid layers needed treatment. The following AARA medications often are helpful when individuals cannot tolerate cortical stimulants.

Clonidine
Catapres. This medication was first used to treat drug or alcohol addiction. Recently it has become helpful in toning down the midbrain triggers for oppositional-defiant disorder and aggression. Catapres has little or no effect on attention span. This powerful medication must be closely monitored by a doctor, who looks for signs of lowered blood pressure or hypoglycemia. Catapres always is taken with food to prevent sudden drops in blood sugar. One in 10 individuals experience extreme drowsiness while taking Catapres. Other possible side effects are headaches, outbursts of aggression, confusion, and depression.

Guanfacine. Tenex is designed to decrease acute hyperactivity (hyperkinesis), excessive impulsivity, rage episodes, and defiance. It has no effect on attention span and is less likely to cause drowsiness than Catapres. It must be closely monitored by a doctor.

When Should We Medicate ADHD and Tag-Along Syndromes?

An excellent guideline for when to medicate comes from Lucy Jo Palladino, a psychologist who specializes in diagnosing and treating learning and behavior disorders: "In diagnostic terms, *interference with daily living* is the critical line that separates personality from pathology" (p. xiv in Hartmann, 2003). During my career, I have been conservative in recommending medication for ADHD or ADD individuals. My rule of thumb is consistent with Palladino's thinking: If the individual's behavior can be managed at home, at school, or at work with advice from others and help staying on task, I do not recommend intervention through medication. I show parents how to examine the diet for any food intolerances that might exist. Whenever it becomes clear that the person cannot function at work, learn at school, or cooperate at home, then I refer families to physicians who understand how ADD, ADHD, or dyslexia can be modified through the right medication.

Strategies for Overcoming ADHD and ADD

8

~ ~

Structure or Chaos?

The universe exists because of an intricate balance between structure and chaos. In the physical, mental, and spiritual worlds we inhabit, the most fundamental requirement for anything to exist is structure. Without structure there is chaos. For human cultures to survive, social structures, often called "law and order," must be maintained or else societies collapse into chaos. Architectural structures hold buildings and bridges in place. By delineating private spaces, social structure sets the boundaries of what belongs to every person. Chronological structure divides time into segments that give meaning to our lives. Every area of human life is governed by structure, or else chaos rules.

The fundamental challenge facing people with ADHD and ADD is a lack of inner structure to discipline impulses and bring order to unstructured mental and emotional activity. In Chapter 5 we met James and Kim, whose lack of internal structure created chaos everywhere they were. We also met Robert, whose lack of inner structure inserted quiet chaos into every area of his life.

Internal Structure Is Missing in ADHD and ADD

In the Introduction, we visited Mrs. Jolly's classroom and watched her struggle to keep Luis, Jacob, and Anna on task and engaged with formal learning. We saw that the basic challenge of ADHD and ADD is a lack of internal structure to self-guide these youngsters without supervision. For Anna, Jacob, and Luis, thought patterns are too loose and unstructured to enable them to stay focused long enough to finish whatever they start to do. Short-term and long-term memory are too spotty and unreliable to let rules and regulations guide their behavior, even for an hour. We witnessed Mrs. Jolly's challenge to provide enough supervised structure to keep these "loose as a goose" youngsters at work without disrupting the other pupils in the classroom.

Parents, teachers, companions, and job supervisors of ADHD and ADD individuals must provide enough structure to enable them to succeed. At the same time, ADHD and ADD persons must be willing to accept help without being resentful or rebellious. When attention deficit symptoms are above Level 5 in severity, those who help and monitor must be the eyes and ears of persons with ADHD or ADD. This requires extraordinary patience on the part of teachers, parents, and workplace leaders. New mercies must be extended again and again without penalizing unstructured persons who cannot stay on task or maintain organization on their own. As hard as it may be for others to believe, ADHD and ADD individuals cannot help being forgetful, disorganized, and too loose to stay on task without assistance.

Structure Strategies for Overcoming ADHD and ADD

Help with Taking Responsibility

Those of us who overcome lifelong challenges do so by learning how to take responsibility for our lives, our decisions, our actions, and our attitudes. The first fundamental lesson we learn is not to feel sorry for ourselves. The second foundational lesson we learn is not to blame others when we falter or fail. The starting place for overcoming ADHD and ADD is learning how to take the first steps in accepting responsibility.

ADHD or ADD Is Not an Excuse

Often it is difficult for individuals with personal challenges not to feel sorry for themselves. For almost 50 years I have observed this struggle in ADHD, ADD, and dyslexic persons. The natural temptation is to use the diagnosis as an excuse. However, Lynn Weiss, who has lived with ADD challenges all her life, gives this wise advice:

> The difference between an excuse and an explanation lies in your motive. If you are simply complaining, helplessly giving in to the rea-

Overcoming Attention Deficit Disorders in Children, Adolescents, and Adults

son for why you are having difficulty, you are using your ADD as an excuse.... If you are actively working with your ADD to make changes in your work habits that will help you to become successful, then chances are you are simply using your ADD to explain your behavior or difficulty in a specific situation.

—Lynn Weiss, 1996, p. 85

Grandmother's First Rule: "Life Is Not Fair"

Most individuals who are challenged by learning differences have moments of wanting to cry out: "Life is not fair!" For 72 years I have lived with the challenges of residual dyslexia, scotopic sensitivity syndrome (described in Chapter 6), awkward visual perception from astigmatism and imbalance of depth perception, and painful fibromyalgia. During my childhood, virtually nothing was known about these frustrating maladies or how to remedy them. My grandmother was a major influence in teaching me a principle that has guided my reaction to challenge all these years. Whenever I slipped into a "pity party" and wailed: "It's not fair!" she let me finish my complaint. Then she said: "No, life is not fair. Fair is where we show cows and pigs and chickens." In her rural life, where people looked forward to the county fair every fall, I learned the lifelong lesson that has guided me to success instead of self-pity. As I entered my early teens, my grandmother added an amendment to the self-pity rule. Whenever I tried to make excuses or blame someone else, she said: "Every tub must sit on its own bottom." I simply could not escape my grandmother's down-to-earth rule about accepting responsibility and getting on with my life. One of the first lessons ADHD and ADD individuals must learn is that life is not always fair, and we have two options. Either we can live in the shallow bitterness of self-pity, or we can learn how to accept our challenges as opportunities to grow and achieve.

249

Grandmother's Second Rule: "Independence Is Achieved Step by Step"

In her book *ADHD and Teens: A Parent's Guide to Making It Through the Tough Years,* Colleen Alexander-Roberts presents her version of the Grandmother Rule:

> Grandmother's Rule is basically a simple arrangement that says, "When you do what is expected, then you may do what you want to do." For example, "When you wash the car, then you may use it." Or "When your homework is finished, then you may call your friend." Grandmother's rule is easy to use and works well for children of all ages. However, never substitute the word "if" for the word "when." Using "if" will only invite your [child] to say, "If I don't do it, what will

happen?" The reason Grandmother's Rule works so well is that you are never saying, "No, you cannot." Grandmother's Rule is a positive way to communicate with your [child].

—Colleen Alexander-Roberts, 1995, p. 73

These and other "Grandmother's Rules" are the beginning steps in the gradual process of teaching ADHD and ADD individuals the priceless lesson of independence. We who live with lifelong challenges achieve success by mastering each step that prepares us for future steps in accepting responsibility, getting on with life's opportunities, and relishing victories over challenges.

Help with Organization

In Chapter 5, I reviewed the organizational challenge that ADHD and ADD individuals face in traditional classrooms and on job sites. Figure 1.15 shows the rigid left-brain linear structure upon which most educational and job situations are based. Being successful inside this "linear box" is a major challenge for ADHD and ADD persons, whose brains are structured for the different style of thinking and learning shown in Figure 1.10. The linear cultures of most classrooms and job sites pose the dilemma of fitting the "round pegs" of attention deficits into the "square holes" of traditional thinking and learning.

Multisensory Structure

To do their best, most ADHD and ADD individuals must engage several sensory modalities at the same time. Simply listening or reading passively does not provide enough sensory stimulation to develop complete mental images of abstract information. Brain imaging research has revealed why typical left-brain linear thinking does not work for most ADHD or ADD persons. Figure 8.1 shows the limited brain activity and mental structure that occur during silent, passive tasks. Figure 8.2 shows the significant increase in brain activity and mental structure during multisensory, interactive activities. Listening to oral information alone is incomplete for most ADHD and ADD individuals. In the same way, silent reading fails to produce complete mental images of what an author presents on the printed page. To be successful inside the left-brain linear box, ADHD and ADD persons must have visual and tactile stimuli to guide them in staying on track within the left-brain linear structure. Unless they also are severely dyslexic, most ADHD and ADD persons read well enough to follow written or printed guidelines. However, the sense of touch must also become part of each ADHD or ADD person's lifestyle to help overcome unstructured attention deficit challenges.

Overcoming Attention Deficit Disorders in Children, Adolescents, and Adults

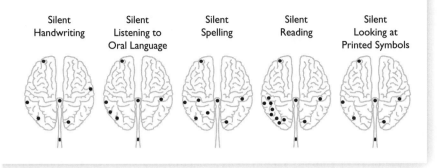

FIGURE 8.1. This composite of brain images taken during passive left-brain linear tasks shows how few regions of the brain are stimulated to work together. Silent, passive learning and thinking do not stimulate the brain enough to hold the attention of individuals who are ADHD or ADD.

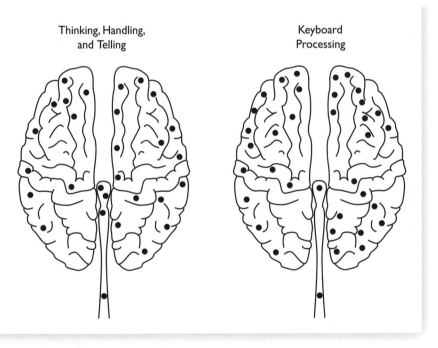

FIGURE 8.2. This composite of brain images taken during interactive, multisensory tasks shows how many more regions of the brain are stimulated to work together. Tasks that incorporate seeing it/saying it/hearing it/touching it stimulate enough brain regions to hold the attention of individuals who are ADHD or ADD.

Overcoming ADHD and ADD

Help with Organizing Important Information

1. *Highlighting while reading.* Cultures that value printed information often condemn the practice of marking pages as individuals read. However, for persons with attention deficits, it is critical to mark the trail as they work through forests of new information. The most direct way to mark the trail is to highlight important details as one reads. Later the reader quickly scans to find specific details and make use of that highlighted data. Using colored highlight markers is an efficient, dependable type of multisensory structure that enables right-brain circular thinkers to succeed inside the left-brain linear format.

2. *Using colored stick-on tags.* Today's culture provides a rich variety of stick-on tags to mark the linear trail for ADHD and ADD individuals. Persons with vivid right-brain color awareness easily figure out color-cue systems that bring them back when attention becomes distracted. They often mark pages or sections of textbooks and job manuals with small colored tags. It is easy to jot a brief note on each stick-on tag to let the person find specific information quickly. When youngsters are trained in using color-cue tags, they develop lifelong visual/tactile structures that carry them successfully into adulthood.

3. *Using linear grids.* Most ADHD and ADD individuals need to see left to right, top to bottom information inside a grid structure similar to the format shown in Figure 8.3. Many computer programs provide spreadsheets that organize financial information, work schedules, and personal calendars within grids. Organizing important data within grids helps right-brain circular thinkers to function inside the linear box. When layers of dyslexia or dysgraphia overlap ADHD or ADD, using a grid greatly improves legibility and ease in editing mistakes, as Figures 8.4 and 8.5 show.

4. *Using electronic pocket organizers.* The 21st century has brought a variety of electronic data processing systems into the lives of most individuals. This revolution in organizing and sharing information provides ideal multisensory, interactive structure for ADHD and ADD individuals. Many schools teach kindergarten and primary grade pupils to use computers to speed up early skills in decoding (reading) and encoding (writing, spelling). Miniature personal computers (called PDAs) that fit into a pocket help individuals of all ages organize the important information of their lives. For example, Palm offers a range of handheld personal organizers called palmOne Zire PDAs. These pocket organizers provide the kind of interactive structure that ADHD and ADD persons need. The palmOne Zire 31 PDA is an excellent entry-level pocket organizer that teaches individuals how to sort and organize dates, schedules, appointments, and deadlines. Hewlett-Packard offers a similar range of handheld pocket computers called HP iPAQ h1945 Pocket PCs. These miniature data pro-

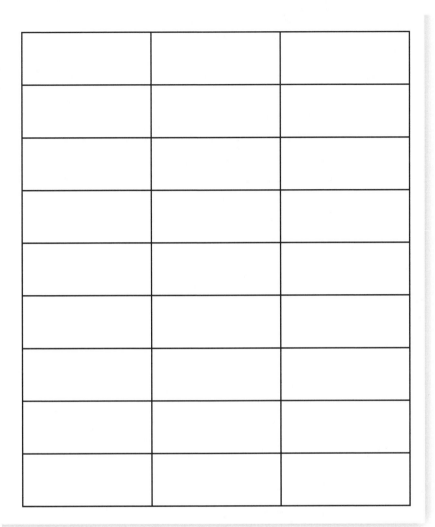

FIGURE 8.3. This kind of linear grid has many uses in helping ADHD, ADD, or dysgraphic individuals control written information. The clearly marked spaces guide the brain in separating chunks of data without crowding too much or running details together.

cessors are designed to remind individuals of daily schedules, future commitments, addresses, phone numbers, and other types of information at the touch of a button. Other types of PDAs are the series offered by Sony and the AXIM X30 series by Dell. As students enter middle school and high school, many ADHD and ADD individuals carry laptop computers everywhere they go to help them stay organized, gather new information, finish assignments on time, and keep up with appointments.

Overcoming ADHD and ADD

What are your best Christmas memories?
Once upona time there waso
bully. Hehad no Friends. There waso
boyhamed Eric. He hadna frienr
ButEric was nice, and unpopular. One
I asked my mom if He couldcame o
My mom said but he is the bully. M
said yes. So I called him and he com
over we played for a while. Then

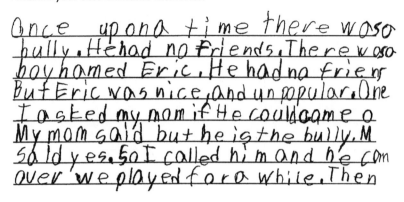

FIGURE 8.4. This 9-year-old boy achieved Full Scale IQ 132 on the *Wechsler Intelligence Scale for Children* (WISC–III) along with reading comprehension at grade level 5.7 on an achievement test. Undiagnosed dysgraphia caused this kind of penmanship struggle on all of his written language assignments.

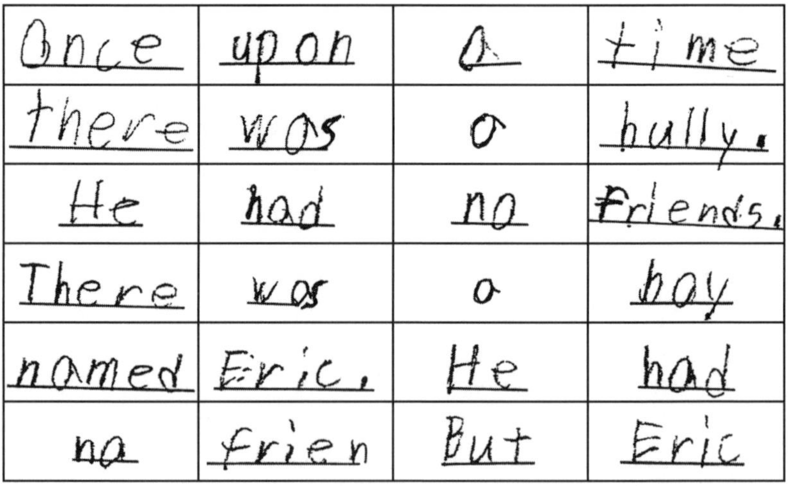

Once
upon
a
time
there
was
a
bully.
He
had
no
Friends.
There
was
a
boy
named
Eric.
He
had
na
frien
But
Eric

FIGURE 8.5. When his teacher separated the words and lines inside this grid, the boy immediately spotted his spelling mistakes. He learned how to compensate for dysgraphia by writing all assignments in a grid like this. Soon he developed good self-editing skills.

Help with Paying Attention

Colleen Alexander-Roberts (1995) describes ADHD attention as "the ability to see the whole picture as if through a wide-angle lens." She points out that this wide-angle perception is a gift of ADHD, except in situations when the person must narrow attentional focus to only one issue long enough to learn new information and think it through. This requires the ADHD or ADD person to structure mental focus by tuning out the edges in order to focus only on the middle. To do so, ADHD and ADD individuals must make a conscious effort to "build mental fences" that shut out everything else in the wide-angle view while attending only to the center of their perceptual field. Of course, this is the ultimate challenge of being ADHD or ADD. How does this person stop seeing, hearing, or feeling everything at the same time?

Each chapter of this book emphasizes the severity scale that must be considered every time we look at ADHD and ADD behaviors:

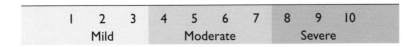

When ADHD or ADD symptoms are above Level 5, individuals cannot pay full attention without help. Those with symptoms above Level 5 usually require low dosage medication along with diet control to stabilize brain chemistry. Without such help, it often is impossible for ADHD or ADD individuals to reduce their wide-angle focus to just the task to be accomplished. When ADHD or ADD symptoms are below Level 5 in severity, it usually is possible to develop self-structure strategies to stay focused long enough to finish a task, or to bring one's wandering attention back into focus without being reminded.

255

Self-Monitoring

For many years Harvey C. Parker has taught parents and teachers how to coach mild and low moderate ADHD and ADD students to self-monitor their challenges in paying full attention. In his book *The ADD Hyperactivity Handbook for Schools* (1996), Parker explains a variety of multisensory, interactive strategies that ADHD and ADD individuals can learn to do as self-monitoring rituals. First, teachers and parents candidly pinpoint the specific behaviors that interfere with learning, participating in groups, doing assignments, and building social skills. These specific challenges are listed so that ADHD or ADD students see the issues that cause problems in their lives. Continually reviewing these lists becomes as important as studying for Friday's spelling test. Parker's point of view is that before an individual can learn self-monitoring skills, he or she must know precisely which behaviors must be improved. This self-structure approach to overcoming ADHD and ADD involves labeling specific behaviors:

1. I often interrupt others.
2. I start to daydream.
3. I stop work before I finish.
4. I forget what I need to do my work.
5. I lose my stuff.
6. I become distracted.

Self-structuring teaches ADHD and ADD students how to use simple checklists several times during the day to frame specific areas of their behavior:

_____ Did I interrupt?
_____ Did I daydream?
_____ Did I stop before I finished?
_____ Did I forget what I needed?
_____ Did I lose my stuff?
_____ Did I become distracted?

As time goes by, this self-structuring ritual builds self-control habits that enable ADHD and ADD individuals to succeed inside the left-brain linear box.

White Sound Background

Recently I was reminded of a self-structure strategy used by many ADHD and ADD individuals to "block out" sensory pathways that intrude when certain kinds of mental work must be done. My wife and I enjoyed a reunion with one of our grownup ADHD boys whom we had helped through overwhelming challenges during his adolescent years. We listened to his victory stories of how he overcame his challenges, once he knew that he was not "dumb" and had a name for why he struggled. We were especially fascinated by Steve's account of how he conquered ADHD challenges well enough to earn a college degree in mechanical engineering, and how he became successful on the job. "I learned that if I listened to classical music," he said, "my body got still and my brain stopped racing. If I put on headphones and listened to Beethoven, I stopped bouncing my legs and my mind stopped jumping all over the place. As long as I listened to classical music, I could concentrate without being distracted. I could read well and finish my work." As Steve works on computer-based engineering projects, he wears headphones to listen to classical music that provides mental structure for focusing on his work. An understanding supervisor encourages Steve to compensate this way to let his creative talents solve complex engineering problems.

Help with Listening

Structured Tactile Pressure

Chapter 4 explained why ADHD or ADD individuals often create doodles. Figure 8.6 shows how an ADD man eliminates distraction through gripping a pencil and doodling. As I conducted a staff training seminar within a state prison, I noticed how eagerly this teacher absorbed new information about ADHD, ADD, and dyslexia in prison inmates. On the final day of the seminar, I passed his work space during an afternoon break. There lay the elaborate doodle shown in Figure 8.6. Later he explained how doodling structures his ability to listen effectively. "If my fingers grip a pencil and I make sketches while I listen, I don't become distracted," he explained. "I can listen all day and learn a lot if I keep my fingers busy doodling." He told me of his lifelong frustration when teachers and instructors have forced him not to doodle. "When I'm not gripping a pencil and doodling," he said, "I can't listen. I become too distracted to understand what the speaker says. Squeezing a pen or pencil drains away the 'noise,' as you call it, from my brain. My brain gets quiet when my fingers are busy like this."

Squeezing and Chewing

ADHD individuals often eliminate distraction by rhythmically squeezing objects as they listen or read. Many classroom teachers provide squeeze objects, or allow students to bring their favorite tactile object to be handled quietly during study time. The rhythmic muscle activity of quietly chewing gum or some other soft substance helps to remove ADHD distraction during periods of quiet concentration and central focus. ADHD and ADD individuals are at the greatest risk of inattention when they are forbidden to do tactile structuring, but instead must sit still and be quiet. Their most productive moments occur when they are free to engage tactile/sensory pathways during left-brain linear tasks.

Help with Managing Time

> Time management does not come naturally to most people because it is not really time management at all. Time cannot be manipulated or managed. Time management is self-management, a skill to be acquired. It takes practice and effort....
> —Russell A. Barkley, 1995, p. 141

> What causes trouble for people with ADD is the division of time into segments, arbitrary segments at that.... Minutes and hours are artificial, arbitrary delineators of time. An ADD mind does not naturally

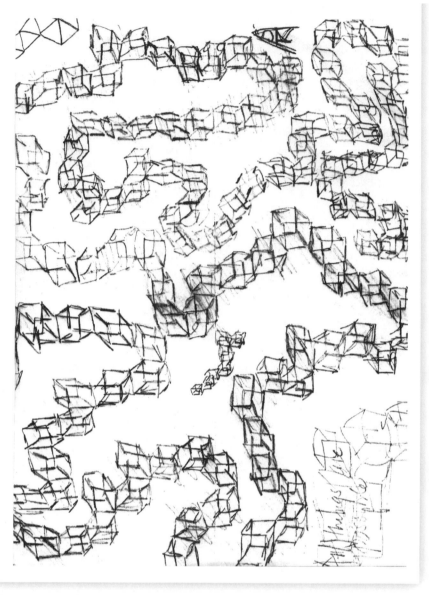

FIGURE 8.6. The tactile sensation of fingers squeezing a pencil or pen to create this kind of doodle often stops random ADHD noise in the brain that interferes with concentration. Most ADHD individuals listen better, comprehend more fully, and build more accurate long-term memories when they engage their sense of touch as they listen.

Overcoming Attention Deficit Disorders in Children, Adolescents, and Adults

think in these terms.... The only aspect of time that many people with ADD are aware of is *now*, the moment in which we are living. Yesterday tends to be forgotten ... and tomorrow never comes to mind.

—Lynn Weiss, 1996, pp. 38–89

Paying Attention to Time Segments

We can see individuals with ADHD and ADD struggle with time by watching an episode in Mrs. Jolly's third-grade classroom. Not long after her students returned from Thanksgiving holiday, she was ready to start a new unit about telling and interpreting time. She gave each child a model of a clock face with moveable hands. Immediately Luis became engrossed with moving the hands to different positions. Then he wanted to see how fast he could make them spin. Within a few minutes he had broken the hour hand by turning it too aggressively. At the same time, he heard what Mrs. Jolly was explaining to the group, but he became bored by her careful, deliberate presentation and stopped listening. As Anna received her clock model, she quietly turned the minute hand, then drifted off into a daydream as she relived a memory of her grandmother using a key to wind her clock so it would chime. Jacob began turning his clock hands backwards as he tried to imitate the clockwise motions Mrs. Jolly was demonstrating. He became so frustrated, he threw his clock face down and began to cry.

Two mothers were visiting Mrs. Jolly's classroom that day to help her teach this interactive lesson about the structure of time. They took charge of the class while Mrs. Jolly led Luis, Jacob, and Anna to the reading corner to work with them as a small group. "Can you tell me how long one minute is?" she asked. With a smile, Anna replied: "It's how long it takes my dad to drive home from work. My mom says that dad will be home any minute." "You're wrong!" Luis exclaimed. "A minute is how long it takes for the football team to win a game." Then Jacob said quietly: "I don't know what a minute is."

[ADHD and ADD individuals] with a poor concept of time are unable to predict how long a task will take. They might think a book report will take only an hour to write, but in reality it will take them two hours. Predicting how long it will take to drive somewhere is easy, but only as long as it is the same route that they have been driving back and forth for months or years. Ask them how long it takes to drive to the post office (a mile away) and they may not be able to give you an accurate time. This poor concept of time interferes greatly in their lives, from writing a book report to missing social appointments.

—Colleen Alexander-Roberts, 1995, p. 34

Overcoming ADHD and ADD

Luis's Perception of Time. For more than 20 years, Thom Hartmann has defined ADHD individuals like himself and Luis as "hunters in a farming society" (Hartmann, 1993, 2000, 2003). Hartmann's hunter concept is based upon the distinctive hyperfocus characteristic of ADHD that causes time to stand still while the brain tunes out distracting issues and focuses intensely on a central theme. For example, a hunter ignores what goes on nearby in order to focus totally on the object of the hunt. Yet the hunter's brain continues to process all that goes on nearby. Without consciously doing so, the hunter's brain keeps track of all the nearby sounds, odors on the breeze, movement of grass and leaves and birds flying over, changes in shadows and light, and so forth. This multitasking talent of hunter ADHD individuals is described by Lynn Weiss, a successful ADHD hunter within the field of counseling psychology:

> Though I didn't know I had ADD when I was a radio talk show host, I discovered a talent that was a result of my ADD. I could think and talk on five levels at once when a caller asked a question. First, I heard the specific question being asked. Simultaneously, I thought about what the motivation of the person might be or what lay behind the question. I was also aware of the needs of the other listeners and the station manager's desires about programming. Finally, I kept track of the mechanics of the show, such as time spent on the line with the caller, proximity to break time, and special communications from my producer and technical director. All five levels operated simultaneously in my head while I was listening and talking. I enjoyed it immensely, and nothing could distract me from my job because the job itself involved so much stimulation.
>
> —Lynn Weiss, 1996, p. 26

Individuals like Luis, Thom Hartmann, and Lynn Weiss do not think in linear time segments. For them, details like minutes and hours tend to be irrelevant. For hunter ADHD individuals, time is elastic, not constant. During events when Luis is hyperfocused like a hunter, time stands still: "A minute is how long it takes for the football team to win a game." Yet when he is bored, a minute stretches to seem like a year. For Luis and other hunter ADHD persons, long-term memory does not consist of a record of time segments. As Luis remembers past events, he recalls the vividly stimulating sensations of those moments, not how long they lasted. When he is hyperfocused like a hunter, it makes no sense for him to be told, "You have three more minutes to finish" or "I want you to work another ten minutes." His brain processes hyperfocused time as *intensely now.* When he is not hyperfocused like a hunter, time is *boringly forever.*

Anna's Perception of Time. In a very different way, Anna's ADD perception of time also is elastic. Like Luis, she does not think in linear terms of minutes, hours, days, weeks, months, or years. While she knows these labels, she does not experience the passing of time by framing her life events within such labels. Anna has good awareness of the overall time segments of "now" and "then." She is aware of what happened before now. If reminded to do so, she can anticipate what will happen later. Yet her ADD point of view centers around timeless emotions and feelings rather than within the structure of linear time segments. For the most part, the center of Anna's world is the magical thinking of daydreams where time is not an issue. Off in her private world of make-believe, time stands still. Ironically, the passive act of daydreaming is as hyperfocused for Anna as the intense activity of being the hunter is for Luis. Yet neither of them thinks in terms of passing minutes or hours as time goes by. Anna does not have an internal clock that marks the passing of time segments. Unless someone reminds her to pay attention to linear time structure, she does not do so on her own.

Jacob's Perception of Time. The dual layers of ADHD and dyslexia trigger intense frustration for Jacob as adults press him to pay attention to linear time structure: "I don't know what a minute is," he admits with a sense of shame. "Everyone else knows what a minute is. What's wrong with me? I don't know what they're talking about." Hartmann has described Jacob's challenge in dealing with time:

> ADD individuals ... have an exaggerated sense of urgency when they're on a task, and an exaggerated sense of boredom when they have nothing to do ... whereas the sense of fast-time when on a project leads to chronic impatience. This elastic sense of time also causes many ADD individuals to describe emotional highs and lows as having a profound impact on them. The lows, particularly, may seem as if they'll last forever, whereas the highs are often perceived as flashing by.
>
> —Thom Hartmann, 1993, p. 3

In observing Jacob's reactions to Mrs. Jolly's expectations, we have seen his overflow of negative, disruptive emotions as he destroyed a worksheet, threw down the clock face, and erupted into tantrums triggered by frustration and shame. Chapter 1 described the fight-or-flight reflex that is triggered whenever the midbrain senses danger or lack of safety in new events. Chapter 5 reviewed the concept of emotional homeostasis that crumbles beneath the shame of too much failure. Jacob's sense of time is smothered under the weight of irregular attention, the dyslexic tendency to do things backward, and the shame of his "messy papers" because of dysgraphia. His lack of knowledge of linear time structure is linked to emotional instability that erupts too easily under the normal stress of classroom performance.

Timepiece Reminders. Individuals who are ADHD or ADD benefit from timepieces that remind them of time segments. Many kinds of digital wristwatches are designed to beep at preset intervals, reminding the person that a time segment has passed. Luis, Anna, and Jacob need this kind of auditory/visual reminder that is always present wherever they are. Each of them needs a sturdy wristwatch that is easy to preset for whatever time segment is important. At the start of a task, they are reminded to set their timers for 3 minutes or 5 minutes to guide them in finishing before they start doing something else. Through patient coaching, they learn not to stop work until they hear the beep. Over time, they learn how to keep on focusing for longer periods before taking a break. Most digital wristwatches also show calendars at the press of a button. As they grow older, Anna, Jacob, and Luis will use this kind of time structure to stay on schedule and meet deadlines without forgetting too often.

Daily Time Diaries. Anna, Jacob, and Luis need to follow a simple time diary that visually structures each day. Figure 8.7 shows a time diary that frames each hour of the day at the same time it shows the linear structure of the days of the week. Later Luis, Anna, and Jacob will learn to use time diaries that divide the day into half-hour or quarter-hour segments. ADHD and ADD individuals must carry a time diary in a pocket or purse to remind them where to be and when to be there.

Help with Keeping Personal Space Tidy

Getting a clutter buddy [is an option] in trading time with another person who also wants to work on reducing clutter. I recently made a deal with a neighbor that if she would sit quietly on my couch for two hours and do something [like paying her bills or writing letters], I would do the same for her. So there she sat—quietly—for two hours. Then the timer went off, and we both went to her apartment, where I sat for two hours and she organized. That's all we needed—another person there to keep us focused.... ADHD people know what to do, but they don't do it. By having another person in the room with them—even sitting quietly—they are more motivated to complete organizational tasks.

—James Lawrence Thomas, 1996, p. 175

	Sunday	Monday	Tuesday	Wednesday	Thursday	Friday	Saturday
7:00 A.M.							
8:00 A.M.							
9:00 A.M.							
10:00 A.M.							
11:00 A.M.							
12:00 P.M.							
1:00 P.M.							
2:00 P.M.							
3:00 P.M.							
4:00 P.M.							
5:00 P.M.							
6:00 P.M.							

FIGURE 8.7. This kind of simple time management grid organizes an individual's day and week at a glance. More mature persons should add half-hour segments to stay on task with more obligations.

Overcoming ADHD and ADD

Keep Structure Simple

ADHD and ADD individuals must do their best to follow a basic life-style guideline: *Keep It Simple.* Those who work or live with an ADD or ADHD person continually cope with clutter that grows and spreads as time goes by. The ADHD or ADD brain does not automatically notice spatial structure that requires objects to fit into given spaces. Luis, Anna, and Jacob must have guidance and supervision that reminds them to notice when too many things are piled together or scattered around. Mrs. Jolly decided to work with them on keeping personal space tidy by engaging her whole class in learning where things should go. Each student decorated two boxes to hold personal things. A small box to contain pencils, crayons, and other classroom work tools would sit on the child's desk, or fit under the chair within easy reach. A larger box would be placed in the classroom Box Center to hold each student's books and larger items. Mrs. Jolly consistently reminds her students to keep their personal spaces tidy. At the end of each school day, they spend 5 minutes putting their things neatly in the right place. At the end of each week, the students spend 15 minutes sorting through their boxes to discard whatever they no longer need to keep. This ensures that on Monday, everything is ready to begin the new week with no clutter to distract attention.

At home, parents of ADHD and ADD children face the challenge of keeping living spaces reasonably tidy. Chapter 5 described how Nate and his mother learned to reduce clutter stress in their home. She agreed not to fuss over the cluttered state of Nate's room, while he agreed not to bring his clutter into the family's living space. Mrs. Jolly guided the parents of Luis, Anna, and Jacob in establishing simple "where things go" structure rules at home. The parents worked daily with their youngsters in memorizing "where things go" rituals. Certain things "go in the drawer." Certain things "go on the floor." Certain things "go on hangers in the closet." Certain things "go on the bed." Mrs. Jolly taught these parents James Thomas's system of being a "clutter buddy." Once a week the parents set aside an hour to be in the same room with Luis, Jacob, and Anna, supervising them in putting things where they go. During this tidy-up hour, these "clutter buddies" helped their children decide "what to keep" and "what not to keep." It is critical that adults not tell ADHD or ADD youngsters to "go clean up your room." It is impossible for Luis, Anna, and Jacob to do so without direct supervision. ADHD and ADD children who receive this kind of simple "where things go" training with the help of a clutter buddy develop lifelong habits of paying attention to where items should go. Without such specific tidy-up training, they move through adolescence into adulthood continuing to clutter their environment, which disrupts the lives of others.

Help with Keeping Track of Things

As ADHD and ADD youngters pass through the developmental years of childhood and adolescence, those who are below Level 5 in severity gradually outgrow most of their ADHD or ADD behaviors. By their early 20s, executive function takes charge of most of their lifestyle issues. As this gradual maturity emerges, it becomes easier for them to develop strategies to keep track of things. By late teen years, most moderately ADHD and ADD individuals become much more efficient in keeping track of their things. Children who are above Level 5 in severity of ADHD and ADD symptoms tend to struggle all their lives keeping track of keys, wallets, purses, school materials, job materials, and so forth. Mrs. Jolly worked with the parents of Anna, Jacob, and Luis to establish simple guidelines for keeping track of their things. Those parents agreed to schedule five minutes each morning and evening to play the Airplane Take Off game with Luis, Jacob, and Anna. Each family created a Take Off Checklist that everyone reviewed together each morning and evening. The routine was to focus full attention on each of these issues, the way a pilot goes down the takeoff checklist before the plane can start its journey:

1. Where are your clothes?
2. Where is your homework?
3. Where are your books?
4. Where is your bookbag?
5. Where is your jacket or sweater?
6. Where is your lunch money?

Families who patiently and consistently do this kind of coaching reduce most of the stress that is triggered when ADHD or ADD individuals cannot find their things when it is time to go.

Help with Schoolwork

Study Buddies
Until they reach executive function maturity in late adolescence, Luis, Jacob, and Anna must have enough one-on-one help with schoolwork to finish each task. Recently I witnessed the powerful incentive that an older study buddy provides for younger learners who need help. As part of a staff training program, I visited an elementary school where students in fourth and fifth grades earn Service Awards by volunteering to be study buddies for pupils in lower grades. Three times each week, older study buddies

spend the last hour of the day with their younger buddies. These special times are devoted to reviewing assignments to make sure everything has been finished. The older buddies listen to the younger partners read stories they have written and illustrated themselves. If younger buddies are stuck with specific skills, the older partner guides practice to strengthen those skills. Study buddies help younger ones prepare for spelling tests. They go over checklists of what to take home for evening practice. At the end of the school term, teachers in this school were amazed at the unexpected progress and success the younger buddies achieved through this study-buddy experience. Having a partner directly helps inattentive persons to stay focused longer and do necessary work without distraction.

Adjusting Help with Homework

John F. Taylor has given wise advice about how supervisors should adjust the amount of one-on-one help they provide:

> Adjusting your help prevents you from becoming overinvolved. Your child can feel his strength while still not being overwhelmed by fears of being left too much on his own. Adjusted help sends the clear message that you have faith in your child's abilities; giving too much help does *not* convey that message. Without physically involving yourself (all the time), you can convey your deep interest in what your child is doing.
>
> —John F. Taylor, 1994, p. 163

Structure with Timers

Wise supervisors coach ADHD or ADD learners in reducing their dependence on help from others. Two important factors are at work in this process. First, some type of timer is used to give a visual or auditory signal when it is OK to pause for a break. Many families discover that a silent sand timer provides the best visual structure of work segments. The goal is for the ADHD or ADD child to keep on working until the sand runs out. Less mature learners do best with a 3-minute timer that is turned over to start a new 3-minute work segment. Others are able to begin with a 5-minute or 10-minute sand timer. Or an auditory timer is set to beep after a certain time has expired. Choosing the kind of timer depends upon the degree of difficulty the child has in tuning out visual or auditory distractions.

Increasing Independence

Wise supervisors coach ADHD or ADD learners in how to reduce their dependence upon help from others. The goal is to reassure the child that help is nearby if or when it is needed. The supervisor frames the structure of working independently by saying "I'm here to help if you get stuck, but first I want you to try by yourself." Without taking charge of the work, the supervisor gives continual support from nearby: "That really was a good job. Now are you ready to do the next one by yourself?" Nervous learners need to hear "I'm watching. I love to watch how well you're doing." Part of this adjusted help structure is for the supervisor to watch for signs of approaching emotional or attentional burnout: "Can you do just one more before we take a break?" When the sand runs out or the timer beeps, the student and supervisor take a structured break. An important part of this adjusted help process is for the child to set a time limit for each break. A useful rule is for the child to work until the time runs out, then take a break for that same length of time. The timer is used to structure each work segment, as well as each break segment.

Reduced Work Quotas

Mrs. Jolly learned to reduce the quota of work on each assignment to fit the emotional and attentional realities of her ADHD and ADD students. She worked out ratios of how much each child could accomplish within the time limits of his or her distractibility. She learned that when he understood what to do, Luis usually could finish five math problems before he lost his focus. Jacob often could do four math problems before he became overly frustrated. With reminding, Anna could finish seven or eight problems before she reached burnout. In spelling tasks, Luis could do ten new words, plus three bonus words, each week. Jacob could learn to spell four new words, if his dyslexic reversals were not counted against his knowledge of spelling. Anna could learn all 10 words on the spelling list if adults reminded her not to daydream. Luis loved to write stories. When he was permitted to engage his hunter ADHD imagination, he often wrote two pages without becoming sidetracked and distracted. Because of his dyslexia and dysgraphia, Jacob labored to write two full sentences before he reached burnout. Anna could complete half of most writing assignments, then illustrate her work with neat doodles and sketches. When work quotas are structured to fit each learner's style and stamina, much less frustration occurs and work stamina is increased.

Help with Becoming One's Self-Advocate

The final goal of the step by step process of becoming independent is to become one's self-advocate.

A student can become his or her own advocate by understanding his or her individual disability from the perspective of his or her

Knowing Why One Struggles

Earlier in this chapter we reviewed Harvey Parker's self-monitoring strategy that lists an individual's challenges that must be overcome to succeed. Because this self-monitoring technique names each stumbling block the student must overcome, this straightforward approach to knowing one's differences is controversial. Many counselors, teachers, and parents fear that this bold strategy might harm a child's self-esteem. Professionals who oppose the practice of labeling learning differences often object to Parker's method of informing individuals by naming and self-monitoring each challenge.

Does frankly naming a person's differences damage his or her self-confidence and self-esteem? As I spent the first half of my life seeking answers for my own chronic challenges, I learned to cherish the emotional freedom and strength that came through knowing the name of what caused me to fail, to feel unwell, and to suffer depression. None of the specialists I consulted could answer my question "Why?" The pain of not knowing why eventually took me to a world-famous diagnostic center where surely I would be told the truth. As day after day of intensive diagnostic activity went by, I came to understand why struggling learners often feel depressed and fearful. Specialist after specialist examined me while showing no emotion. As they probed, gouged, and invaded my body, I heard guarded comments such as "Hmmm!" and "Uh-oh!" and occasionally "Wow!" Yet when I demanded to know what those specialists were thinking, I received guarded smiles and neutral tones that implied I was not intelligent enough to understand. When I tried to read their charts and graphs, I was pushed away and told that "This is confidential." Eventually the final test was performed and the exit conference was scheduled. I nearly burst with eagerness to learn the name of my malaise. "Dr. Jordan, we don't know what is causing your syndrome," they agreed. "For lack of a better term, we call it Stiff Man Syndrome. Because all of your tests are negative for disease, we agree that you should enter psychoanalysis to discover what your problem really is." I had never been so emotionally shattered or intellectually insulted in my life. Those learned doctors dismissed me the way children often are dismissed by adults. I do not have the words to describe the devastation that lack of a name poured over me.

The day after I returned home from that disappointing experience, I visited my extraordinary family physician. While I was away, he had spent many hours researching new data about my malaise. With great tenderness, he said: "I've concluded that you're suffering from fibromyalgia." At last I knew the name of the beast that made my life so miserable. I burst into tears of relief as Dr. M embraced me to contain my anger for not knowing before. In that moment, I knew exactly what every challenged student feels when adults refuse to be open and honest about why he or she is different in the classroom or at home.

Becoming a Self-Advocate

Certainly adults must be careful when helping children understand why they struggle in the classroom, or why they have difficulty making new friends. Yet not giving an honest answer to a child's question "Why?" fosters destructive suspicion that "something must be wrong with me." For most individuals, not knowing why implants the deep-seated belief that "I'm dumb. I must be stupid." As struggling learners become mature enough to understand, frankly naming each layer of challenge prepares their feelings and emotions for open discussion. The final step into independence is being able to talk maturely with others about why certain accommodations are required for job performance and higher education achievement.

An excellent guide for becoming a self-advocate is Patricia Quinn's book *ADD and the College Student: A Guide for High School and College Students with Attention Deficit Disorder* (2001). This guidebook is designed to help parents, teachers, and counselors prepare ADD or ADHD individuals to represent themselves in new situations. This preparation coaches them on using correct terminology, organizing legal information to support their requests for help, and providing data from high school to document their need for accommodations. It is not enough to help challenged learners finish high school, then turn them loose in the adult world not knowing what to do next.

Enhancing Brain Functions

We now recognize that our brain isn't limited by considerations that are applicable to machines. Thoughts, feelings, and actions, rather than mechanical laws, determine the health of our brain. Furthermore, we know that the brain never loses the power to transform itself on the basis of experience, and this transformation can occur over very short intervals. For instance, your brain is different today than it was yesterday. This difference results from the effect on your brain of yesterday's and today's experiences, as well as the thoughts and feelings you've entertained over the past 24 hours.

Overcoming ADHD and ADD

> Think, therefore, of the human brain as a lifetime work in prog-
> ress that retains plasticity—the capacity for change—as long as the
> "owner" is still alive.
>
> —Richard Restak, 2003, pp. 7–8

Our society entered the 21st century with a surge of new techniques to enhance brain functions in learning, thinking, remembering, and expessing
what we know. Chapter 1 explained the neurological process of pruning
that enables the brain to learn new skills and develop long-term memory.
Today a variety of brain training techniques are available to help ADHD
and ADD individuals bypass attention deficits and stimulate new brain
functions. The brain functions through five types of brainwave patterns
that are manipulated through neurofeedback (biofeedback) stimulation.

> *Delta waves* (1 to 4 cycles per second). These are very slow brainwaves
>   that occur mostly during deep sleep.
> *Theta waves* (5 to 7 cycles per second). These slow brainwaves occur
>   during daydreaming, ADD drifting of thoughts and mental images,
>   and twilight states while going to sleep and waking up.
> *Alpha waves* (8 to 12 cycles per second). These moderately faster brain-
>   waves occur during moments when the body and thoughts are
>   awake yet relaxed.
> *SMR (sensorimotor rhythm) waves* (12 to 14 cycles per second). These
>   faster brainwaves occur when the brain is focused yet the body and
>   emotions are relaxed.
> *Beta waves* (13 to 24 cycles per second). These very fast brainwaves occur
>   when the brain is fully engaged in concentration and doing mental
>   work.

Biofeedback (Neurofeedback) Stimulation

Beginning in the mid-1990s, an enormous biofeedback (neurofeedback) in-
dustry emerged to offer a multitude of brain stimulation therapies for the
following disorders.

Addiction	Epilepsy
Anxiety	Fetal Alcohol Syndrome
Attachment Disorder	Learning Disabilities/Dyslexia
ADHD/ADD	Migraine
Autism	Obsessive/Compulsive Disorder
Autoimmune Dysfunction	Pre-Menstrual Syndrome
Chronic Pain	Post-Traumatic Stress Disorder

Chronic Fatigue Syndrome	Sleep Disorders
Conduct Disorders	Stroke
Depression	Tourette's Syndrome
Eating Disorders	Traumatic Brain Injury

Biofeedback treatment measures physical responses such as hand temperature, rate of breathing, sweat gland activity, heartbeat, blood pressure, and brainwave patterns. As these measurements are taken, the person practices making a conscious effort to change these physical activities. Electrodes on the scalp measure changes in the five brainwave patterns described above. This therapy requires intense concentration, which stimulates beta waves. This activates changes in how the brain creates signals for muscle activity. Over time, permanent changes occur in neuron/dendrite pathways within the plastic brain. Pruning is accelerated while new neurons and dendrites build new connections between brain centers. This new technology literally reprograms the brain to relieve certain types of brain-based ailments, as well as to teach the brain how to do new kinds of work.

ADHD/ADD Brain Training Therapy

Several clinics and research centers in the United States offer neurofeedback training to reduce ADHD and ADD symptoms. This is done through speeding up the slow theta brainwaves that foster daydreaming in individuals like Anna and Jacob, whom we met in earlier chapters. For example, Joel F. Lubar and his staff at the Southeastern Biofeedback and Neurobehavioral Institute in Tennessee (www.eegfeedback.org) work with ADHD and ADD individuals through the QEEG analysis and neurofeedback technique. A similar type of brain stimulus therapy developed by Susan and Sigfried Othmer is provided by EEG Spectrum International clinics (www.eegspectrum.com). In most ADHD or ADD individuals, the outcome is significant reduction in daydreaming, distraction, and impulsive behavior.

Language Enhancement Through Brain Stimulation

Sonido, Inc., in Valdosta, Georgia (www.sonidoinc.com) offers a wide variety of computer-based brain training programs that stimulate neuron growth in the language regions of the brain. For example, the Dichonics system of auditory processing therapy is designed to overcome language handicaps related to central auditory processing disorder (CAPD), dyslexia, speech deficits, hearing loss, aphasia, and attention deficits. When these products are used consistently over time, most ADHD and ADD individuals show marked decrease in distractibility and impulsivity along with increased fluency in speaking and listening. The comprehensive language training program Fast ForWord is offered by clinics sponsored by Scientific Learning Corporation (www.scientificlearning.com). The Fast ForWord listening therapy is designed to overcome the "tone deaf" challenges of auditory dyslexia described in Chapter 6. Intensive work with Fast ForWord rewires the medial geniculate nucleus so that tone deaf individuals begin to hear individual speech sounds, especially vowels and soft consonants. Significant gains are seen in spelling and phonetic analysis of words in reading.

Recovery from Brain Injury

The rapidly developing technology of Web-based health care delivery, called e-health, provides a remarkable source of brain stimulus therapy for brain trauma patients who have suffered stroke, head trauma, or onset of dementia. Many individuals develop ADHD, ADD, or dyslexic symptoms following brain trauma incidents. In Oklahoma City, Cognitive Systems (www.cog-systems.com) offers an intriguing teletherapy brain retraining program developed by John and Marie Hatfield. Their research is documenting dramatic recovery of language functions and cognitive skills in brain-injured adults who participate in this brain stimulus program from their homes or rehabilitation centers. Patients with acquired ADHD, ADD, or dyslexia find their symptoms reduced through this teletherapy. This cutting-edge technology shows great promise for future rehabilitation programs, as well as for special education in public and private schools. The growing homeschool movement also will benefit from this home therapy technology.

Jordan Executive Function Index for Children

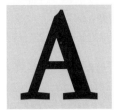

This appendix presents the Jordan Executive Function Index for Children. Two points of view are obtained by having parents fill out the Parent Response page for personal background information, along with the behavior items on the checklists. Also, a teacher who knows the child is asked to fill out the Teacher Response page, along with the checklist items. Then the results are compared to see if behavior is significantly different at home and at school.

Scoring instructions are given at the bottom of each page of the questionnaire. For example, each page yields a total score. Then each total score is entered on the corresponding page of the Summary of Behaviors profile: Attention Behavior, Organization Behavior, Inhibition Behavior. These total scores show how severe each subtype of ADHD/ADD behavior is. Finally, each total score is marked on the Rating Scale Chart to give a quick visual indication of where each of these ADHD/ADD behaviors ranks in severity.

As time goes by, parents and teachers can keep track of the child's emerging maturity and progress. The goal is to see when original Never items move up to Sometimes, when Sometimes items move up to Usually, and when Usually items become Always.

Parent Response

Name _____ Date _____
                                        year   month   day

Grade _____ Retained? _____ Birthdate _____
                                          year   month   day

If retained, what grade? _____ Age _____
                                      year   month   day

Speech Development: Early ☐ On time ☐ Late ☐

Tooth Development: Early ☐ On time ☐ Late ☐

Allergies: None ☐ Mild ☐ Moderate ☐ Severe ☐

Otitis Media: None ☐ Mild ☐ Moderate ☐ Severe ☐

Mother's Pregnancy: Normal ☐ Difficult ☐ Problems off and on ☐

Birth Length _____ Birth Weight _____ _____
                inches   pounds   ounces

Born early? Yes ☐ No ☐ If early, how early? _____

Diagnosed as ADHD? Yes ☐ No ☐ If so, at what age? _____

Diagnosed as ADD? Yes ☐ No ☐ If so, at what age? _____

Diagnosed as LD? Yes ☐ No ☐ If so, at what age? _____

What type of LD? _____

Medication for ADHD or ADD? Yes ☐ No ☐

If so, at what age? _____

What medication? _____ What dosage? _____

For how long? _____

On the next three pages, please mark the column after each statement that is MOST like this student MOST of the time.

Attention Behavior

	Never 0	Sometimes 1	Usually 2	Always 3
Keeps attention focused on the task without darting/drifting off on mental rabbit trails.	___	___	___	___
Tunes out (ignores) what goes on nearby in order to keep on doing necessary work.	___	___	___	___
Keeps on listening to oral information without darting/drifting off on mental rabbit trails.	___	___	___	___
Listens to and understands new information without saying, "Huh?" or "What?" or "What do you mean?"	___	___	___	___
Finishes tasks without wandering off on rabbit trails before work is completed.	___	___	___	___
Does necessary tasks without needing continual reminding and supervision.	___	___	___	___
Can be part of a team or play group without wandering off on mental rabbit trails during the game.	___	___	___	___
Follows the rules of games without having to be reminded over and over.	___	___	___	___
Remembers what to do after school without being reminded or supervised.	___	___	___	___
Remembers phone messages and messages from teachers to parents.	___	___	___	___
Cleans up own room/workspace without supervision.	___	___	___	___
Does routine chores without being reminded or supervised.	___	___	___	___
Pays attention to TV shows/movies without wandering off on mental rabbit trails.	___	___	___	___
Notices how others respond to his/her behavior.	___	___	___	___
Picks up on cues as to how own behavior should be changed.	___	___	___	___
Notices details (how things are alike/different) without being told to notice.	___	___	___	___
Notices how/where objects are placed and tries not to bump/knock them over.	___	___	___	___
Notices how work pages are organized (how lines are numbered, how details are spaced, where written responses should go).	___	___	___	___
Follows conversations without losing it or jumping to a different subject before others finish speaking.	___	___	___	___

Add all of the scores: 0 for Never, 1 for Sometimes, 2 for Usually, 3 for Always

Attention Behavior Total Score ___

Organization Behavior

	Never 0	Sometimes 1	Usually 2	Always 3
Keeps track of own things without losing them.	_____	_____	_____	_____
Gathers up things and gets them back to school without being reminded/supervised.	_____	_____	_____	_____
Keeps track of assignments/school projects without having to be reminded/supervised.	_____	_____	_____	_____
Keeps room/desk/locker space tidy and orderly without supervision.	_____	_____	_____	_____
Keeps clothes/personal belongings organized without being told/supervised.	_____	_____	_____	_____
Keeps work space orderly while doing tasks.	_____	_____	_____	_____
Hears or reads instructions, then does the task in an orderly way without supervision.	_____	_____	_____	_____
Spaces written work well on page without having to do it again.	_____	_____	_____	_____
Plans ahead/budgets time realistically without needing supervision.	_____	_____	_____	_____
Manages own money realistically without supervision.	_____	_____	_____	_____
Has realistic sense of time without needing reminding/supervision.	_____	_____	_____	_____
Plans activities, then explains plans to others without help.	_____	_____	_____	_____
Plans ahead for gifts or cards at holidays and special days without help.	_____	_____	_____	_____
Notices sequence patterns (how things should be arranged) without being told.	_____	_____	_____	_____
Keeps things together in appropriate groups (books on shelves, school papers together, shoes in pairs, tools in sets, knives/forks/spoons in correct places) without being reminded/supervised.	_____	_____	_____	_____
Keeps schoolwork organized in notebooks, folders, files, stacks without supervision.	_____	_____	_____	_____
Plays by the rules. Wants playmates/teammates to follow the rules.	_____	_____	_____	_____
Does tasks in order from start to finish without skipping around.	_____	_____	_____	_____

Add all of the scores: 0 for Never, 1 for Sometimes, 2 for Usually, 3 for Always

Organization Behavior Total Score _____

Inhibition (Self-Control) Behavior

	Never 0	Sometimes 1	Usually 2	Always 3
Thinks of consequences before doing what comes to mind.	___	___	___	___
Puts off pleasure in order to finish necessary work.	___	___	___	___
Follows own sense of right and wrong instead of being influenced by others.	___	___	___	___
Puts needs and welfare of others ahead of own wishes/desires.	___	___	___	___
Says "no" to own impulses when responsibilities must be carried out.	___	___	___	___
Makes an effort to grow up instead of remaining immature and impulsive.	___	___	___	___
Tries to change habits/mannerisms that bother/offend others.	___	___	___	___
Learns from experience. Thinks about lessons learned the hard way.	___	___	___	___
Lives by rules/spiritual principles instead of by whim/impulse.	___	___	___	___
Accepts reponsibility instead of making excuses or blaming others.	___	___	___	___
Asks for help/advice instead of being stubborn.	___	___	___	___
Apologizes/asks forgiveness when behavior has hurt/offended others.	___	___	___	___
Is recognized by peers and leaders as being mature, unselfish, dependable, teachable, cooperative.	___	___	___	___
Stops inappropriate impulses/desires before they emerge so that others will not be bothered/offended.	___	___	___	___
Sticks to promises/agreements without being reminded or supervised.	___	___	___	___
Goes the extra mile for others without complaining or quitting.	___	___	___	___
Absorbs teasing/rudeness without flaring or becoming defensive.	___	___	___	___
Is kind toward others. Avoids sarcasm/hateful remarks/putdowns.	___	___	___	___
Resists urge to take things apart, tear structures down, rip things apart, pick at things with fingers.	___	___	___	___
Is flexible/creative instead of being ritualized/rigid.	___	___	___	___

Add all of the scores: 0 for Never, 1 for Sometimes, 2 for Usually, 3 for Always

Inhibition (Self-Control) Behavior Total Score _____

Summary of Behaviors

Rating Scale

0 to 11	12 to 25	26 to 40	41 to 55	56 to 60
severe	moderately severe	moderate	mild	none

Attention Behavior

Total Score (transfer from bottom of Attention Behavior page)

_____ **0–11 Severe Attention Deficit**

Cannot function in mainstream classroom or group. Must have constant supervision to succeed. Cannot do sustained tasks without one-on-one monitoring. Cannot follow instructions without step-by-step supervision. Has very short work time. Loses the task (off on rabbit trails) after 30 to 90 seconds.

Medication and diet control are required to enable this student to function in academic and social situations.

_____ **12–25 Moderately Severe Attention Deficit**

Can function part-time in nonacademic classrooms and groups (activity classes, art, music) if level of stimulus is controlled. Must have continual supervision to succeed. Can work briefly (2 to 4 minutes) in sustained tasks, but rapidly reaches burnout. Can follow simple one-step instructions with continual reminding and supervision. Must have one-on-one instruction to fill in gaps in skills and new information. Must be told and reminded to notice things.

Medication and diet control should be considered to help this student succeed and earn praise.

_____ **26–40 Moderate Attention Deficit**

Can function in mainstream classroom and groups with frequent reminding and supervision. Is easily distracted. Wanders off on rabbit trails and must be called back to the task. Must have frequent one-on-one help to fill gaps in skills and new information. Must be guided and reminded in following instructions. Notices now and then, but needs a lot of reminding to notice and pay attention.

_____ **41–55 Mild Attention Deficit**

Can function effectively in most situations. Occasionally becomes overly distracted by nearby events. Needs frequent monitoring to finish tasks and stay on schedules. Can be taught to monitor self and bring attention back to tasks.

_____ **56–60 No Attention Deficit**

Overcoming Attention Deficit Disorders in Children, Adolescents, and Adults

Organization Behavior
Total Score (transfer from bottom of Organization Behavior page)

_____ 0–11 **Severe Organizational Deficit**
Cannot manage own things without help and supervision. Cannot remember where things are, what things are needed for certain tasks, where things were put when last used. Cannot gather up own things without supervision. Cannot remember what to take home or bring back to school. Loses things on school bus, at home, in the classroom, in the lunchroom, on the playground. Loses clothes, books, bookbag, shoes, jackets, wraps. Cannot recall where they were left. Leaves tools and playthings in yard overnight. Cannot clean up own room or desk without direct supervision. Must be guided/supervised/monitored in order to finish any task. Often is called "lazy" and "careless." Is in continual conflict with adults who do not understand organizational deficits.

_____ 12–25 **Moderately Severe Organizational Deficit**
Must have supervision and help to organize. Can do better if steps are written on notes. Must be reminded to go back to notes/outlines to make sure everything has been finished. Cannot clean up room or do chores without supervision. Cannot manage school things without being reminded. Can learn to follow checklists and outlines if someone provides supervision and continual reminding. Must not be expected to organize or stay on schedule without help.

_____ 26–40 **Moderate Organizational Deficit**
Ability to organize is spotty and unpredictable. Needs a lot of reminding and supervision. Responds well to written reminders (notes, outlines). Must be reminded to refer back to notes and outlines to make sure each step has been followed. Tends to be absentminded. Tends to mislay things. Keeps things in loose piles or stacks that become mixed together. Must have help cleaning out desk/locker/work space. Has cycles of better organization/poorer organization.

_____ 41–55 **Mild Organizational Deficit**
Can develop effective strategies for staying organized and on schedule. Responds well to keeping calendars, outlines of tasks, schedules on paper. Needs to be reminded frequently. Tends to wander off on rabbit trails and forget. Appears to be absentminded and careless.

_____ 56–60 **No Organizational Deficit**

Appendix A

Inhibition (Self-Control) Behavior
Total Score (transfer from bottom of Inhibition Behavior page)

_____ 0–11 **Severe Problems with Self-Control**
Cannot function successfully in relationships. Is severely self-focused/self-centered. Does not notice needs or wishes of others. Places self first. Thinks mostly of satisfying own desires. All of personal energy goes toward fulfilling own self-needs. Does not extend affection without demanding something in return. Cannot respond normally to the give-and-take of friendships/family relationships/social relationships. Is irritable, quick-tempered, judgmental of others. Attitude is demanding, short-tempered, critical of others. Refuses to share except when sharing will serve his/her purposes. Demands to be first. Wants biggest piece or share for self. Makes insatiable demands on others. Destroys the good will of others. Often is rejected by others. Moves from one friend to the next after short term of friendship. Cannot share space peacefully. Usually creates conflict with others. Cannot fit into groups. Lives in a state of unhappiness. Complains, gripes, finds fault when others see no problem. This person creates continual conflict for leaders. Must be handled firmly. Cannot respond to normal suggestions that depend upon noticing others. Continually argues, challenges, blames others, indulges in self-pity. Uses others without showing regret or concern. Must have medication to succeed.

_____ 12–25 **Moderately Severe Problems with Self-Control**
Has trouble functioning in relationships, but can do so if others are patient and forgiving enough. Must be closely supervised in groups. Triggers frequent arguments/conflicts with peers. Is disliked by most leaders. Often is rejected by peers and/or adults. Can respond temporarily to coaching in how to treat others more kindly, but such lessons do not last. Does not have a natural bent for extending kindness and positive attention to others. Leaders must intervene frequently to stop conflict or restore peace. This person requires extra effort from leaders to keep things going smoothly. Triggers a lot of dislike from peers. Spends much time planning revenge and getting even. Needs medication and diet control to succeed.

_____ 26–40 **Moderate Problems with Self-Control**
Responds to reminding about manners and appropriate behavior. Requires frequent one-on-one guidance in how to behave more appropriately and less selfishly. Can respond well to reminder cues. Responds to guidance/counseling strategies that teach this person how to notice others. Triggers some conflict within groups. Has good days/bad days in relationships. Argues a lot over trivial

Overcoming Attention Deficit Disorders in Children, Adolescents, and Adults

issues. Tends to split hairs over things others take in stride. Seldom is a fully cooperative member of groups. Seeks subtle ways to get even.

_____ 41–55 **Mild Problems with Self-Control**
Needs frequent reminding about how to interact with others. Responds to guidance about noticing needs/wishes of others. Can learn to put own needs last or postpone wishes until later. Has good day/bad day cycles in relationships. Needs a lot of forgiveness and forgiving.

_____ 56–60 **No Problems with Self-Control**

Comparison Rating Scale

Mark each of the three total scores on this scale to compare the difference between the child's attention, organization, and inhibition behaviors at home.

Severe		
10	**9**	**8**
0 1 2 3	4 5 6 7	8 9 10 11

Moderately Severe	
7	**6**
12 13 14 15 16 17 18	19 20 21 22 23 24 25

Moderate	
5	**4**
26 27 28 29 30 31 32	33 34 35 36 37 38 39 40

Mild		
3	**2**	**1**
41 42 43 44 45	46 47 48 49 50	51 52 53 54 55

None
0
56 57 58 59 60

Teacher Response

Student's Name _____ Age _____ Grade _____

Classroom Performance

High Achiever	Average Achiever	Low Achiever

No Struggle	Moderate Struggle	Severe Struggle

High Motivation (always motivated)	Average Motivation (comes and goes)	Low Motivation (seldom motivated)

Classroom Behavior

Fits in well. Liked by peers. Little or no peer conflict.	Some conflict. Not always liked by peers. Usually fits in with help from adults.	Continual conflict. Is disliked by peers. Doesn't fit in even with help from adults.
Usually cheerful and happy.	Often moody, touchy, grouchy, irritable.	Seldom cheerful. Usually unhappy. Usually overly sensitive and touchy.
Outgoing. Active. Eager to cooperate. Ready to participate or lead. Willing to follow.	Quiet. Passive. Needs to be prompted to participate. Willing to cooperate and follow. Shy about leading.	Withdrawn. Does not want to cooperate. Usually unconnected from the group.
Creative. Actively involved with group planning. Shows good imagination.	Sometimes creative. Often daydreams and needs to be called back to participation.	Continually elsewhere in daydreams. Short attention span. Must be called back again and again.

On the next three pages, please mark the item after each statement that is MOST like this student MOST of the time.

Overcoming Attention Deficit Disorders in Children, Adolescents, and Adults

Attention Behavior

	Never 0	Sometimes 1	Usually 2	Always 3
Keeps attention focused on the task without darting/ drifting off on mental rabbit trails.	____	____	____	____
Tunes out (ignores) what goes on nearby in order to keep on doing necessary work.	____	____	____	____
Keeps on listening to oral information without darting/drifting off on mental rabbit trails.	____	____	____	____
Listens to/understands new information without saying, "Huh?" or "What?" or "What do you mean?"	____	____	____	____
Finishes tasks without wandering off on mental trails before work is completed.	____	____	____	____
Does necessary tasks without needing continual reminding and supervision.	____	____	____	____
Can be part of a team or play group without wandering off on rabbit trails during the game or activity.	____	____	____	____
Follows game rules without having to be reminded.	____	____	____	____
Takes part in group activities without being called back to attention over and over.	____	____	____	____
Remembers what to take home without being supervised.	____	____	____	____
Remembers messages from teachers to parents.	____	____	____	____
Cleans up own work space without supervision.	____	____	____	____
Does routine classroom chores without being supervised.	____	____	____	____
Pays attention to video presentations without wandering off on mental rabbit trails.	____	____	____	____
Notices how others respond to his/her behavior. Heeds cues as to how own behavior should change.	____	____	____	____
Notices details (how things are alike/different) without being told to notice.	____	____	____	____
Notices how/where objects are placed and tries not to bump/knock them over.	____	____	____	____
Notices how work pages are organized (how lines are numbered, details are spaced, where to write).	____	____	____	____
Follows conversations without losing the meaning or jumping to a different subject before others finish speaking.	____	____	____	____

Add all of the scores: 0 for Never, 1 for Sometimes, 2 for Usually, 3 for Always

Attention Behavior Total Score _____

Organization Behavior

	Never 0	Sometimes 1	Usually 2	Always 3
Keeps track of own things without losing them.	___	___	___	___
Gathers up things and gets them home and back to school without supervision.	___	___	___	___
Keeps track of assignments/projects without supervision.	___	___	___	___
Keeps room/desk/locker tidy without supervision.	___	___	___	___
Keeps personal belongings organized without supervision.	___	___	___	___
Keeps work space tidy/orderly while doing tasks.	___	___	___	___
Hears/reads instructions, then does the task in an orderly way without supervision.	___	___	___	___
Uses things, then puts them away without supervision.	___	___	___	___
Cleans up work space when tasks are finished without supervision.	___	___	___	___
Spaces written work well on the page without having to do it again.	___	___	___	___
Plans ahead realistically without supervision.	___	___	___	___
Manages time realistically without supervision.	___	___	___	___
Has realistic sense of time without supervision.	___	___	___	___
Plans activities, then explains to others without help.	___	___	___	___
Is aware of coming holidays and special days without being reminded.	___	___	___	___
Notices sequence patterns (how things should be arranged, how things fit together) without being told.	___	___	___	___
Keeps things together in appropriate groups (books on shelves, school papers/classroom materials together) without supervision.	___	___	___	___
Keeps schoolwork organized in notebooks, bookbag, folders, stacks, files without supervision.	___	___	___	___
Plays by the rules. Expects others to follow the rules.	___	___	___	___
Does tasks in order from start to finish without skipping around or losing the sequence.	___	___	___	___

Add all of the scores: 0 for Never, 1 for Sometimes, 2 for Usually, 3 for Always

Organization Behavior Total Score _____

Inhibition (Self-Control) Behavior

	Never 0	Sometimes 1	Usually 2	Always 3
Thinks of consequences before acting.				
Puts off pleasure in order to finish work.				
Follows own sense of right and wrong instead of being influenced by others.				
Puts needs and welfare of others ahead of own wishes/desires.				
Says "no" to impulses when responsibilities must be carried out.				
Makes an effort to grow up instead of remaining immature or impulsive.				
Tries to change habits/mannerisms that bother or offend others.				
Learns from experience. Thinks about lessons learned the hard way.				
Lives by rules/spiritual principles instead of by whim/impulse.				
Accepts responsibility instead of making excuses or blaming others.				
Asks for help/advice instead of being stubborn.				
Apologizes when behavior has hurt/offended others.				
Is recognized by others as being mature, friendly, unselfish, dependable, teachable, cooperative.				
Stops inappropriate impulses/desires so that others will not be bothered or offended.				
Sticks to promises/agreements without supervision.				
Goes the extra mile for others without complaining or feeling self-pity.				
Sets and works toward long-term goals without complaining or quitting.				
Absorbs teasing/rudeness without flaring or becoming defensive.				
Is kind toward others. Avoids sarcasm/hateful remarks.				
Resists urge to take things apart, tear structures down, rip things apart, pick at things with fingers.				
Is flexible and creative instead of being ritualized and rigid.				

Add all of the scores: 0 for Never, 1 for Sometimes, 2 for Usually, 3 for Always

Inhibition (Self-Control) Behavior Total Score _____

285

Appendix A

Summary of Behaviors

Rating Scale

0 to 11	12 to 25	26 to 40	41 to 55	56 to 60
severe	moderately severe	moderate	mild	none

Attention Behavior
Total Score (transfer from bottom of Attention Behavior page)

_____ 0–11 **Severe Attention Deficit**
Cannot function in mainstream classroom or group. Must have constant supervision to succeed. Cannot do sustained tasks without one-on-one monitoring. Cannot follow instructions without step-by-step supervision. Has very short work time. Loses the task (off on rabbit trails) after 30 to 90 seconds. Medication and diet control are required before this student can function in academic and social situations.

_____ 12–25 **Moderately Severe Attention Deficit**
Can function part-time in nonacademic classrooms and groups (activity classes, art, music) if level of stimulus is controlled. Must have continual supervision to succeed. Can work briefly (2 to 4 minutes) in sustained tasks, but rapidly reaches burnout. Can follow simple one-step instructions with continual reminding and supervision. Must have one-on-one instruction to fill in gaps in skills and new information. Must be told and reminded to notice things. Medication and diet control should be considered to help this student succeed and earn praise.

_____ 26–40 **Moderate Attention Deficit**
Can function in mainstream classrooms and groups with frequent reminding and supervision. Is easily distracted. Wanders off on daydream rabbit trails and must be called back to task. Must have frequent one-on-one help to fill in gaps in skills and new information. Must be guided and reminded in following instructions. Notices now and then, but needs a lot of reminding to notice and pay attention.

_____ 41–55 **Mild Attention Deficit**
Can function effectively in most situations. Occasionally becomes overly distracted by nearby events. Needs frequent monitoring to finish tasks and stay on schedules. Can be taught to monitor self and bring attention back to tasks.

_____ 56–60 **No Attention Deficit**

Overcoming Attention Deficit Disorders in Children, Adolescents, and Adults

Organization Behavior
Total Score (transfer from bottom of Organization Behavior page)

_____ 0–11 **Severe Organizational Deficit**
Cannot manage own things without help and supervision. Cannot remember where things were put when last used. Cannot gather up own things without supervision. Cannot remember what to take home or what to bring back to school. Loses things on school bus, in the classroom, in the lunchroom, on the playground. Loses books, bookbag, clothing articles. Cannot recall where they were left. Cannot clean up own desk area or locker without direct supervision. Must be guided/supervised/monitored to finish tasks. Is in continual conflict with adult expectations.

_____ 12–25 **Moderately Severe Organizational Deficit**
Must have supervision and help with organizing. Can do better if steps are written on notes and outlines. Must be reminded to go back to notes and outlines to make sure everything has been finished. Needs supervision to clean up desk area or locker. Cannot manage classroom materials without supervision. Can learn to follow checklists and outlines if adults maintain supervision with frequent reminding. Must not be expected to organize or stay on schedule without help.

_____ 26–40 **Moderate Organizational Deficit**
Ability to organize is spotty and unpredictable. Needs frequent reminding and monitoring to stay organized. Responds well to written reminders (notes, outlines, calendar schedules). Must be reminded to go back to notes and outlines to make sure each step has been followed. Tends to be absentminded with frequent daydreaming. Tends to mislay things. Keeps things in loose piles or stacks that often become mixed together and out of order. Must have help cleaning desk area, locker, or work space. Has cycles of good days/bad days in keeping things adequately organized.

_____ 41–55 **Mild Organizational Deficit**
Can develop effective strategies for staying organized and on schedule. Responds well to keeping calendars, outlines of tasks, and schedules on paper. Must be reminded frequently to review the calendar, outlines, and schedules. Tends to wander off on mental rabbit trails and forget. Appears to be absentminded and careless when left to work alone.

_____ 56–60 **No Organizational Deficit**

Inhibition (Self-Control) Behavior
Total Score (transfer from bottom of Inhibition [Self-Control] Behavior page)

_____ 0–11 **Severe Problems with Self-Control**
Cannot function successfully in relationships. Is severely self-focused/self-centered. Does not notice needs or wishes of others. Places self first. Thinks mostly of satisfying own desires. All of personal energy goes toward fulfilling self-needs. Does not extend affection without demanding something in return. Cannot respond normally to the give-and-take of friendships/social relationships. Is irritable, quick-tempered, critical of others. Refuses to share except when sharing will serve his/her purposes. Demands to be first. Wants biggest piece for self. Makes insatiable demands on others. Often bullies others. Destroys the good will of others. Often is rejected by others. Cannot share space peacefully. Triggers conflict with others. Lives in a state of unhappiness. Complains, gripes, whines, finds fault where others see no problem. This person creates continual conflict for leaders. Must be handled firmly. Cannot respond normally to suggestions or instructions. Continually argues. Challenges authority. Blames others. Indulges in self-pity. Always another person's fault. Shows little or no regret when own behavior hurts or offends others.

_____ 12–25 **Moderately Severe Problems with Self-Control**
Has trouble functioning in relationships. Can do so if others are patient and forgiving enough. Must be closely supervised in groups. Triggers frequent arguments/conflicts with peers. Often is disliked by peers and some leaders. Often is rejected by peers. Can respond temporarily to coaching in how to treat others more kindly, but such lessons do not last. Does not naturally extend kindness or pay positive attention to others. Leaders must intervene frequently to stop conflict and restore peace. This person requires extra effort from leaders to keep things going smoothly.

_____ 26–40 **Moderate Problems with Self-Control**
Responds to reminding about manners and appropriate behavior. Requires frequent one-on-one guidance in behaving more appropriately and less selfishly. Can respond well to reminder cues. Responds to guidance/counseling strategies that teach how to notice and relate to others. Triggers occasional group conflict. Has good days/bad days in relationships. Argues a lot over trivial issues. Tends to split hairs over things others take in stride. Seldom is fully cooperative in group activities. Seeks subtle ways to get even with others.

_____ 41–55 **Mild Problems with Self-Control**
Needs frequent reminding about how to interact with others. Responds to guidance about noticing needs/wishes of others. Can learn to put own needs last or postpone wishes until later. Has good day/bad day cycles in relationships. Needs a lot of forgiveness with reminders on how to forgive others.

_____ 56–60 **No Problems with Self-Control**

Comparison Rating Scale

On this scale, mark each of the three total scores to compare the differences between the child's attention, organization, and inhibition behaviors in the classroom.

Severe		
10	9	8
0 1 2 3	4 5 6 7	8 9 10 11

Moderately Severe	
7	6
12 13 14 15 16 17 18	19 20 21 22 23 24 25

Moderate	
5	4
26 27 28 29 30 31 32	33 34 35 36 37 38 39 40

Mild		
3	2	1
41 42 43 44 45	46 47 48 49 50	51 52 53 54 55

None
0
56 57 58 59 60

Jordan Executive Function Index for Adults

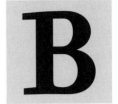

This appendix presents the Jordan Executive Function Index for Adults. This can be a self-administered questionnaire for adults who read well, if the person is mature enough to respond honestly to each item. For those who struggle to read or who are less mature, the questionnaire can be an oral activity with the instructor, spouse, or other adult reading each item aloud, and the client helping to choose which column to mark. Often it is effective to do this as an interview similar to one-on-one interviews seen on television programs.

Scoring is done exactly as described on the Jordan Executive Function Index for Children (see Appendix A). A spouse, companion, parent, or other adult helps the individual to provide the background information on the Self-Response page. The same procedure is followed on the Counselor or Instructor Response page by someone who knows the client well.

Self-Response

Name _____ Date _____
　　　　　　　　　　　　　　　　　　　year　　　month　　　day

Last grade in school _____ Birthdate _____
　　　　　　　　　　　　　　　　　　　year　　　month　　　day

Retained? _____ What grade? _____ Age _____
　　　　　　　　　　　　　　　　　　　year　　　month　　　day

Speech Development: Early ☐ On time ☐ Late ☐

Tooth Development: Early ☐ On time ☐ Late ☐

Physical coordination _____
(standing, walking, skipping, running, drawing, writing)

Physical therapy? Yes ☐ No ☐

Allergies? None ☐ Mild ☐ Moderate ☐ Severe ☐

Early ear infections: Yes ☐ No ☐
(Otitis Media)

Mother's Pregnancy: Normal ☐ Difficult ☐

Birth Length _____ Birth Weight _____ _____
　　　　　　　inches　　　　　　　　　　pounds　　　　ounces

Born early? Yes ☐ No ☐ If early, how early? _____

Born late? Yes ☐ No ☐ If late, how late? _____

Diagnosed as LD? Yes ☐ No ☐ What age? _____

What type of LD? _____

Diagnosed as ADHD? Yes ☐ No ☐ What age? _____

Medication? _____

Diagnosed as ADD? Yes ☐ No ☐ What age? _____

Medication? _____

Special school program? Yes ☐ No ☐

What kind of help? _____

Did you begin to outgrow early LD, ADHD, or ADD? Yes ☐ No ☐

What age? _____

Other relatives with similar history? Yes ☐ No ☐

What relation? _____

On the next three pages, please mark the item after each statement that is MOST like this person MOST of the time.

Overcoming Attention Deficit Disorders in Children, Adolescents, and Adults

Attention Behavior

	Never 0	Sometimes 1	Usually 2	Always 3
Keeps attention focused on the task without being distracted by what happens nearby.	___	___	___	___
Keeps attention focused without drifting off into daydreams or mentally darting off to something else.	___	___	___	___
Keeps on listening to oral information without drifting/darting off to something else.	___	___	___	___
Listens to/understands new information without saying "Huh?" or "What?" or "What do you mean?"	___	___	___	___
Finishes tasks without changing to something else before first job is finished.	___	___	___	___
Does necessary work without needing to be reminded or supervised.	___	___	___	___
Can be part of a team or group without mentally wandering off during group activity.	___	___	___	___
Follows rules without having to be reminded.	___	___	___	___
Takes part in group activities without having to be called back to attention.	___	___	___	___
Remembers what to do after work or school without being reminded or supervised.	___	___	___	___
Remembers phone messages and other oral information.	___	___	___	___
Cleans up own living or work space without having to be reminded or supervised.	___	___	___	___
Does routine chores without having to be reminded or supervised.	___	___	___	___
Pays attention to video presentations without wandering off on mental rabbit trails.	___	___	___	___
Notices how others respond to his/her behavior. Picks up cues as to how own behavior should be changed.	___	___	___	___
Notices details (how things are alike/different) without being told to notice.	___	___	___	___
Notices how and where things are placed and tries not to bump or knock them over.	___	___	___	___
Notices how materials are organized (how lines are numbered, how details are spaced, where writing should go).	___	___	___	___
Follows conversations without losing the thought or jumping to a different subject before others finish speaking.	___	___	___	___

Add all of the scores: 0 for Never, 1 for Sometimes, 2 for Usually, 3 for Always

Attention Behavior Total Score _____

293

Appendix B

Organization Behavior

	Never 0	Sometimes 1	Usually 2	Always 3
Keeps track of own things without losing them.	___	___	___	___
Gathers up and returns things to correct places without being reminded or supervised.	___	___	___	___
Keeps track of assignments/work projects without having to be reminded or supervised.	___	___	___	___
Keeps own living space/work space clean and orderly without being reminded.	___	___	___	___
Keeps clothes, tools, and personal things organized without being reminded or supervised.	___	___	___	___
Keeps work space orderly while doing tasks.	___	___	___	___
Hears or reads instructions, then does the task in an orderly way without needing supervision.	___	___	___	___
Gets out tools and materials, then puts them away in correct places without being supervised.	___	___	___	___
Keeps living space tidy without being cluttered or messy.	___	___	___	___
Spaces handwriting well on the lines without crowding or being messy.	___	___	___	___
Plans ahead/budgets time realistically without being reminded.	___	___	___	___
Has realistic sense of time without needing to be reminded or supervised.	___	___	___	___
Manages money realistically without needing to be reminded or supervised.	___	___	___	___
Plans activities, then explains plans to others without needing help.	___	___	___	___
Plans ahead for gifts or cards for holidays and special days.	___	___	___	___
Notices sequence patterns (how things should be be arranged) without being told to notice.	___	___	___	___
Keeps things together in appropriate groups (books on shelves, papers together, shoes in pairs, tools in sets, silverware in correct place) without having to be reminded or supervised.	___	___	___	___
Keeps papers organized in notebooks, folders, files, neat stacks without supervision.	___	___	___	___
Follows the rules. Wants others to follow rules.	___	___	___	___
Does tasks in order from start to finish without skipping around.	___	___	___	___

Add all of the scores: 0 for Never, 1 for Sometimes, 2 for Usually, 3 for Always

Organization Behavior Total Score _____

Overcoming Attention Deficit Disorders in Children, Adolescents, and Adults

Inhibition (Self-Control) Behavior

	Never 0	Sometimes 1	Usually 2	Always 3
Thinks of consequences before doing what comes to mind.	___	___	___	___
Puts off pleasure in order to finish work.	___	___	___	___
Follows own sense of right/wrong instead of being influenced by others.	___	___	___	___
Puts needs/welfare of others ahead of own wishes/desires.	___	___	___	___
Says "no" to impulses when responsibilities must be carried out.	___	___	___	___
Makes an effort to grow up instead of remaining impulsive or immature.	___	___	___	___
Tries to change habits/mannerisms that bother or offend others.	___	___	___	___
Learns from experience. Thinks about lessons learned the hard way.	___	___	___	___
Lives by rules/spiritual principles instead of by whim or impulse.	___	___	___	___
Accepts responsibility instead of making excuses or blaming others.	___	___	___	___
Asks for help instead of being stubborn.	___	___	___	___
Apologizes/asks forgiveness when behavior has hurt or offended others.	___	___	___	___
Is recognized by peers and leaders as being mature, unselfish, dependable, teachable, cooperative.	___	___	___	___
Stops inappropriate impulses/desires before they emerge so others will not be bothered/offended.	___	___	___	___
Sticks to promises/agreements without having to be reminded or supervised.	___	___	___	___
Goes the extra mile for others without complaining or feeling self-pity.	___	___	___	___
Sets long-term goals and works toward them without complaining or quitting.	___	___	___	___
Absorbs teasing/rudeness without flaring or becoming defensive.	___	___	___	___
Is kind toward others. Avoids sarcasm or hateful/putdown remarks.	___	___	___	___
Resists urge to take things apart, pick at things with fingers.	___	___	___	___
Is flexible/creative instead of being rigid/ritualized.	___	___	___	___

Add all of the scores: 0 for Never, 1 for Sometimes, 2 for Usually, 3 for Always

Inhibition (Self-Control) Behavior Total Score _____

Summary of Executive Function Behaviors
Rating Scale

0 to 11	12 to 25	26 to 40	41 to 55	56 to 60
severe	moderately severe	moderate	mild	none

Attention Behavior
Total Score (transfer from bottom of Attention Behavior page)

_____ **0–11 Severe Attention Deficit**
Cannot function in mainstream classroom or work group. Must have constant supervision to succeed. Cannot do sustained tasks without one-on-one monitoring. Cannot follow instructions without step-by-step supervision. Very short work time. Loses the task, off on mental rabbit trails after 60 to 90 seconds. Medication and diet control required for this person to function in academic, workplace, or social situations.

_____ **12–25 Moderately Severe Attention Deficit**
Can function part-time in nonacademic groups if level of stimulus/distraction is controlled. Must have continual supervision/monitoring to succeed. Can work in brief segments (5 to 10 minutes) in sustained tasks, but reaches rapid burnout and must take a brief break. Can follow simple one-step instructions with consistent reminding and supervision. Must have one-on-one instruction to fill in gaps in skills and understand new information. Must be told/reminded to notice details. Medication and diet control should be considered to help this person succeed and earn praise.

_____ **26–40 Moderate Attention Deficit**
Can function in mainstream classroom and work groups with frequent reminding and supervision. Easily distracted. Wanders off on mental rabbit trails and must be called back to the task. Must have frequent one-on-one help to fill gaps in skills and to understand new information. Must be guided in following through on instructions and procedures. Notices details now and then, but needs a lot of reminding to notice and pay attention.

_____ **41–55 Mild Attention Deficit**
Can function effectively in most situations. Occasionally becomes overly distracted by nearby events, or drifts away in daydreams. Needs frequent monitoring to finish tasks and stay on schedules. Can be taught to monitor self and bring own attention back to task.

_____ **56–60 No Attention Deficit**

Organization Behavior

Total Score (transfer from bottom of Organization Behavior page)

_____ 0–11 **Severe Organizational Deficit**
Cannot manage own things without help and supervision. Cannot remember where things are, what things are needed for certain tasks, where things were put when last used. Cannot gather up own things without supervision. Cannot remember what to take home or what to bring back to work or school. Loses things on the bus, at home, at work, while shopping. Loses keys, wallet, purse, books, important papers, clothing items. Leaves tools and work things in the yard overnight. Cannot clean up own living space or work space without help. Must be guided, monitored, supervised to finish tasks. Often called "lazy" and and "careless." Is in continual conflict with others because of organizational deficits.

_____ 12–25 **Moderately Severe Organizational Deficit**
Must have help to organize at home. Must be supervised at work. Can do better if steps are written on notes or outlines. Must be reminded to go back to notes and outlines to make sure everything has been finished. Cannot maintain tidy work space or living space without help. Cannot manage own things without help. Can learn to follow checklists and outlines if others continually remind. Must not be expected to organize, stay on schedules, or tidy up without help.

_____ 26–40 **Moderate Organizational Deficit**
Ability to organize is spotty and unpredictable. Needs frequent reminding. Responds well to written reminders (notes, outlines, calendars). Must be reminded to refer to notes/outlines/calendars to make sure all steps have been followed. Tends to be absentminded. Drifts into daydreams. Tends to mislay things. Keeps things in loose piles or stacks that often become mixed together. Must have help cleaning up desk/locker/work area/living space. Has cycles of better organization/poorer organization.

_____ 41–55 **Mild Organizational Deficit**
Can develop effective strategies for staying organized and on schedule. Responds well to keeping calendars, outlines of tasks, reminders on stick-on notes. Needs to be reminded frequently. Tends to wander off on mental rabbit trails and forget.

_____ 56–60 **No Organizational Deficit**

Inhibition (Self-Control) Behavior

Total Score (transfer from bottom of Inhibition [Self-Control] Behavior page

_____ 0–11 **Severe Problems with Self-Control**
Cannot function successfully in relationships. Is severely self-focused and self-centered. Does not notice the needs/wishes of others. Places self first. Personal energy goes toward fulfilling own self-needs. Does not extend affection without demanding something in return. Cannot respond normally to the give-and-take of friendships/family relationships/social relationships. Is irritable, quick-tempered, judgmental when pressed to pay attention to others. Lifestyle attitude is demanding, short-tempered, critical of others. Refuses to share except when he/she gets something in return. Makes insatiable demands on others. Self-focused lifestyle triggers rejection by others. Cannot share space peacefully. Triggers conflict in others. Cannot fit into groups. Is unhappy much of the time. Complains, gripes, whines, finds faults when others see no problem. Continually argues, challenges authority, blames others, indulges in self-pity. Resorts to bullying behavior that intimidates others into letting this person have his/her own way.

_____ 12–25 **Moderately Severe Problems with Self-Control**
Has trouble functioning in relationships, but can do so if others are patient and forgiving enough. Must be closely supervised in groups. Triggers frequent arguments/conflicts with peers and leaders. Does not have a natural bent for extending kindness, generosity, or positive attention to others. Triggers much dislike from peers. Spends much time and energy planning revenge and getting even. Leaders must intervene to stop cycles of conflict to restore peace and order.

_____ 26–40 **Moderate Problems with Self-Control**
Responds to reminding about appropriate behavior. Requires frequent one-on-one guidance in how to behave more appropriately. Can respond to reminder cues. Responds to guidance/counseling strategies that teach this person how to notice others in positive ways. Often triggers conflict within groups. Has good day/ not-so-good day cycles in relationships. Argues a lot over trivial issues. Tends to split hairs over issues that others take in stride. Seldom is a fully cooperative group member. Seeks subtle ways to get even with others.

_____ 41–55 **Mild Problems with Self-Control**
Needs frequent reminding about how to interact with others. Responds to guidance about noticing wishes/needs of others. Can learn to put own needs last or postpone wishes until later. Has

good day/not-so-good day cycles in relationships. Needs a lot of forgiveness and forgiving.

_____ 56–60   **No Problems with Self-Control**

Comparison Rating Scale

Mark each of the three total scores on this scale to compare the differences between this person's attention, organization, and inhibition behaviors.

Severe		
10	**9**	**8**
0 1 2 3	4 5 6 7	8 9 10 11

Moderately Severe	
7	**6**
12 13 14 15 16 17 18	19 20 21 22 23 24 25

Moderate	
5	**4**
26 27 28 29 30 31 32	33 34 35 36 37 38 39 40

Mild		
3	**2**	**1**
41 42 43 44 45	46 47 48 49 50	51 52 53 54 55

None
0
56 57 58 59 60

Instructor/Supervisor Response

Name _____ Date _____

Classroom? Yes ☐ No ☐ Workplace? Yes ☐ No ☐ Other? _____

Above average effort (always does his/her best)	Average effort (good days/bad days)	Below average effort (usually could do better)
High motivation (always motivated)	Average motivation (good days/bad days)	Below average motivation (seldom motivated)
Well organized (neat, tidy, orderly)	Not always organized (often untidy, disorganized)	Poorly organized (always untidy, disorganized)
Fits in well. Liked by peers.	Some conflict. Not always liked by peers.	Usually in conflict. Is misfit with peers.
Positive attitude (usually cheerful, happy)	Positive days/negative days	Negative attitude (grouchy, complaining, finds fault, makes excuses)
Thoughtful of others (looks out for needs of others).	Not always thoughtful (sometimes looks out for needs of others).	Is not thoughtful of others (self-focused— does not look out for needs of others).
Dependable. Works well without supervision.	Not always dependable. Needs a lot of supervision.	Undependable. Cannot work without supervision.
Creative. Comes up with good ideas.	Seldom creative. Follows what others suggest.	Does not contribute new ideas. Complains about ideas from others.
Good at following instructions.	Must be monitored to follow instructions.	Cannot follow instructions without supervision.
Positive influence. Makes others feel better.	Sometimes positive influence. Mood swings effect others.	Negative influence. Triggers conflicts. Argues. Sabotages authority.
Generous. Shares. Volunteers to help.	Sometimes generous, sharing. Helps others when they ask.	Does not share or help. Complains when asked to help.
Follows rules and regulations. Goes extra mile.	Sometimes takes short cuts. Does what is required.	Looks for ways not to follow rules. Looks for easy way out. Rules "aren't fair."

On the next three pages, please mark the item after each question that is MOST like this person MOST of the time.

Overcoming Attention Deficit Disorders in Children, Adolescents, and Adults

Attention Behavior

	Never 0	Sometimes 1	Usually 2	Always 3
Keeps attention focused on the task without being distracted by what happens nearby.	___	___	___	___
Keeps on listening to oral information without drifting/darting off to something else.	___	___	___	___
Listens to/understands new information without saying "Huh?" or "What?" or "What do you mean?"	___	___	___	___
Follows instructions without needing them repeated.	___	___	___	___
Finishes tasks without changing to something else before first job is finished.	___	___	___	___
Does necessary work without needing to be reminded or supervised.	___	___	___	___
Can be part of a team or group without mentally wandering off during group activities.	___	___	___	___
Follows rules without having to be reminded.	___	___	___	___
Takes part in group activities without having to be called back to attention.	___	___	___	___
Remembers what to do after work or school without being reminded or supervised.	___	___	___	___
Remembers phone or other oral messages.	___	___	___	___
Cleans up own space without having to be reminded or supervised.	___	___	___	___
Does routine chores without having to be reminded or supervised.	___	___	___	___
Pays attention to video presentations without wandering off on mental rabbit trails or talking to others.	___	___	___	___
Notices how others respond to his/her behavior. Picks up cues on how own behavior should be changed.	___	___	___	___
Notices details (how things are alike/different) without being told to notice.	___	___	___	___
Notices how/where things are placed and tries not to bump or knock them over.	___	___	___	___
Notices how work materials are organized (where parts should go, which tools go together, where materials should be stacked, etc.).	___	___	___	___
Follows conversations without losing it or jumping to another subject before others finish speaking.	___	___	___	___

Add all of the scores: 0 for Never, 1 for Sometimes, 2 for Usually, 3 for Always

Attention Behavior Total Score _____

Organization Behavior

	Never 0	Sometimes 1	Usually 2	Always 3
Keeps track of own things without losing them.	_____	_____	_____	_____
Gathers up/returns things to correct places without being reminded or supervised.	_____	_____	_____	_____
Keeps track of assignments/work projects without having to be reminded or supervised.	_____	_____	_____	_____
Keeps own work space clean and orderly without having to reminded or supervised.	_____	_____	_____	_____
Keeps tools and supplies organized without being reminded or supervised.	_____	_____	_____	_____
Keeps tools/materials inside own space without cluttering space of others.	_____	_____	_____	_____
Hears/reads instructions, then does the task without being reminded or supervised.	_____	_____	_____	_____
Gets out tools/materials, then puts them away in correct places without being reminded or supervised.	_____	_____	_____	_____
Follows instructions in correct sequence without being reminded or supervised.	_____	_____	_____	_____
Makes sure that handwriting is legible on reports and memos.	_____	_____	_____	_____
Plans ahead/budgets work time realistically without being reminded or supervised.	_____	_____	_____	_____
Has realistic sense of time passing without being reminded or supervised.	_____	_____	_____	_____
Is punctual/on time without being reminded or supervised.	_____	_____	_____	_____
Manages supplies realistically without being reminded or supervised.	_____	_____	_____	_____
Plans ahead for special events without being reminded or supervised.	_____	_____	_____	_____
Notices sequence patterns (how things should be arranged) without being told to notice.	_____	_____	_____	_____
Keeps things together in appropriate groups (tools in sets, materials sorted) without having to be reminded or supervised.	_____	_____	_____	_____
Keeps paperwork organized in a notebook, folder, or file without being reminded or supervised.	_____	_____	_____	_____
Follows rules and wants others to follow rules.	_____	_____	_____	_____
Does tasks in order from start to finish without skipping around or leaving out steps.	_____	_____	_____	_____

Add all of the scores: 0 for Never, 1 for Sometimes, 2 for Usually, 3 for Always

Organization Behavior Total Score _____

Overcoming Attention Deficit Disorders in Children, Adolescents, and Adults

Inhibition (Self-Control) Behavior

	Never 0	Sometimes 1	Usually 2	Always 3
Thinks of consequences before doing what comes to mind.	____	____	____	____
Puts off pleasure in order to finish work.	____	____	____	____
Follows own sense of right/wrong instead of being influenced by others.	____	____	____	____
Puts needs/welfare of others ahead of own wishes/desires.	____	____	____	____
Says "no" to impulses when responsibilities must be carried out.	____	____	____	____
Makes an effort not to bother others.	____	____	____	____
Tries to change habits/mannerisms that bother or offend others.	____	____	____	____
Learns from experience. Thinks about lessons learned the hard way.	____	____	____	____
Lives by rules/spiritual principles instead of by whim or impulse.	____	____	____	____
Accepts responsibility instead of making excuses or blaming others.	____	____	____	____
Asks for help instead of being stubborn.	____	____	____	____
Apologizes/asks forgiveness when behavior has hurt or offended others.	____	____	____	____
Is recognized by peers and leaders as being mature, unselfish, dependable, teachable, cooperative.	____	____	____	____
Stops inappropriate impulses before they emerge so others will not be bothered/offended.	____	____	____	____
Sticks to promises/agreements without having to be reminded or supervised.	____	____	____	____
Goes the extra mile for others without complaining or feeling self-pity.	____	____	____	____
Sets long-term goals and works toward them without complaining or quitting.	____	____	____	____
Absorbs teasing/rudeness without flaring or becoming defensive.	____	____	____	____
Is kind toward others. Avoids sarcasm or hateful/putdown remarks.	____	____	____	____
Resists urge to dismantle things when curiosity is inappropriate.	____	____	____	____
Is flexible/creative instead of being rigid or ritualized.	____	____	____	____

Add all of the scores: 0 for Never, 1 for Sometimes, 2 for Usually, 3 for Always

Inhibition (Self-Control) Behavior Total Score _____

Summary of Executive Function Behaviors
Rating Scale

0 to 11	12 to 25	26 to 40	41 to 55	56 to 60
severe	moderately severe	moderate	mild	none

Attention Behavior
Total Score (transfer from bottom of Attention Behavior page)

_____ 0–11 **Severe Attention Deficit**
Cannot function in groups. Must have constant supervision to succeed. Cannot do sustained tasks without one-on-one monitoring. Cannot follow instructions without step-by-step supervision. Has very short work time. Loses the task (off on mental rabbit trails) after 60 to 90 seconds. Medication and diet control are required before this person can function in academic, social, or work situations.

_____ 12–25 **Moderately Severe Attention Deficit**
Can function part-time in groups if level of stimulus is controlled. Must have continual supervision to succeed. Can work briefly (3 to 5 minutes) in sustained tasks, but reaches rapid burnout. Can follow simple one-step instructions with continual reminding and supervision. Must have one-on-one instructions to fill in gaps in skills and new information. Must be told and reminded to notice details. Medication and diet control should be considered to help this person succeed and earn praise.

_____ 26–40 **Moderate Attention Deficit**
Can function in mainstream classroom and work groups with frequent reminding and supervision. Is easily distracted by what goes on nearby. Frequently wanders off on mental rabbit trails and must be called back to the task. Must have frequent one-on-one help to fill in gaps in skills and new information. Must be guided in following through on instructions. Notices details now and then, but needs a lot of reminding to notice and pay attention.

_____ 41–55 **Mild Attention Deficit**
Can function effectively in most situations. Occasionally becomes overly distracted by nearby events. Needs frequent monitoring to finish tasks and stay on schedules. Can be taught to monitor self and bring attention back to task.

_____ 56–60 **No Attention Deficit**

Organization Behavior
Total Score (transfer from bottom of Organization Behavior page)

_____ 0–11 **Severe Organizational Deficit**
Cannot manage own things without help and supervision. Cannot remember where things are, what things are needed for certain tasks, where things were put when last used. Cannot gather up own things without supervision. Cannot remember what to take home or what to bring back to school or work. Loses things on the bus, at home, at work. Loses clothes, books, wallet, purse, keys, important papers. Cannot recall where they were left. Leaves tools and work things outdoors overnight. Cannot clean up own space without direct supervision. Must be guided/supervised/monitored in order to finish any task. Often is called "lazy" and "careless." Lives in continual conflict with others who do not understand organizational deficits.

_____ 12–25 **Moderately Severe Organizational Deficit**
Must have supervision and help to organize. Can do better if steps are written on notes or in outlines. Must be reminded to go back to notes/outlines to make sure everything has been finished. Cannot clean up own space or do routine chores without supervision. Cannot manage own things without being reminded. Can learn to follow checklists and outlines if others continue to remind. Must not be expected to organize or stay on schedule without help.

_____ 26–40 **Moderate Organizational Deficit**
Ability to organize is spotty and unpredictable. Needs a lot of reminding. Responds well to written reminders (sticker notes, outlines). Must be reminded to refer back to notes/outlines to make sure each step has been followed. Tends to be absentminded. Tends to mislay things. Keeps things in loose piles or stacks that often become mixed together. Must have help cleaning out desk/locker/work space. Has cycles of better organization/poorer organization.

_____ 41–55 **Mild Organizational Deficit**
Can develop effective strategies for staying organized and on schedule. Responds well to keeping calendars, outlines of tasks, schedules on paper. Needs to be reminded frequently. Tends to wander off on mental rabbit trails and forget. Appears to be absentminded and careless.

_____ 56–60 **No Organizational Deficit**

305

Appendix B

Inhibition (Self-Control) Behavior
Total Score (Transfer from bottom of Inhibition [Self-Control] Behavior page)

_____ 0–11 **Severe Deficit in Self-Control**
Cannot function successfully in relationships or groups. Is severely self-focused and self-centered. Does not notice the needs or wishes of others. Places self first. Most of personal energy goes toward fulfilling own self-needs. Does not extend affection without demanding something in return. Cannot respond normally to the give-and-take of friendships/family relationships/social relationships. Is irritable, quick tempered, demanding, judgmental when pressed to pay attention to others. Refuses to share unless something is received in return. Makes insatiable demands on others. Sabotages good will from others. Cannot share space peacefully. Continually triggers conflict with others. Cannot fit into groups. Is usually unhappy. Complains, gripes, finds faults when others see no problem. Creates continual conflict for leaders. Must be handled firmly by leaders. Continually argues, challenges authority, blames others, makes excuses, indulges in self-pity. Denies own mistakes. Rationalizes why others are to blame.

_____ 12–25 **Moderately Severe Deficit in Self-Control**
Has trouble functioning in relationships, but can do so if others are patient and forgiving enough. Must be closely supervised in groups. Triggers frequent arguments/conflicts with peers. Often is disliked by peers and leaders. Often is rejected by others. Can respond to coaching in how to treat others more kindly, but such lessons do not last. Does not have a natural bent for extending kindness and positive attention to others. Leaders must intervene frequently to stop conflict and restore peace. This person requires extra effort from leaders to keep things going smoothly. This person triggers a lot of dislike from peers. Much of his/her time is spent planning revenge/trying to get even.

_____ 26–40 **Moderate Deficit in Self-Control**
Responds to reminding about manners and appropriate behavior. Requires frequent one-on-one guidance in how to behave more appropriately and less selfishly. Can respond well to reminder cues. Responds to guidance/counseling strategies that teach how to notice others. Triggers some conflict in groups. Has good days/not-so-good days in relationships. Argues a lot over trivial issues. Tends to split hairs over things others take in stride. Is seldom a fully cooperative member of a group. Seeks subtle ways to get even with others.

_____ 41–55 **Mild Deficit in Self-Control**
Needs frequent reminding about how to interact with others. Reponds to guidance about noticing needs/wishes of others. Can learn to put own needs last or postpone until later. Has good day/not-so-good day cycles in relationships. Needs a lot of forgiveness and forgiving.

_____ 56–60 **No Deficit in Self-Control**

Comparison Rating Scale

Mark each of the three total scores to compare the differences between the person's attention, organization, and inhibition behaviors at school or at work.

Severe		
10	**9**	**8**
0 1 2 3	4 5 6 7	8 9 10 11

Moderately Severe	
7	**6**
12 13 14 15 16 17 18	19 20 21 22 23 24 25

Moderate	
5	**4**
26 27 28 29 30 31 32	33 34 35 36 37 38 39 40

Mild		
3	**2**	**1**
41 42 43 44 45	46 47 48 49 50	51 52 53 54 55

None
0
56 57 58 59 60

Jordan Attention Deficit Scale

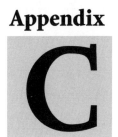

Chapters 2 through 5 describe the many layers of ADHD and ADD. The Jordan Attention Deficit Scale is designed to separate these layers to let you see clearly the many faces of ADHD or ADD. This questionnaire will answer the question: "Is this person ADHD or ADD?" If so, the Jordan Attention Deficit Scale will show you whether symptoms are borderline, moderate, or severe. The results of this evaluation will help you organize your observations of individuals who have trouble paying attention, staying on task, and ignoring distraction. This kind of organized information about how individuals pay attention will help you decide when to make a referral for professional treatment through medication or counseling. These checklists and the rating scale will help you discuss classroom or workplace behavior with parents, companions, or workplace supervisors. This information also will guide you in developing accommodations and strategies to help ADHD or ADD children, adolescents, or adults succeed at school, at work, and in personal relationships.

As time goes by, you can use the Jordan Attention Deficit Scale to chart an ADHD or ADD person's progress. As behavior symptoms go down from Always to Usually, or from Usually to Sometimes, you can keep track of which layers of ADHD or ADD are overcome through increasing maturity and helpful accommodations.

Jordan Attention Deficit Scale

Mark the level of each item that is MOST like this person MOST of the time.

	Never 0	Sometimes 1	Usually 2	Always 3

1. Hyperactivity   _____ _____ _____ _____
Constant excessive body activity. Cannot leave things alone. Cannot keep still or stay quiet. Cannot say "no" to impulses. Cannot leave others alone. Cannot spend time alone without feeling nervous or left out.

2. Passive Behavior   _____ _____ _____ _____
Below normal level of body activity. Is reluctant to become involved with group activity. Tries not be involved in group discussion. Avoids answering questions or giving oral responses. Does not volunteer information. Prefers to stay alone during play situations. Avoids being included in games. Spends long periods of time off in own private world doing make-believe/fantasy thinking. Uses fewest possible words when required to talk.

3. Short Attention   _____ _____ _____ _____
Cannot keep thoughts focused longer than 60 to 90 seconds. Is continually off on mental rabbit trails. Must continually be called back to tasks. Attention drifts or darts away from task before finishing.

4. Loose Thought Patterns   _____ _____ _____ _____
Cannot maintain organized mental images. Continually loses important details. Cannot do a series of things without starting to make mistakes. Cannot remember a series of events, facts, or details. Must have continual help to tell what has happened. Cannot remember a sequence of instructions. Cannot remember assignments over time. Cannot remember rules of games. Keeps forgetting names of people and things.

5. Poor Organization   _____ _____ _____ _____
Cannot keep life organized without help. Continually loses things. Cannot stay on schedule without supervision. Lives/works in a cluttered space. Cannot tidy up own space without help. Cannot do classroom work, homework, or job work without supervision.

	Never	Sometimes	Usually	Always
	0	1	2	3

6. Change of First Impressions

First impressions do not stay the same. Mental images immediately change. Continually erases and changes as writing is done. Continually backs up to change what was first done. Has the impression that others are "playing tricks" because things seem to shift and change. Is continually surprised or startled as mental images change. Word patterns, spelling patterns, math problems, dimensions, how things fit together seem to change.

7. Poor Listening Comprehension

Cannot get the full meaning of what others say. Continually says "What?" or "Huh?" or "What do you mean?" Does not get the full meaning without hearing it again. Needs oral information to be repeated and explained again. Does not keep on listening. Attention drifts or fades away before speaker finishes speaking. Later insists, "You didn't say that" or "I didn't hear you say that." Cannot remember later what a speaker said.

8. Time Lag

Long pauses before person reacts. Does not start assignments without being pushed or guided to start. Long periods of time go by with no work done. Long pauses while he or she searches memory for information. Continually falls behind the pace of group activities. Does not stay on set schedules.

9. Overly Sensitive

Is immediately defensive toward criticism or correction. Blames others. Spends much emotional energy defending self and blaming others. Flies into tantrums when criticized. Jumps the gun, does not wait to receive all of the information before becoming angry or defensive. Leaders must spend a lot of time restoring calm and soothing hurt feelings.

	Never	Sometimes	Usually	Always
	0	1	2	3

10. Leaves Tasks Unfinished

Does not finish tasks without supervision. Leaves
several unfinished tasks scattered around. Thinks
work is finished when there is more to do. Does not
realize when more is yet to be done.

11. Trouble Fitting in Socially

Cannot fit into groups without conflict. Whines or
clamors for his/her own way. Complains about rules
being unfair. Storms out of games when not winning.
Wants to quit and do something else before others are
finished. Is aggressive and domineering in order to
get own way. Cannot carry on small talk as part of social events. Wanders about, avoiding personal involvement in social gatherings. Is insensitive to normal
manners and social protocol. Tends to be abrupt,
rude, impolite in expressing opinions. Is overly critical of how social events are managed. Keeps conflicts
going over unimportant issues. Displays self-focused
attitude instead of noticing needs or wishes of others.

12. Too Easily Distracted

Attention continually darts or drifts to what happens
nearby. Cannot ignore what others are doing. Is overly
aware of nearby sound, odor, movement. Cannot
ignore own body sensations. Must scratch every itch,
adjust clothing, touch or feel nearby objects.

13. Immature

Behavior is obviously less mature than expected for
that age. Behaves like a much younger person. Cannot get along well with age-mates. Prefers to play or
be with younger persons. Has interests and thought
patterns of younger individuals. Does not make effort
to "grow up." Refuses to accept responsibility or to be
responsible. Behavior is impulsive/compulsive. Acts
on spur of the moment instead of thinking things
through. Insists on immediate satisfaction of wishes
and desires. Puts self ahead of others. Blames others
for own mistakes. Triggers displeasure of companions. Often is disliked by others.

	Never	Sometimes	Usually	Always
	0	1	2	3

14. Insatiable

Desires never are satisfied fully. Clamors for more.
Cannot leave others alone. Demands attention. Becomes bored quickly and wants something different.
Complains that others get larger share. Drains emotions of those who must be involved with this person's
life. Triggers desire in others to push this person
away. Often is dreaded by others. Becomes target of
rejection by others.

15. Impulsive

Does not plan ahead. Acts on spur of the moment.
Does whatever comes to mind. Shows no common
sense in making decisions. Does not think of consequences. Demands immediate satisfaction of wishes
and desires. Is a "now" person. Cannot put off desires
or wishes.

16. Disruptive

Is a disruptive influence in a group. Keeps things
stirred up. Triggers conflicts within groups. Disturbs
neighbors during study or work time. Causes others
to complain about how this person is behaving. Others are relieved when this person is absent.

17. Body Energy Overflow

Some part of the body is in continual motion. Cannot
sit still. Cannot be quiet. Can hold body motions under
control briefly, but energy overflow starts again soon.
Fingers fiddle with things. Feet scrub the floor and
bump furniture. Body squirms around. Feet and legs
jiggle. Mouth continually makes irritating sounds.

18. Emotional Overflow

Emotions always are near the surface. Cries too easily. Laughs too loudly. Squeals too much. Giggles too
often. Protests too frequently. Clamors in an emotional way. Is triggered easily into a state of hysteria.
Tantrums always are near the surface. Flares into
anger over trivial issues that others ignore. Misreads
behavior of others into thinking they are criticizing
or being rude. Continually blames or finds fault with
others.

Appendix C

	Never	Sometimes	Usually	Always
	0	1	2	3

19. Lack of Continuity _____ _____ _____ _____

Lifestyle has no continuity. This person's life is lived in unconnected segments. One event does not flow into the next. Must have supervision and guidance to stay with a course of action. In this person's mind, a present activity is not connected with what happened previously or what will follow. Daily patterns and routines do not register. Continually, this person is surprised by each task requirement.

20. Poor Telling and Describing _____ _____ _____ _____

Stumbles over words, names, and specific details while telling or describing. Speech jumps around without following an organized theme. Speech is made of fragments instead of whole statements. Many pauses while telling or describing. "Loses the words" while telling or describing.

Add all the marks in each column to find the subscore for each column.

Subscore _____ _____ _____ _____

Add the subscores to find the **Total Score** _____

314

Enter the Total Score in the appropriate place on the Attention Deficit Profile.

Attention Deficit Profile

_____ 0-10   **No Attention Deficit**

_____ 11-25   **Borderline Attention Deficit**

This individual can succeed in a mainstream classroom or workplace with extra attention to keep him or her on schedule and focused on the task. Leaders must make sure that all oral information has been understood. This person must be reminded frequently to finish all steps before leaving each task. Companions, parents, instructors, and job supervisors must do consistent reminding while repeating oral information enough to help this individual comprehend fully. Occasional one-on-one tutoring or reviewing will be necessary to fill in gaps in what the person understands and remembers.

_____ 26-35   **Moderate Attention Deficit**

This person requires a system that provides enough supervision to keep him or her on task. This individual must be reminded continually about observing details, following step-by-step, and going from start to finish before leaving tasks. Oral information must be given in segments, then repeated, to make sure it is comprehended fully. Written notes or outlines must be posted nearby to give visual cues of what is expeced. This "loose thinker" must have help keeping track of materials and supplies on the job, at school, and at home. Someone in this person's life must be a supervisor to monitor forgetfulness, remind of important deadlines, and help organize his or her life so that attention deficit does not sabotage success. This individual cannot function effectively alone. He or she can be successful with consistent help.

_____ Above 35   **Severe Attention Deficit**

This individual cannot function in traditional classrooms or most workplace situations unless special intervention and supervision are provided. Severe ADHD or ADD require cortical stimulant medication and diet control to maintain stable brain chemistry. Without medication and elimination of trigger food substances, this person's feelings and emotions are overwhelmed by conflict and confusion. Along with medical and dietary intervention, accommodations for ADHD or ADD must be made in classroom and workplace expectations. This person must have written guidelines to review frequently. Must have a study buddy and workplace partner who remind him or her to slow down, think about it first, and review finished work for mistakes. This individual must have a lot of one-on-one instruction to fill in gaps in skills and information.

Sources for Further Help and Information

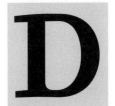

~ ~

Easy-to-Read Books

These books provide a broad overview of the different points of view that surround ADHD and ADD. These books are a rich source of easy-to-read information about how genetics, brain structure, body chemistry, and layers of tag-along syndromes determine the scope and shape of ADHD and ADD.

> *ADHD: The Great Misdiagnosis,* by Julian S. Haber (Taylor Trade Publishing, 2000).
> Pediatrician Julian Haber gives the reader a behind-the-scenes look at diagnostic methods, development and use of medications, and commonsense guidelines for parents of ADHD or ADD children. Dr. Haber writes frankly about controversial issues related to the diagnosis and treatment of attention deficit disorders.

> *ADHD: Attention-Deficit Hyperactivity Disorder in Children, Adolescents, and Adults,* by Paul H. Wender (Oxford University Press, 2000).
> In simple language, pediatrician Paul Wender explains the physician's point of view in guiding parents of ADHD or ADD children. He discusses the pros and cons of medication, diet control, and simple strategies for parenting attention deficit youngsters.

Healing ADD: The Breakthrough Program That Allows You to See and Heal the 6 Types of ADD, by Daniel G. Amen (Berkley Books, 2001).

Psychiatrist Daniel Amen (www.amenclinic.com) describes his revolutionary methods of diagnosing attention deficit disorders through SPECT brain scan and body chemistry analysis. He describes the 6 types of ADD that others see as subtypes of mental health or personality disorders. He gives detailed information about how each type of ADD is treated through brain stimulus therapy, diet control, medication, and talk therapy.

Attention Deficit Disorder: A Different Perception—The Hunter in A Farmer's World, by Thom Hartmann (Underwood Books, 1993). *The Edison Gene: ADHD and the Gift of the Hunter Child*, by Thom Hartmann (Park Street Press, 2003).

These books are part of the Thom Hartmann series that describe a type of hyperfocused lifestyle he calls "the hunter personality." Hartmann presents a comprehensive summary of how brain development and genetic heritage distinguish hyperfocused individuals from those typically diagnosed as ADHD.

The ADHD Autism Connection: A Step Toward More Accurate Diagnosis and Effective Treatment, by Diane M. Kennedy (Waterbrook Press, 2002).

This comprehensive study shows how ADHD and ADD fit into the broad spectrum of neurological differences called autism. Kennedy explains the genetic and neurotransmitter links between autism, Asperger's syndrome, ADHD, and ADD. This book makes a strong argument that ADHD should be considered a subtype of the autistic brain syndrome.

What's Going On In There? How the Brain and Mind Develop in the First Five Years of Life, by Lise Eliot (Bantam Books, 1999).

In simple language, neuroscientist Lise Eliot tells the fascinating story of how a new brain develops from the moment of conception to age 5. Her easy-to-read style leads the reader through every stage of brain development, explaining how each region of the brain functions and how the regions work together. This book is a rich source of information of how each new brain is prepared for its lifelong work.

ADHD & Teens: A Parent's Guide to Making It Through the Tough Years, by Colleen Alexander-Roberts (Taylor Publishing Company, 1995).

This book is an encyclopedia of practical ideas that show parents how to guide ADHD or ADD adolescent children safely into adulthood.

This mother of two ADHD children has "been there/done that." Her wisdom and common sense help other parents to see light at the end of the adolescent tunnel.

ADD and the College Student: A Guide for High School and College Students with Attention Deficit Disorder, by Patricia O. Quinn (Magination Press, 2001).
This book is a valuable step-by-step guide to help parents and ADHD students find the help they need in high school and higher education. Dr. Quinn's down-to-earth, commonsense approach to problem solving is practical and effective. This book shows how to negotiate for accommodations and how to self-advocate with school officials.

Family Therapy for ADHD: Treating Children, Adolescents, and Adults, by Craig and Sandra Everett (Guilford Press, 1999).
From their private practice at the Arizona Institute of Family Therapy in Tucson, Craig and Sandra Everett have prepared this thoughtful guidebook to show families how to resolve problems related to ADHD. This book presents a comprehensive review of how families can conquer challenges related to medication, emotional imbalance, and at-risk relationships between parents and child, as well as between spouses themselves.

A.D.D. On the Job: Making Your A.D.D. Work for You, by Lynn Weiss (Taylor Publishing Company, 1996).
From her personal experience of overcoming ADD, psychologist Lynn Weiss offers a wealth of commonsense advice for overcoming one's ADD or ADHD in the workplace. This book is filled with positive hope. Weiss explains how she learned to regard her ADD as a gift, not a burden. She frankly discusses ADD behaviors that are potential workplace liabilities unless ADD individuals learn how to turn them into assets.

Homeschooling Almanac 2002–2003: Your Complete Homeschooling Resource, by Mary and Michael Leppert (Prima Publishing Company, 2001).
This book is an encyclopedia of "everything you want to know" about homeschooling. The Lepperts (www.homeschoolnewslink.com) take readers from start to finish in how to establish the right kind of home education, which materials are best to use, how to assemble a computer-based curriculum, where to find educational software of every kind, how to interface with homeschool groups everywhere in the United States, and much more. This catalog of how-to-do-it guidelines is a must-read book for families who are concerned about homeschooling children with special needs.

Organizations

Attention Deficit Information Network, Inc.
475 Hillside Ave.
Needham, MA 02194
781/455-9895
Fax 781/444-5466
www.addinfonetwork.com

Children and Adults with Attention Deficit Disorders (CHADD)
8181 Professional Place
Suite 201
Landover, MD 20785
800/233-4050
301/306-7070
Fax 301/306-7090
http://www.chadd.org

Learning Disabilities Association (LDA)
4156 Library Rd.
Pittsburgh, PA 15234-1349
412/341-1515
Fax 412/344-0224
www.ldanatl.org

National Attention Deficit Disorder Association
1788 Second St.
Suite 200
Highland Park, IL 60035
www.add.org

ADD Warehouse
Clearinghouse for books and materials related to ADD/ADHD
300 N.W. 70th Ave.
Suite 102
Plantation, FL 33317
(800)233-9273

References

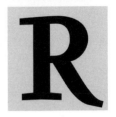

Alexander-Roberts, C. (1995). *ADHD and teens: A parent's guide to making it through the tough years.* Dallas, TX: Taylor.

Amen, D. G. (2001). *Healing ADD: The breakthrough program that allows you to see and heal the 6 types of ADD.* New York: Berkley Publishing Group.

American Psychiatric Association. (1968). *Diagnostic and statistical manual of mental disorders* (2nd ed.). Washington, DC: Author.

American Psychiatric Association. (1980). *Diagnostic and statistical manual of mental disorders* (3rd ed.). Washington, DC: Author.

American Psychiatric Association. (1987). *Diagnostic and statistical manual of mental disorders* (3rd ed., rev.). Washington, DC: Author.

American Psychiatric Association. (1994). *Diagnostic and statistical manual of mental disorders* (4th ed.). Washington, DC: Author.

American Psychiatric Association. (2000). *Diagnostic and statistical manual of mental disorders* (4th ed., text revision). Washington, DC: Author.

Andreasen, N. C. (2001). *Brave new brain: Conquering mental illness in the era of the genome.* New York: Oxford University Press.

Attwood, T. (1998). *Asperger's syndrome: A guide for parents and professionals.* Philadelphia: Jessica Kingsley Publishers.

Bain, L. J. (1991). *A parent's guide to attention deficit disorders.* New York: Dell.

Barkley, R. A. (1990). *Attention-deficit hyperactivity disorder: A handbook for diagnosis and treatment.* New York: Guilford.

Barkley, R. A. (1995). *Taking charge of ADHD: The complete, authoritative guide for parents.* New York: Guilford.

Barnard, K. E., & Brazelton, T. B. (Eds.). (1990). *Touch, the foundation of experience.* Madison, CT: International Universities.

Bastian, C. H. (1869). On various forms of loss of speech in cerebral disease. *The British Medico-Chirurgical Review, 43,* 209–236, 470–494.

Bender, L. (1942). Postencephalitic behavior disorders in children. In J. B. Neal (Ed.), *Encephalitis: A clinical study.* New York: Grune & Stratton

Berlin, R. (1887). *Einebosondere art der wortblindheit: Dyslexie* [A special type of word-blindness: Dyslexia]. Wiesbaden, Germany: J. F. Bergmann.

Blakemore-Brown, L. (2002). *Reweaving the autistic tapestry.* London: Jessica Kingsley Publishers.

321

Block, N., Flanagan, O., & Guzeldere, G. (Eds.). (1997). *The nature of consciousness: Philosophical debates.* Cambridge, MA: MIT Press.

Bradley, W. (1937). The behavior of children receiving benzedrine. *American Journal of Psychiatry, 94,* 577–585.

Brazelton, T. B. (1992). *Touchpoints, the essential reference: Your child's emotional and behavioral development.* New York: Addison-Wesley.

Broadbent, W. H. (1872). On the cerebral mechanism of speech and thought. *Transactions of the Royal Medical and Chirurgical Society, 15,* 145–194.

Brody, B. A. (1987). Sequence of central nervous system myelination in human infancy: 1. An autopsy study of myelination. *Journal of Neuropathology and Experimental Neurology, 46,* 282–301.

Carlson, B. M. (1994). *Human embryology and developmental biology.* St. Louis. MO: Mosby.

Chaguni, H. T. (1999). Metabolic imaging: A window on brain development and plasticity. *Neuroscientist 5,* 29–40.

Clements, S. D., & Peters, J. E. (1962). Minimal brain dysfunction in the school aged child. *Archives of General Psychiatry, 6,* 185–197.

Cohen, D. J., Paul, R., & Volkmar, F. R. (1968). Issues in the classification of pervasive and other developmental disorders: Toward DSM-IV. *Journal of Child Psychology and Psychiatry, 24,* 443–455.

Conners, C. K. (1986). *Hyperkinetic children: A neuropsychosocial approach.* Beverly Hills, CA: Sage.

Conners, C. K. (1989). *Feeding the brain: How foods affect children.* New York: Plenum Press.

Crook, W. G. (1986). *The yeast connection: A medical breakthrough.* Jackson, TN: Professional Books.

Crook, W. G. (1991). *Help for the hyperactive child.* Jackson, TN: Professional Books.

Damasio, A. R. (1994). *Descartes' error: emotion, reason, and the human brain.* New York: Avon Books.

Damasio, A. R. (1999). *The feeling of what happens: Body and emotion in the making of consciousness.* New York: Harcourt Brace.

Denckla, M. B. (1972). Clinical syndromes in learning disabilities. The case for "splitting" versus "lumping," *Journal of Learning Disabilities, 5,* 405–406.

Denckla, M. B. (1978). Minimal brain dysfunction. In J. S. Chall & A. F. Mirshy (Eds.), *Education and the brain* (pp. 223–268). Chicago: University of Chicago Press.

Denckla, M. B. (1985). Issues of overlap and heterogeneity in dyslexia. In D. B. Gray & J. F. Kavanaugh (Eds.), *Biobehavioral measures of dyslexia* (pp. 41–46). Parkton, MD: York Press.

Denckla, M. B. (1991, March). *The neurology of social competence.* Paper presented at the Learning Disabilities Association national conference, Chicago.

Dennet, D. (1991). *Consciousness explained.* Boston: Little, Brown.

Dinklage, D., & Guevremont, D. (1990). Children's atypical developmental scale (CADS). In R. A. Barkley, *Attention-deficit hyperactivity disorder: A handbook for diagnosis and treatment* (pp. 196–205). New York: Guilford.

Duane, D. (1985, March). *Psychiatric implications of neurological difficulties.* Paper presented at symposium conducted at the Menninger Foundation, Topeka, KS.

Eden, G. E. (1996, November). *Visualizing vision in dyslexic brains.* Paper presented at symposium conducted by the Society for Neroscience, San Francisco.

Eliot, L. (1999). *What's going on in there: How the brain and mind develop in the first five years of life.* New York: Bantam.

Elliott, P. T. (2002), Afterword in D. M. Kennedy, *The ADHD/autism connection: A step toward more accurate diagnosis and effective treatment.* Colorado Springs, CO: Waterbrook Press.

Everett, C. A., & Everett, S. V. (1999). *Family therapy and ADHD: Treating children, adolescents, and adults.* New York: Guilford.

Feingold, B. E. (1975). *Why your child is hyperactive.* New York: Random House.

Fisher, S. E., & DeFries, J. C. (2002). Developmental dyslexia: Genetic dissection of a complex cognitive trait in *Nature Reviews Neuroscience, 30,* 767–780.

Geffner, R. A., Loring, M., & Young, C. (2001). *Bullying behavior: Current issues, research, and interventions.* New York: Haworth Press.

Gilger, J. W., Pennington, B. F., & DeFries, J. C. (1992). A twin study of the etiology of comorbidity: Attention deficit hyperactivity disorder and dyslexia. *Journal of the American Academy of Child and Adolescent Psychiatry, 31,* 357–68.

Gilligan, J. (1996). *Violence: Reflections on a national epidemic.* New York: Random House.

Grandin, T. (2002). Foreword in D. M. Kennedy, *The ADHD/autism connection: A step toward more accurate diagnosis and effective treatment* (p. xi). Colorado Springs, CO: Waterbrook Press.

Green, C., & Chee, K. (1994). *Understanding ADD: Attention deficit disorder.* New York: Doubleday.

Haber, J. S. (2003). *ADHD: The great misdiagnosis.* New York: Taylor.

Hallowell, E. M., & Ratey, J. J. (1994a). *Driven to distraction.* New York: Pantheon.

Hallowell, E. M., & Ratey, J. J. (1994b). *Answers to distraction.* New York: Pantheon.

Hampton-Turner, C. (1981). *Maps of the mind.* New York: Macmillan.

Hartmann, T. (1993). *Attention deficit disorder: A different perception.* Grass Valley, CA: Underwood Books.

Hartmann, T. (2000). *Thom Hartmann's complete guide to ADHD.* Grass Valley, CA: Underwood Books.

Hartmann, T. (2003). *The Edison gene: ADHD and the gift of the hunter child.* Rochester, VT: Park Street Press.

Hinshelwood, J. (1896). A case of dyslexia: A peculiar form of word-blindness. *The Lancet,* 1451–1454.

Hinshelwood, J. (1900). Congenital word-blindness. *The Lancet, 1,* 1506–1508.

Huttenlocher, P. R. (1990). Morphometric study of human cerebral cortex development. *Neuropsychologia, 30,* 517–527.

Ingersoll, B. D., & Goldstein, S. (1993). *Attention deficit disorder and learning disabilities: Realities, myths and controversial treatments.* New York: Doubleday.

Inhelder, B., & Piaget, J. (1974). *The early growth of logic in the child.* New York: Harper & Row.

Irlen, H. (1991). *Reading by the colors: Overcoming dyslexia and other reading disabilities through the Irlen method.* Garden City, NY: Avery.

Jacobson, M. (1991). *Developmental neurology* (3rd ed.). New York: Plenum.

James, W. (1890). *The principles of psychology.* New York: Henry Holt.

Jamison, K. R. (1995). *An unquiet mind.* New York: Random House.

Jordan, D. R. (1972). *Dyslexia in the classroom* (1st ed.). Columbus, OH: Merrill.

Jordan, D. R. (1988a). *Attention deficit disorder.* Austin, TX: PRO-ED.

Jordan, D. R. (1988b). *Jordan prescriptive/tutorial reading program for moderate and severe dyslexics.* Austin, TX: PRO-ED.

Jordan, D. R. (1996a). *Overcoming dyslexia in children, adolescents, and adults* (2nd ed.). Austin, TX: PRO-ED.

Jordan, D. R. (1996b). *Teaching adults with learning disabilities.* Malabar, FL: Krieger.

References

Jordan, D. R. (1998). *Attention deficit disorder: ADHD and ADD syndromes* (3rd ed.). Austin, TX: PRO-ED.

Jordan, D. R. (2000a). *Understanding and managing learning disabilities in adults.* Malabar, FL: Krieger.

Jordan, D. R. (2000b). *Jordan dyslexia assessment/reading program* (2nd ed.). Austin, TX: PRO-ED.

Jordan, D. R. (2002). *Overcoming dyslexia in children, adolescents, and adults* (3rd ed.). Austin, TX: PRO-ED.

Joseph, R. (1988). The right cerebral hemisphere. Emotion, music, visual-spatial skills, body image, dreams, and awareness. *Journal of Clinical Psychology, 44,* 632–673.

Judevine Center for Autism. (2004, February 16). Retrieved from www.judevine.org/autism.htm

Kahn, E., & Cohen, L. H. (1934). Organic drivenness: A brain stem syndrome and an experience. *New England Journal of Medicine, 210,* 748–756.

Kennedy, D. M. (2002). *The ADHD-autism connection: A step toward more accurate diagnosis and effective treatment.* Colorado Springs, CO: Waterbrook Press.

Killackey, H. P. (1995). The formation of a cortical somatosensory map. *Trends in Neuroscience, 18,* 402–407.

Klin, A., Volkmar, F. R., & Sparrow, S. S. (Eds.). (2000). *Asperger Syndrome.* New York: Guilford.

LaHoste, G. J., Swanson, J. M., & Wigal, S. B. (1996). Dopamine genes and ADHD. *Molecular Psychiatry, 1,* 121–124.

Laufer, M., Denhoff, E., & Solomons, G. (1957). Hyperkinetic impulse disorder in children's behavior problems. *Psychosomatic Medicine, 19,* 38–49.

Lehmkuhle, S., Garzia, R. P., Turner, L., Hash, T., & Baro, J. A. (1993). A defective visual pathway in children with reading disability. *New England Journal of Medicine, 328,* 989–996.

Livingstone, M. S., Rosen, G. D., Dislane, F. W., & Galaburda, A. M. (1991). Physiological and anatomical evidence for a magnicellular deficit in developmental dyslexia. *Proceedings of the National Academy of Science, USA, 88,* 7943–7947.

Livingstone, M. D. (1993, October). Personal correspondence.

Llinas, R. (1993). Coherent 40-Hz oscillation characterizes dream state in humans. *Proceedings of the National Academy of Science, 90,* 2078- 2081.

Lyon, G. R. (2000, January/February). Why reading is not a natural process. *LDA Newbriefs, 35*(19), 12–17.

McGinn, C. (1991). *The problem of consciousness.* Oxford, England: Basil Blackwell.

McGuinness, D. (1997). *Why our children can't read.* New York: Touchstone.

Moses, M. (1998, September). *Dyslexia and related disorders: Texas state law, state board of education rule, and the revised procedures concerning dyslexia.* Austin: Texas Education Agency.

Olson, R. K. (1999). Genes, environment and reading disabilities. In R. J. Sternberg & L. Spear-Swerling (Eds.). *Perspectives on learning disabilities.* Boulder, CO: Westview Press.

Olweus, D. (1994). Annotation: Bullying at school: Basic facts and effects of a school-based intervention program. *Journal of Child Psychology and Psychiatry, 35,* 1171–1190.

O'Rahilly, R., & Muller, F. (1996). Neurolation in the normal human embryo. In B. Bock & J. Marsh (Eds.), *Neural tube defects* (pp. 70–89). CIBA Foundation, Symposium 181. Chichester, England: Wiley.

Orton, S. T. (1925). "Word-blindness" in children. *Archives of Neurology and psychiatry, 14,* 581–615.

References

Orton, S. T. (1928). Specific reading disability—strephosymbolia. *Journal of the American Medical Association, 90,* 1095–1099.

Orton. S. T. (1937). *Reading, writing and speech problems in children.* Armenia, NY: Academy of Orton-Gillingham Practitioners and Educators.

Osman, B. B., & Blinder, H. (1982). *Nobody to play with: The social side of learning disabilities.* New York: Random House.

Palladino, L. J. (2003). Foreword in T. Hartmann, *The Edison gene: ADHD and the gift of the hunter child* (p. xiii). Rochester, VT: Park Street Press.

Parker, H. C. (1989). *The ADD hyperactivity workbook for parents, teachers, and kids.* Plantation, FL: Impact Publications.

Parker, H. C. (1996). *The ADD hyperactivity handbook for schools* (2nd ed.). Plantation, FL: Specialty Press, Inc.

Pearce, J. C. (2002). *The biology of transcendence: A blueprint of the human spirit.* Rochester, VT: Park Street Press.

Pennington, B. F., Gilger, J. W., Paul, D., Smith, S. A., Smith, S. D., & DeFries, J. C. (1991). Evidence for major gene transmission of developmental dyslexia. *Journal of the American Medical Association, 266*(11), 1527–1534.

Pennington, B. F., & Gilger. J. (1996). How is dyslexia transmitted? In C. H. Chase, G. D. Rosen, & G. Sherman (Eds.). *Developmental dyslexia.* Timonium, MD: York Press.

Penrose, R. (1994). *The shadows of the mind.* New York: Oxford University Press.

Pollan, C., & Williams, D. (1992). Learning disabilities in adolescents and young adult school dropouts. Unpublished raw data.

Quinn, P. O. (Ed.). (2001). *ADD and the college student: A guide for high school and college students with attention deficit disorder* (2nd ed.). Washington, DC: Magination Press.

Ramachandran, V. S. (1993). Behavioral and magnetoencephalographic correlates of plasticity in the adult human brain. *Proceedings of the National Academy of Science, USA, 90,* 10413–10420.

Rapp, D. J. (1991). *Is this your child? Discovering and treating unrecognized allergies.* New York: William Morrow.

Ratey, J. J., & Johnson, C. (1997). *Shadow syndromes.* New York: Pantheon.

Restak, R. M. (2002). *The secret life of the brain.* New York: The Dana Press and Joseph Henry Press.

Restak, R. M. (2003). *The new brain: How the modern age is rewiring your mind.* Emmaus, PA: Rodale Press.

Rimland, B. (2002). Introduction in D. M. Kennedy, *The ADHD autism connection: A step toward more accurate diagnosis and effective treatment* (p. ix). Colorado Springs, CO: Waterbrook Press.

Rowe, D. C., Stever, C., & Giedinghagen, L. N. (1998). Dopamine D4 receptor gene polymorphism is associated with attention deficit hyperactivity disorder. *Molecular Psychiatry 3,* 419–426.

Scarborough, H. S. (1998). Early identification of children at risk for reading disabilities: Phonological awareness and some other promising predictions. In B. K. Shapiro, P. J. Accordo, & A. J. Capute (Eds.). *Specific Reading Disability.* Timonium, MD: York Press.

Schacter, D. L. (1996). *Searching for memory.* New York: Basic Books.

Searle, J. (1997). *The mystery of consciousness.* New York: New York Review of Books.

Shapiro, B. K., Accordo, P. J., & Capute, A. J. (1998). *Specific reading disability.* Timonium, MD: York Press.

Shaywitz, S. (1996, November). Dyslexia: A new model. *Scientific American,* 2–8.

325

Shaywitz, S. (2003). *Overcoming dyslexia: A new and complete science-based program for reading problems at any level*. New York: Alfred A. Knopf.

Slingerland, B. H. (1984). *Slingerland Screening Tests for Identifying Children with Specific Language Disability*. Cambridge, MA: Educators Publishing Service.

Smalley, S. L., Bailey, J. N., Palmer, C. G. (1998). Evidence that the dopamine D4 receptor is a susceptibility gene in attention deficit hyperactivity disorder. *Molecular Psychiatry, 3*, 427–430.

Smith, L. (1976). *Improving your child's behavior chemistry*. New York: Prentice Hall.

Smith, L. (1979). *Feed your kids right*. New York: McGraw-Hill.

Sternberg, R. J., & Spear-Swerling, L. (Eds.). (1999). *Perspectives on learning disabilities*. Boulder, CO: Westview Press.

Still, G. F. (1902). Some abnormal psychical conditions in children. *The Lancet, i*, 1008–1012, 1077–1082, 1163–1168.

St. Amand, R. P. (1999). *What your doctor may not tell you about fibromyalgia: The revolutionary treatment that can reverse the disease*. New York: Time Warner.

Strauss, A. A., & Kephart, N. C. (1955). *Psychopathology and education of the brain-injured child: Vol. 2, Progress in theory and clinic*. New York: Grune & Stratton.

Sutherland, N. S. (1992). *Irrationality: The enemy within*. London: Constable.

Swanson, J. M., Sunohara, G. A., & Kennedy, J. L. (1998). Association of the dopamine receptor D4 (DRD4) gene with a refined phenotype of attention deficit hyperactivity disorder (ADHD): A family-based approach. *Molecular Psychiatry, 3*, 38–41.

Swearer, S. M., & Doll, B. (2001). Bullying in schools: An ecological framework. In Geffner, Loring, & Young (Eds.) *Bullying behavior: Current issues, research, and interventions* (pp. 7–23). Binghampton, NY: Haworth.

Tallal, P., Miller, S., & Fitch, R. (1993). Neurobiological basis of speech: A case for the preeminence of temporal processing. *Annals of New York Academy of Sciences, 682(6)*, 74–81.

Taylor, J. F. (1994) *Helping your hyperactive/attention deficit child* (2nd ed.). Rocklin, CA: Prima Publishing.

Thomas, J. L. (1996). *Do you have attention deficit disorder?* New York: Dell.

Tredgold, A. F. (1908). *Mental deficiency (amentia)*. New York: W. Wood.

Ungerleider, L. G., & Haxby, J. V. (1994). "What" and "where" in the human brain. *Current Opinion in Neurology, 4*, 157–165.

Wacker, J. (1975). *The dyslogic syndrome*. Dallas: Texas Association for Children with Learning Disabilities.

Warren, P., & Capehart, J. (1995). *You and your A.D.D. child: How to understand and help kids with attention deficit disorder*. Nashville, TN: Thomas Nelson Publishers.

Wechsler, D. (1974). *Wechsler Intelligence Scale for Children, Revised*. San Antonio, TX: Psychological Corporation.

Wechsler, D. (1994). *Wechsler Intelligence Scale for Children* (3rd ed.). San Antonio, TX: Psychological Corporation.

Weisel, L. (1992). *POWERPath to adult basic learning*. Columbus, OH: The TLP Group.

Weisel. L. (2001). *POWERPath to adult basic learning* (2nd ed.). Columbus, OH: The TLP Group.

Weiss, G., & Hechtmann, L. T. (1993). *Hyperactive children grown up* (2nd ed.). New York: Guilford.

Weiss, L. (1992). *Attention deficit disorder in adults: A practical guide for sufferers and their spouses* (2nd ed.). Dallas, TX: Taylor.

Weiss, L. (1996). *A.D.D. on the job: Making your A.D.D. work for you*. Dallas, TX: Taylor.

References

Wender, P. H. (2000). *ADHD: Attention-deficit hyperactivity disorder in children, adolescents, and adults.* New York: Oxford.

Wing, L. (1997). *The autistic spectrum: A guide for parents and professionals.* London: Constable and Company.

Wing, L. (2001). *The autistic spectrum* (2nd ed.). Berkeley, CA: Ulysses Press.

Wood, F. (1991, February). *Brain imaging and learning disabilities.* Paper presented at the Learning Disabilities Association national conference, Chicago.

Zaidel, E., & Zaidel, D. (1979). Self-recognition and social awareness in the disconnected minor hemisphere. *Neuropsychologia, 8,* 41–55.

Zametkin, A. J., Nordahl, T. E., Gross, M., King, A. C., Semple, W. E., Rumsey, J., Hamburger, S., & Cohen, R. M. (1990). Cerebral glucose metabolism in adults with hyperactivity of childhood onset. *New England Journal of Medicine, 323,* 1361–1367.

References

Index

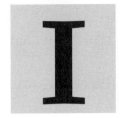

333

tantrums, xiv–xv, 72, 108, 120, 139–142, 151–152, 224
  volatile emotions, 58, 72, 139–143
  withdrawal, 99–100
Distraction. *See* Disruptive behaviors
Doodling, viii, xvii, 96–98
Drug holiday. *See* Medications
Dual diagnosis. *See* Diagnosis
Duane, Drake, 200
Dyscalculia. *See* Dyslexia; Language disorders
Dysgraphia. *See* Dyslexia; Language disorders
Dyslexia
  auditory dyslexia, 205, 207–211, 222
  dyscalculia, 205, 218–223
  dysgraphia, xiv–xv, 10, 20, 123–124, 151, 205, 211–218, 254, 262
  dysnomia, 205, 220
  visual dyslexia, 205–207
Dyslogical behavior. *See* Executive dysfunction
Dysnomia. *See* Dyslexia; Language disorders
Dysthymia. *See* Mental health disorders

Eating disorders, 99, 244
Edison gene. *See* Genetics
Edison Gene: ADHD and the Gift of the Hunter Child, The, ix, 56
Educators Publishing Service, xvi, 124, 209
EEG Spectrum International clinics, 271
Elation. *See* Bipolar disorder; Mental health disorders
Electronic organizers. *See* Accommodations
Eliot, Lise, 4–6, 72
Elliott, Paul T., 188
Emotional expression
  emotions and feelings, 6, 11, 25, 29, 36–42, 71, 99–102
  homeostasis, 11, 17, 36, 42, 113, 116
  optimism, 108, 166–167, 178
  pessimism, 108, 166–167, 178
Encephalitis lethargica, 148
Enhancing brain functions. *See* Brain training
Epilepsy. *See* Neurological disorders
Executive dysfunction, 13, 51–54
  cannot wait, 64

checklist, 79–86
  dyslogical behavior, 17, 139–142
  impulsivity, 29, 70–71, 139–142
  inappropriate behavior, 134–136
  inattention, 74–75
  noisy brain, 43–44, 64, 89–90, 111, 172, 257–258
  overly sensitive to criticism, 74, 139–142
  underarousal, 12, 24, 28–29, 35–51, 236–237
Executive function, 12, 24, 28–29, 35–51, 236–237
  arousal, 65, 236–237
  commonsense reasoning, 29, 39
  logic, 23, 29, 36, 39
  patience, 24, 248
  restraint/wait, 29, 39
  self-control, 24, 29
  socially constructive emotions, 29, 39

Failure, 115–116, 129
Family life
  impact of ADHD and ADD on, 129–143
  marriage, 173–174
  religious belief, 28, 102, 130
Fast ForWord. *See* Brain training
Feedback. *See* Accommodations
Feed Your Kids Right, 228
Feeding the Brain: How Foods Affect Children, 228
Feingold, Benjamin, 226
Feingold Kaiser-Permanente Diet. *See* Diet
Fetal development
  conception, 1–3, 6
  gestation, 6, 9–10, 21
Fibromyalgia, 230–231. *See also* Autoimmune disorders
Fight-or-flight reflex. *See* Brain functions
Filtering. *See* Brain functions
Following instructions, 117–121
Food intolerance. *See* Diet
Forgiveness, 24, 154–155
Frankness, 255–256, 268–269
Frederick II, King of Prussia, 30
Functional literacy. *See* Literacy skills

Gastrointestinal disorders, 229–231, 242. *See also* Chron's disease
Genetics
  alleles, 1–2, 186–187

Overcoming Attention Deficit Disorders in Children, Adolescents, and Adults

Edison gene, ix–x, xvi, 23, 50, 62, 108
    genetic codes, 1–2, 10, 18, 36, 186–187, 204
    genome research, 1–2, 186–187, 204
    inherited genes, 1–2, 10–11, 15, 204
Gilligan, James, 42, 112
Glucose metabolism. *See* Brain functions
Goldstein, Sam, 225
Gone with the Wind, 175
Grammar. *See* Language skills
Grandin, Temple, 185
Green, Christopher, 35, 226
Gripping, 257. *See also* Accommodations
Grooming. *See* Personal care
Guevremont, David, 158

Haber, Julian S., 35, 55, 63, 231, 238
Hallowell, Edward, 108, 173
Handwriting. *See* Literacy skills
Hartmann, Thom, ix–x, xvi, 23, 50, 56, 62–63, 108, 229, 234, 260
Hatfield, John, 272
Hatfield, Marie, 272
Healing ADD: The Breakthrough Program that Lets You See and Heal 6 Types of ADD, 57
Hectmann, Lily T., 166
Help for the Hyperactive Child, 228
Highlighting. *See* Accommodations
Homeostasis. *See* Emotional expression
Home schooling, 50, 272
Hope, 108, 183
Hopelessness. *See* Disruptive emotions and feelings
Hunters. *See* Personality style
Hygiene. *See* Personal care
Hyperactivity. *See* Disruptive behaviors
Hyperfocus. *See* Attention deficit disorder
Hyperkinetic Children: A Neuropsychosocial Approach, 228
Hyperkinetic impulse disorder (HID), 87, 149
Hyperlexia. *See* Disruptive behaviors
Hypersensitivity. *See* Disruptive emotions and feelings
Hypoglycemia, 230–232. *See also* Autoimmune disorders
Hypolexia. *See* Language disorders
Hypomania. *See* Bipolar disorder; Mental health disorders

Improving Your Child's Behavior Chemistry, 228
Impulsivity. *See* Disruptive behaviors
Ingersoll, Barbara, 225
Inner voice. *See* Brain language
Insatiability. *See* Disruptive behaviors
Intelligence, 76, 172–173, 185, 189, 207–208, 225, 254
    giftedness, 204
    intuition, 19, 23, 25
    IQ, 36, 172–173, 185, 189, 207–208, 225, 254
    nonverbal, 21, 23
    potential, 28, 204
    talent, 204
    verbal, 23
Interactive learning. *See* Learning style
Intervention, 99–102
Irlen, Helen, 195
Irlen syndrome. *See* Visual perception disorders
Is This Your Child? Discovering and Treating Unrecognized Allergies, 228
Isolation, 110–111

James, William, 148
Jameson, Kay R., 173, 177
Jaska, Peter, x
Johns Hopkins University School of Medicine, 36
Johnson, Catherine, 42–43, 138, 151, 166–167, 173
Jordan Attention Deficit Scale, xviii, 309–315
Jordan Dyslexia Assessment Inventory, 59
Jordan Dyslexia Assessment/Reading Program, xviii, 201, 206–207, 211, 225
Jordan Executive Function Index for Adults, xviii, 36, 49, 59, 291–307
Jordan Executive Function Index for Children, xviii, 36, 49, 59, 273–289
Jordan Social–Emotional LD Mood Index, 166, 168–169
Judevine Center for Autism, 187

Keeping track of things. *See* Accommodations
Kennedy, Diane, 63, 151, 158, 185

Index

Overcoming Attention Deficit Disorders in Children, Adolescents, and Adults

337

338

339

White sound background. *See*
    Accommodations
Williams, Dorothy, 200, 235
Wood, Frank, 67
Wordblindness. *See* Visual perception
    disorders
Workplace, 138–145
Work quotas. *See* Accommodations

Writing skills. *See* Language skills

Yale University Center for the Study of
    Learning and Attention, 32
*Yeast Connection: A Medical Breakthrough,
    The,* 228

Zametkin, Alan, 66–67

Author

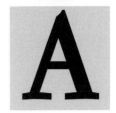

✔ ✔

In 1957, Dale R. Jordan began his career as an elementary classroom teacher with children who could not read or write. That experience with struggling learners led him to earn a PhD degree in educational psychology. For 47 years, Jordan has been active in teacher education at several universities while maintaining private practice in diagnosing dyslexia, attention deficit disorders, and other types of learning disorders. During his doctoral studies, Jordan began to research dyslexia in prison populations, the military, and the workplace. Throughout his career, he has been a prolific author and workshop presenter. In 1972 he published the landmark study *Dyslexia in the Classroom*, one of the first comprehensive descriptions of the subtypes of dyslexia most teachers encounter in mainstream classrooms. In 1976 he was co-developer of the popular D'Nealian handwriting program for Scott, Foresman, and Company. Jordan's professional work has included working with struggling learners of all ages. He has been featured in numerous adult education film and video programs developed by Indiana University, Ohio State University, Marshall University, Kentucky Educational Television, and Arkansas Educational Telecommunications Network.

Jordan's current publications include *Overcoming Dyslexia in Children, Adolescents, and Adults; Jordan Dyslexia Assessment/Reading Program;* and *Overcoming ADHD and ADD in Children, Adolescents, and Adults,* published by PRO-ED, Inc. He also is author of *Teaching Adults with Learning Disabilities* and *Understanding and Managing Learning Disabilities in Adults,* published by Krieger Publishing Company.

Now in retirement in northeast Oklahoma, Jordan continues to diagnose children with learning difficulties and consult with schools in accommodating special learning needs.